Grady Baby

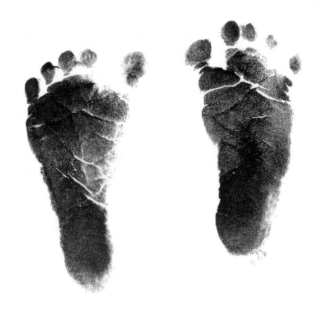

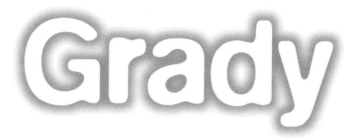

Grady

A Year in the Life of
Atlanta's Grady Hospital

Baby

Jerry Gentry

University Press of Mississippi
Jackson

http://www.upress.state.ms.us

07 06 05 04 03 02 01 00 99   4 3 2 1
∞

Library of Congress Cataloging-in-Publication Data

Gentry, Jerry.
    Grady baby : a year in the life of Atlanta's Grady Hospital /
Jerry Gentry.
        p.   cm.
    ISBN 1-57806-157-1 (cl. : alk. paper)
    1. Hospitals—Maternity services—Georgia—Atlanta—History.
2. Grady Memorial Hospital (Atlanta, Ga.)—History.   I. Grady
Memorial Hospital (Atlanta, Ga.)   II. Title.
RG501.U6G46   1999
362.1′982′009758231—dc21   99-30385
                                                          CIP

British Library Cataloging-in-Publication Data available

Contents

Preface

All events in this book are true. Some minor chronological changes were made for the sake of smooth readability. Likewise, some minor changes were made to conversations, such as compressing several into one, also to facilitate smooth storytelling. I used pseudonyms except in the chapter on Grady's desegregation, which is a matter of historical record, and in the chapter on the medical mercy trip to Mexico. (The Grady PA, Walt Robinson, of course, on that trip retained his pseudonym.) Conversations and interviews I either wrote by hand on paper or recorded on audio tape and later transcribed. A few quotations and comments I recalled later and wrote down. Any reported thoughts of individuals were told to me later by that person. A few very minor characters are composites, such as hospital staff who appeared briefly in some scenes and were not crucial to the central stories.

Grady Memorial Hospital graciously allowed me exceptional access to the Maternal/Child Health Department, under the condition that no confidential patient information would be passed to me except by individual patients. The only such information in this book was shared with me by women who agreed in writing to participate in the project, or concerns patients about whom I have no identifying information; they were discussed strictly on an anonymous basis. I was paid no stipend or salary by Grady Hospital and was not considered in any way an employee or contract employee of Grady. Any implied opinions in the book are those of the author, and not of Grady Memorial Hospital.

I explained my book project to each Grady patient before she signed a release allowing me to use conversations and interviews in the book. In rare cases, some individuals requested that I not include certain information I learned in their presence, and I honored those requests.

Many people are due gratitude for their help on this project. I wish I could name them all. I thank, first, the administrators at Grady Memorial Hospital for allowing me access to an institution with such incredibly diverse stories. I appreciate the tolerance and cooperation of the Grady OB/GYN staff, who allowed me to follow them around and ask all manner of nosy questions. I admire the dignity with which they treated their patients. Most of all, I thank the Grady patients who shared with me their lives. I am honored that you trusted me to tell your stories.

I thank my editor, Craig Gill, for his confidence in this book, and Evan Young for his careful and helpful copyediting. Also, thanks to the anonymous external reviewer. My precious wife, Tina Pippin, encouraged me when I felt discouraged and bewildered. For that, I owe her much gratitude.

This book is dedicated to Jacy Gentry Pippin—not a Grady baby, but a source of great joy and love.

Grady Baby

Prologue

On a February morning, Robin James walked with her daughter, Cheryl, into the new five-story, marble-tile-walled atrium at Grady Memorial Hospital in downtown Atlanta. Outside, the chilling wind whipped through the city, the cloudless sky a deep blue. Pedestrians—horrified southerners who rarely faced frigid weather—covered every possible inch of skin, pulling hoods down over their faces. Big oily machines roared and clanged loudly in front of the adjacent main hospital building, which was being renovated. The atrium's automatic doors stayed open as people scurried inside, letting in the cold. The receptionist at the round information desk wore her scarf tied tightly around her neck and head. She reached up with her gloved hand as she gave directions, pulling the scarf tighter. A cursing man stalked out of the Walk-In Clinic, which was by the desk. "Those stupid damn bitches," he muttered.

Robin is a Grady baby. Grady has for decades been the medical center of last resort for poor Atlantans, both before there was Medicaid and later, when most doctors would not accept Medicaid patients. "I'm a Grady baby" is said with pride in Atlanta—not the pride of someone born into status, but that of someone who has been through it and survived. Many Grady babies return to Grady for medical care for the rest of their lives. The enormous institution has served its community as a sixteen-story substitute for a family doctor.

Robin nearly died at Grady in 1977. Or 1978. She is not sure which. She barely remembers that visit. She does remember briefly glimpsing what is in store for her after her death. Telling this story a few months after the visit to Grady on that frigid day, Robin stared at the ceiling of her apartment's living room, mightily recalling little details that were still in a haze. She guessed that someone found her confused and helpless, perhaps unconscious. "Take her to Grady": the first thought of anyone in Atlanta finding someone in Robin's condition.

"I remember waiting in this little cold room," she recalled. Her voice was high-pitched but strong—a peep from an iron bird. "There was a old white lady and a old white man in there." She remembered sitting on a bench and wearing hospital shoes. The mental picture of the scene slowly assembled in her memory. "They had a tag on my toe that said, 'Jane Doe.' But I was alive. They told me to count backwards from a hundred, and I remember lying there, hesitating, trying to figure out why they want me to start counting backwards. The nurse asked me, 'Do you understand me?' And I said yes, like that, I nodded. So she started counting with me. I remember her saying, 'One hundred.' And I said"—her voice softened again as she imitated herself following the nurse's instructions—"'One hundred.' And then I said, 'Ninety-nine, ninety-eight, ninety-seven.' "

Sometime past ninety-seven Robin drifted into a consciousness that hovered between this world and the next. Robin likely became one more Grady story, a story added to others that emergency room workers in large city public hospitals cannot resist telling, at home, over drinks with friends. "We had a woman today who didn't even know how she *got* there. . . ." Standing on a solid tile floor, the nurse helping Robin count herself to sleep could not have known where Robin went next. This part of Robin's story is exclusively her own.

"The next thing I knew I was standing on clouds, and I was looking around. I saw two big lights coming at me, but these lights were train lights, and I wondered, 'Where that train coming from?' They had the big wheels, but the train didn't have no culumpity-culunk sound. And as the train got closer I saw people on the train, and they were sitting like normal people, but the expression they had on their faces, was like they was going to work, when you ride the bus early in the morning, this look on their face like, uh, 'Wonder what the day going to bring,' or 'Wonder if so-and-so going to start some junk.' Like a deep thankful thought about what was going to happen that day.

"I was so amazed when I seen the cloud, I noticed the absence of the weight that wasn't up under the bottom of my feet. And I said, 'Lord, I'm not standing on solid ground.' And the Lord laughed. That tickled me. And I asked him where, how, and why. And I didn't hear no answer, but the nurse said, 'We got you! We almost lost you,' and I closed my eyes real quick because I wanted to go back so bad, not really because of the train or standing on the cloud, but because of the peace. Everything could just go silent, and you would still not be able to hear the silence that I heard. It was just so peaceful."

Like many others who have been brought to Grady's ER, Robin had good reasons for desiring the peace she thought she would find only by boarding the train rolling silently through the clouds. Drug abuse had so clouded her life that she does not remember anything for weeks before she was taken to Grady. She does, however, remember vividly the day, the hour, when she began using drugs, a decision that would take her back to Grady over and over. It began with a little deception, to impress her friends, that she later regretted.

"Help me, Lord, I was ill. I was twenty-three when I took my first drink. I didn't smoke cigarettes until I was thirty, but between the ages of twenty-three and twenty-six is when I lied, I lied. I had been around people that was doing drugs, and I told them that I had done drugs before, that I knew all about it." She had not yet used drugs, but she had seen too much, said too much, been there for transactions, and, she said about the man making those transactions, "I kinda liked the guy." She had to use or attract suspicion. "They caught up with me and put me in a very bad predicament and it was from that time when I snorted that stuff."

Robin's arms were strong, her build stocky; her bodily strength seeped into her voice. When she shouted instructions to her grandson in another room, her high voice carried solidly through her apartment. She willingly showed the scars on her wrists, where she tried to kill herself sometime during the years when drugs controlled her life. Another trip to Grady, another Grady story. The scars, symbols of emotional weakness on such strong arms, emphasized the despair she felt, just as her suddenly lowered voice emphasized her emotion when she spoke again, softly this time.

"I've sought for that peace. I've isolated myself. I've went to the uttermost parts trying to find that peace. But it's not here. That peace only comes when we went into the spiritual. It was not a dream because, like sometimes you dream something and you might get real scared, and you might say, 'Ooh, I was scared.' But then eventually the fear that was with the dream, it fades. But the peace that I felt it does not fade. It's like it's a part of me. I don't worry about dying no more because I know there's life after death. I know that when I left here, I know I died. Just like I know my name is Robin because my mom-n-em told me my name was Robin. If somebody say, 'Well, your name Mary,' my name might be Mary, but my name will always be Robin. It's imprinted like a blueprint on my mind. And so is life after death. That's how close I came. I closed my eyes real quick because I wanted to go back. It was the wonderful quiet that I felt that was so deep.

"Now, I'm going on two years clean," she claimed, then retreated a little. "I'm saying two years, but I'm gon' say one year, really clean, because in the first year you be thinking about it, you be dreaming about it, you be déjà vu about it, and that's a real real danger zone."

When Robin entered the new atrium years later with Cheryl, they were visiting Robin's eldest daughter, Pauline, who was expecting another Grady baby. Pauline's frail body had been able to conceive, but not fully nurture, prior fetuses. She had already lost two babies. Robin rode the elevator to the second floor and walked to the special OB clinic, to see about her daughter and the tiny fetus that was dying inside her womb.

Roughly about that time, all this happened:

Jan Dorman got a job. Her boyfriend had suggested she become a dancer at a strip club; for a month she resisted, thinking, "He's trying to pimp me," but she finally agreed. He told her it was a chance to be independent.

"He let me know that whatever money I made was mine," she said later. "He didn't want none of it. He just said, 'I want you to have your own job and your own money. I want you to know you can make it on your own.' He said, 'You don't have to pay me no rent, nothing. All I ask you to do is make your own money, and feel confident and independent.' I was ashamed of my body, so when I was dancing I had to get sloppy drunk, where I couldn't even stand up. Heh heh. I could dance but I couldn't walk. Just the thought of stripping your clothes off in front of people you don't know. For a good month and a half, I wouldn't even let him see my body. If we did anything it was in the dark and under the covers. So it took me a while."

Her courage was bolstered by her newly-flat stomach: "I keep a little bulge, and somehow I managed to find an exercise that flattened it out. It took me three years to do it, but I finally found a special exercise." She worked at the club only a few weeks. One day she noticed the bulge was back. "I knew what it was that time because I had been exercising every day and dancing. I knew what it was."

Lisa Dean went to the Grady emergency room. A cut on her head required three stitches. She told the nurse that she was playing with her son and boyfriend, became dizzy and fell. Much later, she would tell the truth. The ER nurse asked her if she might be pregnant, and Lisa said she did not think so. The nurse asked when she had her last period, and Lisa said November—two and a half months before. "Why did you think you hadn't had your cycle?" the nurse asked, skeptical. Lisa mumbled and finally said, "I thought it was waiting for the new year." The nurse, who had heard it all, gave her a look and laughed.

Azi Torres returned to Atlanta from Brazil. Three months earlier, she had left Atlanta, after she found out she was pregnant, just as she and her boyfriend, Jeff, were breaking up. Jeff had arrived in Brazil five days after she did, eager to see this new country, but she was too busy throwing up to show him the sights. Two weeks they were together, both miserable. She was sick; he was bored. Azi was glad, however, that Jeff could see that she was not a poor, desperate Brazilian who went to America for money. She knew his family, who were worth millions, distrusted her, assumed she wanted access to their abundant American dollars. Yet, carrying in her womb an heir to so much money, Azi returned to America and found herself at Grady, Atlanta's hospital for the indigent.

Blood Pressure and Weight

Thirty-two years old, slim, Pauline James worried if she would ever have a baby. Her mother Robin with her, again she walked to the clinic for high-risk pregnancies. She had prayed, if it's going to end like the others, let it end early, not go seven months like the last one, and be born and not live.

Waiting for her appointment, she recalled her previous pregnancy: "I really wanted him. I loved his father. I have pictures and everything. They thought he was under one pound, but he was much bigger. They kinda encouraged it. They put me in the hospital the last four months, my legs propped up and everything because my water was leaking. I was hurting all the time. They were trying to seal it over. They thought I couldn't carry it the whole time."

They were right. Her body delivered the baby before it was fully developed, at the beginning of her seventh month. "They asked me when I went into labor if we can try to keep it alive, but the heart and lungs weren't really mature enough to survive on its own. The person explaining really didn't do such a good job. When the baby came out, he wasn't dead like they thought. I was drugged up because I had been in so much pain. They were asking me, Do you want us to try to keep him alive? but they were telling me it's really hard when it's under one pound, but he was over two pounds. And when he came out, they said, 'Oh no'; he was heavy enough that we could have tried to kept him. He might have been sick, but his dad was a millionaire, so he could have paid the bills. I was really caught up in a hard spot, choosing to have him. They were saying he could have mental and physical disabilities. They had me so nervous about him being so little.

"They didn't try to keep him alive. They just let the heart and lungs collapse because they asked me. I told 'em, yeah, that was OK because they kept saying it was so hard to save a premature baby that small. But right away, when we saw the baby—He was moving around and everything. They said, 'Are you sure you don't want to hold it?' I was in so much pain from the delivery, that I was begging for something to take the pain away. When they gave me the medicine, it really drugged me up, and I didn't know what I was saying or doing. I just wanted the pain to be over with."

The millionaire father of the child was Scott Marvin, a professional football player formerly with the Atlanta Falcons then with the Los Angeles Raiders. "I really loved him," she said. "Even now. We really loved each other. We tried to do all the right things, but it just didn't work out. Now, in a way, I feel kinda responsible that I didn't just take a chance when they asked if I wanted to try to keep the baby alive, or did I think it's better to let nature take its course. I should have tried to keep it alive. Since I've been reading books and things, babies that weighed less than he did survived, and they're OK now. They don't even go to the doctor all the time like people said they would."

She had been with her current boyfriend, the father of the child inside her, for two years, but she never forgot Scott Marvin. "I don't love him nowhere near as much as I love Scott. It's like you have a love that you can never let go. He is the only person that I would consider cooking and cleaning for, the kind of things that wives have to do."

A Grady nurse had taken a Polaroid picture of the baby whose inadequately-developed lungs and heart quit soon after he was born. Pauline kept that picture and a picture of Scott safely tucked in a large Bible in her home. From time to time, she removed them, stared at the picture of Scott and gently moved her fingers over the picture of the baby.

Before Scott, there was a husband, with whom she conceived, and whom she suspects was the cause of her first miscarriage. "In the beginning he was good, but he started drinking a lot. I got pregnant and then one day he threw me down the stairs, and I was about five months. I didn't have a miscarriage that day, but it wasn't long after."

Pauline was called to an exam room, and, again, she learned she would have no child. It was already dead inside her. Labor was induced, and her dead baby was delivered. She held it, and Robin held it. Then Pauline held it again, not wanting to let go. By the end of the year, however, Pauline would be thinking, "Maybe this was not the right father. Only God knows that, so He just went ahead and took it away before I had to find it out on my own. I don't feel bad about losing that one. I thought I was in love with that guy, but there's something about him that I don't love."

Nancy Forrest's job, in the blood pressure room of the OB clinic, was simple enough. Take their blood pressure; weigh them. Take their blood pressure; weigh them. These two easily-measured vital signs were watched carefully by the OB clinic staff. A mysterious condition called pregnancy-induced hypertension can interfere with proper delivery of oxygen through the blood and can thus be fatal to the woman or the fetus. And they wanted each pregnant woman to gain around thirty pounds. Pregnant women usually hated gaining weight, but it provided nutrition and a safe little home for the baby.

"Slip off your shoes and step up on the scales," Forrest told a patient.

"Take off my shoes?"

"We want the real you."

She waddled to the scales, used the front tip of her right foot to push down the back of her left shoe, and withdrew her left foot. She used the socked foot to remove her right shoe and stepped on the scales. She was not pleased.

"Oh, my God!"

"Now you know this is no quick-weight-loss clinic."

The patient chuckled and shook her head. Forrest used this quip about ten times daily, and it worked almost every time. Patients usually laughed at themselves and got over their horror. To the right of the scales, the wall was stained with smudged fingerprints by patient after patient stepping onto the scales and reaching out for balance, touching the wall.

After weighing, they touched the wall for balance again as they put their shoes back on.

The next patient wore a T-shirt imprinted in large gold sparkling letters, "Jesus Messiah King of Kings." She stepped on the scale and thrice muttered, "Oh Lord." A young man holding a baby entered the room and looked around, seeking the baby's mother. Noticing he held the baby awkwardly, Forrest got up and showed him how to hold a baby. "I can't do this," he said, shaking his head.

"Yes, you can. Hold your hand right here, like this. If his head bounces back, you got it. Go sit down. Don't walk around so much. You'll do fine." The man walked out of the room, gently holding the baby, as instructed.

A woman walked in with a young son behind her. She stood on the scales, and the son looked at the dial and cried, "Oohwee, mom." His eyes widened, and he shook his head.

Forrest recognized the next patient and asked how she was doing.

"My boyfriend's been fighting me, and I've been having flashbacks to his fighting me before."

Forrest walked to the liaison nurse office, and returned to tell the patient that the nurse could see her now.

"We've been trying to get her away from him," Forrest said after the patient left.

A woman's voice announced over the hospital-wide intercom, "Anyone with knowledge of Vietnamese, please call the operator."

The next patient weighed herself, put her shoes back on, and sat in the chair next to Forrest, who wrapped the black cuff around the patient's right arm and tightened it with Velcro strips. She held the flat metal end of her stethoscope against the inside of the patient's elbow. Using the side of her thumb to turn a small metal knob, she tightened the air valve. She squeezed the little black rubber bulb. The cuff enlarged in puffy increments, the air whistling through the rubber tube. When the cuff was full, she loosened the valve with her thumb, gradually releasing the air and the constriction on the blood vessel. She turned her eyes toward the meter to watch the needle return to zero. She listened through her stethoscope for a thump—the compressed vessel suddenly opening as a rush of blood pushed through it. She wrote down the number that coincided with the thump, continued to release air and wrote down the number at the last thump, when the blood resumed its flow. She removed the cuff, the Velcro sounding like it was tearing apart.

"Put your Grady card away," Forrest warned. "You can't afford to lose that." The card was gold with black letters. The patient's name, birth date, and Grady number were embossed on the plastic. The patient carefully slipped the card into a slot in her purse, and zipped it shut.

The patient's little daughter leaned against her mother's leg and squeezed her Barney the dinosaur doll in her small arms. Forrest smiled at the little girl and said, "You just love Barney to death. You're giving him a big hug. You're taking care of Barney." Behind Forrest's smile and delight with the girl was a memory of a child who broke her heart, a memory that, nineteen years before, forced her to leave the hospital unit she had loved.

"I got tired of watching children die," she recalled.

Forrest was a Grady baby. Her first return to the place of her birth was as an employee, where she worked as a nurse's aid in the pediatric unit. Children from age three to sixteen came with leukemia, sickle-cell anemia, and other diseases that end fragile young lives. "I had specifically requested pediatrics when I first came to Grady. I hadn't been back to Grady since. We always had insurance. As a kid, I always thought Grady was a place where you went and died because they always took people with strokes there. When they took my grandmother to Grady I said, 'I bet she's going to die.' My mom was surprised at what I said." She imitated her mother's shocked expression, gaping her mouth and widening her eyes. "I said that a neighbor had been taken there, and *she* died, and a man up the street was in a car accident and died at Grady. 'So try and tell me Grady isn't a place where you go to die.' My mom said some went to Grady to see a doctor and get well. I said no doctors are at Grady. 'You go there to die.'"

After high school, Forrest had attended a nurse's assistant program at Atlanta Area Tech. Divorced from her first husband, she had one child.

She rode the bus to her mother's house, dropped off her child, took the bus to school, then rode the bus to the hospital.

"It was hectic, but my high school biology teacher had said, 'Don't start it if you're not going to finish it.' I wanted to quit. I had to get on that bus early. I finally graduated, and Emory, Grady, and South Fulton all called, but Grady gave me pediatrics. I could have gone to Emory, but the bus went by there only once an hour until ten a.m., then no more 'til two. If my baby got sick, how would I get back? I could have taken a cab to the bus station, but I didn't have the money every day."

She called Grady for an appointment. "This lady asked me why I was interested in pediatrics. I told her I loved small children. She said they had an eleven-to-seven shift and asked if I had someone to keep my child. I told her yes, my mother. 'How will you get here?' 'The bus.' 'You must be really determined; you can start Monday.' I worked in pediatrics the first five years. I would get off work, sleep 'til one, get up and clean up, go to my mother's for my child, play with her some, go home, and put her to bed, then start over again."

She remembered how much she enjoyed caring for the ill children, and how sad the work could be. "We would hold them and play with them as they came in and out of the hospital. Some would look better for so long. You would feel optimistic that you were helping them. They would call for you and ask you to play with them. You'd be busy, but you'd play with them anyway. When you're ready to leave at the end of a shift, to a dying child it feels like everyone is leaving. Kids know when they're dying, and they ask you to be there with them a lot. They hold you. They have IVs in their arms, and they look at you with those eyes that say, 'I need your help.' You feel like your hands are tied. Then a child goes to sleep one night and never wakes up. You feel like you know when they're dying and you can't help.

"All the time you're thinking *this* is the child that'll make it. You've seen two or three who have. Children sometimes bounce back better than adults. I loved pediatrics, but it wears you down. One diabetic girl was in and out of Grady so many times. She eventually died. I couldn't believe it because I'd seen her in her worst times, and I thought she'd never make it, but she always did. Then when she died, I didn't think she looked that bad."

One sick little boy she remembered more than any of them.

"There was one boy, Andy, six years old, who was in and out a lot. Sometimes I'd work a double shift, if I knew I could do private duty with Andy. He needed private duty a lot. He asked for peanut butter crackers one day. I heard him crying because I hadn't gotten any for him yet. It was nine o'clock. I told him, 'At nine-fifteen I'll be on break and I'll get them for you, when the short hand is on the nine and the long hand is on the three. Are you going to call me before then?' 'I think not,' he said.

"At nine-fifteen I got him some peanut butter crackers. I came back and saw several nurses at his door. I said, 'What happened? Did he call me?' Someone said, 'He didn't call no one.' I told them it was nine-fifteen and I had brought these crackers for him. A nurse said I should have brought them at nine-oh-five. He had passed."

Forrest immediately decided to leave the pediatrics unit.

"I went to the pre-term nursery for a while, but the babies were so small, and you try to save them, but they die. Then you wrap them and take them to the morgue. Some days I had to take two down."

Forrest arranged a transfer to the OB clinic where, at last, she would no longer hold dying or dead children in her arms.

"Next, you go to the lab," she instructed the patient with the child clutching Barney the dinosaur, "and give some urine. The lab is past these two double doors, on the right. Then come back to this waiting room right here." She pointed outside the door. "Not that one over there." She changed the angle of her point. "They look just alike, but over there you won't hear your name called. They'll also give you your blood sugar test. Drink the soda they give you, then go back in an hour. No matter where you are you say, 'I got to go to the lab.' Or we'll have to start over. I'm counting on you to do that part."

Nancy Forrest was busy with patients in the blood pressure room all morning until around 10:30, when the crowd eased. The waiting room was quiet, even though several children played with each other, sometimes running around the room. Three children slept curled up in chairs.

A Hispanic woman walked into the blood pressure room and smiled at Forrest, who greeted her, but the woman did not respond, apparently knowing no English but knowing the routine. She leaned against the wall and reached down to take off her shoes. She stepped on the scale, Forrest wrote down her weight, and she sat in the chair for her blood pressure to be taken.

"Now go to the lab."

She nodded and went the right direction.

A young woman carrying a baby walked into the blood pressure room.

"Hey, Mrs. Forrest, look at my baby."

She put the baby carrier on Forrest's desk. Forrest pulled back the small striped blanket.

"Oh, look at the baby. He's cute. Who does he look like?"

"His father." She laughed, saying, "My mama said to him, 'It looks just like your mug shot.' "

At the front desk, the security officer who sat outside the OB clinic said to clinic aide Emily McGriff, whom everyone called Ms. Griff, "There's a woman out there in labor. Can you take her to the fourth floor?" Plump Ms. Griff was a grandmother with a child's impish round face lurking beneath small wrinkles spreading from her eyes. She followed him out the door. He pointed at a woman sitting in an open area between the OB and GYN clinics and the elevators. The atrium arose above it on two sides.

"Have you been seen?" Ms. Griff asked her.

The woman nodded.

"Did she say you had dilated?"

"She said the head was right there."

"But have you dilated? If you haven't dilated enough, it's best to go home, sit in warm water, and relax. If you go up there and you haven't dilated, you'll have to undress, walk for two hours, and they'll send you home." To a young woman sitting nearby, Ms. Griff said, to confirm the validity of her judgment, "I been doing this a long time, haven't I?"

"Yeah, a long time," the young woman answered.

"If you want to go, I'll take you, but it's a waste of time, and it will cost more. When they examine you, you feel uncomfortable and you think you're in labor. Your stomach's not used to being stretched. I can tell it's close. Your fingers and face are swollen. But it's not today. If you really want to go, I'll take you, but it's best if you go home and relax. Look at the things you got for your baby. Think about the blessed event that's about to happen."

"OK."

A mischievous expression on her face, the other woman said, "Drink castor oil."

Ms. Griff pounced. "Don't say that! I'm going to beat you up for saying that." She said rapidly, "Don't listen to her. Castor oil could make you doo-doo. Your lungs could collapse. It could make your baby turn. It could mean a C-section. Or the baby could die. God takes care of fools like her, but you be smart." She turned back and said, "I can't believe you said that."

Walking back to the clinic, Ms. Griff muttered, "I can't believe that. She's one of my children. I mean, she grew up in my neighborhood and was one of a lot of children who was always over at my house."

Lisa Dean arrived for her prenatal visit with her midwife, Lauren Foley. She checked in and walked to the blood pressure room. She weighed two hundred ten pounds. Lisa walked to the waiting room and sat in a chair against the wall. She carried her large-framed body well. Her broad face was accented with light brown freckles. Her toothy smile was classic, wide and deep. Her laughs came from the back of her throat. Her body joined in each laugh, shifting in her chair, her head swinging from side to side.

Lisa learned she was pregnant in January when she came to the Grady ER for stitches in the side of her head. "I was wearing slippery shoes," she explained, "and I fell and hit the corner of a brick wall. They always ask about your cycle. I told her my last one was November the twenty-fourth, so they gave me a pregnancy test. I found out before I even got my stitches. I couldn't say anything. It's been almost five years. This is the last one."

Lisa wanted this delivery to be all natural. "I do not want an epidural," she said firmly. She pursed her lips, which she did when she wanted you to know she meant what she said. She walked to the back, through the double doors, to the exam room areas and asked Ms. Griff if she had time to go to McDonald's. Ms. Griff said OK.

"Good, I got to meet my boyfriend there." Lisa turned, stopped and looked back and asked, "Can he go in the exam room with me?"

"Yes," Ms. Griff replied.

She returned with Dwayne. She sat and waggled her foot nervously. They occasionally snuggled and laughed, or looked bored waiting. Foley called her name, and they both went through the double doors, down the hall and into the exam room. Foley noted that Lisa had gained seven pounds in the last month and told her she should gain about thirty pounds total. "Watch what you eat," she advised. When Foley asked Lisa to undress for the exam, Dwayne left.

Lisa's apartment was in Floral Acres, a small public housing community near the Atlanta airport. It was a tiny place with one bedroom, a bathroom, kitchen, and living room. The kitchen sink faucet steadily dripped large drops of water. She shared the upstairs bedroom with her four-year-old son, Rob; her brother Franklin slept on the couch. ("And Dwayne practically lives here," she often said.) The walls were made of painted cinder blocks. She and her neighbor heard much of what happened in each other's homes. She picked this public housing community because she thought it would have lots of flowers. It did not. "I didn't know what the hell Floral Acres was," she said. The ground around the apartments was mostly weeds and bare Georgia red clay, which shimmered after a rain, looking as if a bright orange-red was painted onto the ground. A metal garbage dumpster sat in the parking lot just across from the sidewalk in front of her door. A handwritten sign on a neighbor's door said, "ALL PHONE CALLS, 75 CENTS, NO EXCEPTIONS, SORRY, EVEN IF YOUR OUR KEN."

Planes landing at the airport flew low overhead. It seemed odd to notice details—black stains, the angle of a wing—on a plane still in the air. They looked shockingly large, floating through the air, and they roared thunderously. The volume of conversations fluctuated with each passing jet, a vocal roller coaster. It came natural after a while.

Children ran and laughed outside. One boy shot his buddies with a cap pistol. Spying Lisa, he sidled up to the wall and peered around the brick corner of her apartment, carefully aimed at her and pulled the trigger several times. Half the caps clicked dully instead of popping. He turned and ran after his buddies.

She went into her living room, which was down a short stairwell from the kitchen, sat on a soft brown sofa, and talked about her pregnancy and about going to Grady.

"My son was born at Grady. I didn't have any epidurals or anything. I was seventeen, and you used to see different doctors because they weren't as organized. I didn't like that because I was like, 'I don't want all of them poking with me.' You'd answer questions with one, and you'd have to answer them again with another one. But now I like it. I went to see my friend; she had her baby, and the baby gets to be in the room with you now. More like a private hospital. I had my baby on the thirteenth floor and I was up in the recovery room, and I don't know where they took my son. I guess they took him to the, whatcha call that room? The nursery for kids. Then they took me to the eleventh floor. They moved you a lot."

She said when she went back to Grady for this pregnancy, Ms. Griff remembered her. "She was like, 'Hi, howya doing? Well, we didn't see you the next year.' She asked if it's my second baby. I said yes. She said, 'That's good. I thought you were ready to say this is your third or fourth. A lot of the girls come back for their six-week and they're pregnant again.' They were like, 'You did good.' When I had my son five years ago, when I came back for my six-week checkup, she said, 'I don't want to see you back next year.' I was seventeen.

"Before I had kids, I went to Grady with a broken arm when I was fourteen. I had a venereal disease when I was sixteen, the first time I had sex. My son, I took him once when he had the pink eye. Other than that—"

"Mama! Mama!" her son, Rob, called from upstairs in their bedroom.

"Yes!" she shouted back.

"I don't know how to get it on the tartoons."

"You better put it on that last channel!" She chuckled and muttered, "'Tartoons,' that boy is funny."

He shouted that he still could not get the tartoons.

"I'll come up there and do it. What time is it?"

"Two-fifteen."

"He's got fifteen minutes before cartoons come on."

"Mama! Mama!" Rob appeared on the stairs. He had a roundish hand-some face and a strong physique for a four-year-old. He stood with his back straight.

"Yes."

"Take these socks off?"

"No. Why do you want to take your socks off? He is a mess."

"Mama!"

"Yes."

"Can I have these cookies?"

"Eat them bananas, please."

"I like to sit around and play with my son," Lisa continued. "Me and him have school together. I make out little work sheets for him. And we go over those. So he'll be prepared when he goes to kindergarten. He's very smart. He's very stubborn, and he won't work with you that long. He'll say 'I don't want it.'" When she imitated Rob, she raised her voice, spoke softly in almost a song and slowly shook her head. "But when he's by hisself, I'll say, 'I thought you didn't want to,' and he'll say, 'I want to, but mom you just *make* me keep saying it.' He knows he's stubborn."

She looked around the room. "You know, I could write a book on my life. It would be something else. Maybe a movie."

"It's had ups and downs? And. . . ."

"Uh-huh." She paused. "Yes it has. Things are all right now. It's all right. It's just, you know, just life. Go through a lot in life. Could I say this off the record?"

"Sure."

It was cool and sunny in the morning, the temperature around thirty-seven degrees. It would reach the high sixties in the afternoon. It was a sparkling spring day, the brisk morning reminding one of the recent winter and the afternoon of the warm days ahead. The dreaded, sultry, humid Atlanta summer seemed far off, though it was not. Spring would often end abruptly in Atlanta, bringing on the heat and mosquitoes, the comfortable mild seventies gone for months.

A pregnant woman with three children entered the blood pressure room in the OB clinic. The oldest daughter, about ten years old, said, "Mommy's got a big tummy. My daddy pretends he's got a big stomach. He does this." She poked out her little stomach as far as she could. "He's funny." When their mother had finished with her weight and blood pressure, all three waved at Nancy Forrest and said, "Good-bye." The middle child peeked through the door after they had left and waved one last time.

It was also Teen Clinic day. The atmosphere in the Teen Clinic could vary dramatically. They saw flippant teens, and they saw very serious teens. Some brought boyfriends; some did not. Some boys swaggered through the waiting room as if they were at the school gym. Some were quiet. Forrest measured them up in a few moments, then spoke gently with some teens, firmly with others.

The next patient, not a teen, was alone. Six months pregnant, she waddled to the seat to have her blood pressure taken and plopped down. She pointed at her large belly and said, "Men should have to do this." Her name was Azi Torres, and she had come a long way, from Brazil. "My boyfriend is no help," she said. "Anything I get from him I think a miracle." She finished and walked to the lab. She reached into a red milk crate and picked up an empty plastic specimen cup with a light blue top. She walked into the bathroom and emerged a few minutes later holding the cup out from her body, barely a quarter of an inch of yellow liquid in the bottom. She walked to the waiting room and sat. She moved uncomfortably in her seat and caressed her swollen belly.

When she learned she was pregnant, Azi said she was confused. Speaking, Azi maintained the grammatical sequences of her native Portuguese: putting "no" before verbs, omitting those aggravating, ubiquitous, indefinite pronouns that populate the English language like pesky gnats. "I was happy and sad at same time. Depressed intense. I don't know what to do. I say to myself, who blame? Not blame me or him. We were about to break up when I got pregnant. I said to myself, 'Something'—she snapped her fingers—'about this month feel different.' Then after six days, seven days that it was late, I make a test. I went to a place I think also is a clinic for abortions. They ask if I want to keep the baby, and I said of course. I didn't understand why they asked. I knew right away, for sure, no one could convince me to take the baby out, make abortion. This is me, inside me, is important to me. When I made him I was making love, not sex. When making love, you have to respect it. If I was raped, would take it out because have nothing to do with my feelings. He is two years of my life, a very hard relationship, but I make with love. We used rubber the whole time, but he asked is it OK, and I said yes because I counted and thought it was safe.

"It was too, too messy to me. You just don't know what you feel. When you are stable, when you have a house and a husband, you have something to share with, but you think what are you going to do now? I no have place to live. I am in foreign country. It's like a hell."

Then came the vomiting, which, for the first three months, Jeff did, too. "He was sick all the time," she said, "but no even close to me."

Azi came to Grady because she had already experienced a private hospital as a foreigner with little money and no insurance. A year before, she said, she went to Piedmont Hospital with severe stomach pains. "They knew that I didn't have insurance anything, and one of the doctors said you can go to Grady Hospital. At Grady they receive me, they treat me better, as a human. They treat me better than Piedmont. At Piedmont, they are very cold, mechanical. They know I am foreign. They know they probably have problem to charge. They left me hours waiting after I get inside the room. They checked me, and then I wait one hour to get back, then I wait one hour again, then I wait one more hour for the doctor to come and see me. I was five hours in the emergency room."

"I'm scared," she said, and chuckled. "I'm afraid I will spank my baby later. He'll say, 'Why, Mom, you do that?' I'll say because you pushed and kicked me during pregnancy." She paused and added, "I have six sisters, and they all had C-sections. I'm worried I might have one, too."

"Azi Torres to exam room 1, please."

After her exam, Azi walked to the car she had borrowed from a friend.

She said, "I'm working every bit I can, babysitting. I want to save some money and buy a car and rent a room for me and the baby. Right now I'm sharing a room with someone else. That's all I can afford." She also said she was afraid she might have to sue her boyfriend, Jeff, for support. That night she dreamed she had a boy, and he looked like his father. His nose, eyes and forehead—exactly like a young Jeff. She was walking along with her son and said to him, "You look like your dad a lot, golly." When she woke up she recalled that she never dreamed of her child as an infant, that it was always a boy, that he always resembled Jeff, and that none of her sister's nephews looked much like their mothers.

At her apartment in Floral Acres, a worried Lisa Dean felt what every pregnant woman dreads: nothing. She called her mother and said, through sobs, "I think my baby quit moving. It hadn't moved for four days." Her mother started crying, too. Lisa's sister joined them on the phone, crying.

"Call the hospital," her mother said.

She called Lauren Foley and, sobbing, she told Foley, who told her to come in. Lisa asked her best friend, Marian Thurston, to go with her. They nervously entered the OB clinic and told the clerk that Foley said for her to come on back to see her. "Through the double doors," she said, but they were already through them when she finished.

Lisa lay on the exam table, and Foley squeezed gel on her belly. She positioned the fetal monitor's head, the transducer, with her hand, and Lisa heard the sweet watery sound of a fetal heartbeat. She let out a big breath.

"It's just fine," Foley said. "Maybe she's content and happy in there, sucking her thumb or something."

"I felt it move more when I was only three months. I guess this baby is going to be lazy," Lisa said.

At Lisa's next OB visit, she checked in and went to the blood pressure room. "Slip off your shoes and step up on the scale," Nancy Forrest said. Lisa stood on the scale and intoned, "Whoo-ee." She weighed two-sixteen.

"This is not no quick-weight-loss program," Forrest said. "You're supposed to gain weight."

"Last time I didn't gain any weight."

Forrest gave her a skeptical look.

Lisa went to the waiting room and sat. A teenage boy across from her wore a T-shirt that said, "If You Don't Like My Attitude Quit Talking To Me." Her friend Tameeka Nesbitt, who lived in the same apartment complex, came in and sat next to Lisa.

"I want a little girl this time," Lisa said. "I'll dress her up so pretty. My boy, he thinks it's gonna be his baby." She imitated her son with a soft high voice. "'I'm ready for my baby. When my baby coming home? I'll help feed him. I'll hold him.'"

In her south Georgia twang, Lauren Foley called Lisa to exam room 6 over the intercom. "Everything's fine," Lisa said, exiting 6 after her exam. She did, however, have a prescription for an infection, and she had a plan for maneuvering through Grady. "First I'm going to get my name on the WIC list, then I'm going to the third-floor pharmacy. Maybe it has a shorter line. It's in the old Grady. When I'm through, maybe it'll be my turn at the WIC office." Lisa signed her name and walked to the old building. As the pharmacy line moved on, she reached a row of chairs, the middle of the line. Moving forward, she hopped up and over the arm between chairs. The beginning and end of the line shuffled forward; the middle hopped.

"Number fifteen, I got fifteen," a man behind the second counter said. A woman stepped forward and received the brown bag holding her medicine. The bag was folded neatly at the top.

Waiting in a chair, Lisa said, "I'm glad my sister is a virgin. She's sixteen. I talk to her all the time. I don't say, 'Don't,' because then she'll do it. I say do it because you *want* to not because your friends pressure you. I hope she doesn't have children 'til later in life, after she's married. I want her to do better than me. She says she doesn't want kids, and I say, 'You say that now. . . .'"

She received her medication and went back to the WIC office in the new clinic building. She looked at the list of names. Three X's were by her name: they had called her three times already. She told the clerk her name; the clerk looked at the list and told her to sit in the office, not out in the waiting area. "You're next," she said. Lisa's plan had worked.

Lisa remembered the registration clerk from when she got her last Grady card. "She asked how many kids I had, I said one, and she said that was good. She asked me how old I was, and I said twenty-two. She said, 'You did real good.' But, no. When I get back in school and finish, *then* I'll say I did real good."

That afternoon, Dr. Charles Holcomb, who saw HIV-positive pregnant women, held his prenatal clinic. Not the special clinic where they were told of their infection—these women already knew. Indistinguishable from the other patients, they had the same routine: check in, blood pressure and weight, to the lab, wait in the waiting room until your name is called.

"We treat them all the same," Nancy Forrest said in the blood pressure room. "Each clinic assistant works with the HIV patients two months out of the year. We rotate. Dr. Holcomb is the one who tells them. I put myself in the patient's place. How would I feel being told? Most of them don't know they were at risk." She said at the clinic when they are first told, no other clinics are scheduled. "Sometimes they are twenty-two, twenty-three years old, have a child who's five, been to college, got a good job, and you're lowering the boom. Some scream and cry. Some are just shocked. I always put extra Kleenex in there. It's hard on me. Because I know. They ask, 'Why is that lady calling me so much? Is something wrong?' When I see them waiting, they're usually playing with their kids, talking. Sometimes they'll ask each other why they're at this clinic, and they won't know either."

Forrest pumped up the blood pressure cuff for the next patient, a teen, who put her shoes back on while Forrest was trying to register her blood pressure. Using her gentle voice, Forrest said, "Quit moving, ma'am. Put your foot down. Thank you." After her blood pressure was recorded, Forrest instructed her, "Go to the lab, give some urine, and come back to the waiting room." She finished all the patients in the blood pressure room, and just as the room cleared, another patient entered.

"Take your shoes off, put your coat down, and get ready to step up on the scale."

The phone rang, and Forrest answered it. It was her sister's son.

"Cooking? What are you cooking?" Forrest asked him. "Spaghetti? What's your mama cooking? . . . Tell her you can't expect to do things in front of kids and not expect them to do it, too. You can't stay out all night and raise children." She hung up the phone and said, "I tell the patients that come in here, 'Being a good parent is hard work.' They say, 'No, it's not. Look at you.' But between back then when I had them and now, I've come a long way."

Forrest asked the next patient, "When you going to quit smoking?"

"I wish I could tell you."

"Cut back some first."

"I have."

"See if you can make it one less a day for one week. If you can cut back one less a day, that's good."

The patient left, and Forrest said she was going to quit working Thursday nights after the next month. Thursday night was "New OB" clinic. New pregnant patients came for their initial physical exam and would thereafter see their resident, midwife, or physician assistant during a day clinic. New OB was tiring. They had worked all day and would be back early the next morning. They might not have very many residents available to do the physicals on a given Thursday night, which would extend the evening further. Residents were paid extra for working New OB, but it was still an unpopular shift. Ms. Griff would often go up to Labor and Delivery and scrounge up residents for New OB, using her hangdog expression. Her round eyes would droop, and she would smile tentatively, her voice soft and pleading. She often did not even have to ask. "Can't work New OB, sorry, Ms. Griff," a resident might say before Ms Griff could even speak, if she appeared on a Thursday afternoon. With too many of those responses, New OB could be a long night. But that was not why Forrest quit working Thursday nights.

"My daughter starts night class on Thursdays," she said. "Friday's a school day, so she needs someone to pick up her daughter at six o'clock. Her husband doesn't get home 'til eight or eight-thirty."

Forrest was doing for her daughter what her mother had done for her.

You Gonna Love 'em Anyway

A bewildered-looking young woman entered the Grady OB waiting room and glanced around. She walked to the desk and said, "They told me to ask for Ms. Andrews." She pulled out a piece of paper on which she had scribbled notes. "They said Dr. Holcomb would be my doctor." The clerk called Ms. Griff, who walked through the double doors from the exam room hall. Another patient slept in a chair, leaning awkwardly back and to her left, her leg stretched out in front of her.

It was the day of Dr. Holcomb's special clinic, when patients first met Holcomb, and some learned for the first time of their HIV infection.

"I'll go witcha," Ms. Griff said cheerily, and walked with her to the liaison nurse office, where Andrews sat at a desk. After about ten minutes, Andrews walked the patient back to the waiting room and told her to have a seat until she was called. She sat and was soon joined by her boyfriend and her older sister. Her sister teased her about her weight gain, and all three laughed. Ms. Griff returned after a while and said Dr. Holcomb was ready to see her. Ms. Griff escorted her back to the only exam room being used.

The patient's sister said to the patient's boyfriend, "It seems like you could just take all the blood out and put in new blood. I know if it was that simple, somebody would have thought of it, but think about it. If they can take out a heart and put in a new one, why can't they take out the blood and put in new blood?" They laughed at the idea. Ms. Griff came back and asked the boyfriend to speak with Holcomb.

The sister tapped his arm and joked, "I knew you'd finally be useful."

Ms. Griff escorted the young man back to Holcomb's room, then sat at the clinic assistant's desk across the hall. To the patient and her boy-friend, she had been kind and dotingly helpful. She had come a long way since AIDS first hit Atlanta and Grady.

"I was a typical stereotype," she said. "I had a phobia about it. I thought it was a white gay thing in San Francisco. When we had to work with AIDS patients, I thought they were pushing it down our throat. They kept saying, 'patient rights,' but as a human being I have rights, too. I talked to a lawyer. But I learned. We had seminars and you get educated and learn to change your mind. I did the special clinic, and I found out other things, but I still thought it was mainly gay white men. Then a friend experimented with drugs and tested positive for HIV. She was a black female, from Atlanta. Atlanta born and Atlanta bred. At first you judge with your eyes and not your heart, and you're not supposed to do that.

"I treat 'em all the same. My brother did drugs, and that could be my brother, and I wouldn't want anyone to slight my brother. No matter what bad he does, he's still my brother. Some of them know they did some wrong things, and they don't need you to tell them again. I just double glove and treat them just like everyone else. One patient looked at me and laughed after I took her blood pressure. She said, 'You didn't wipe off the cuff.'

"One mother was fussing at her daughter for being pregnant. She didn't know the half of it. And I couldn't tell her. There was one who was saving her money, preparing for the special time in her life. She was thirty-three and having her first child. I might could work the special clinic all the time, when they're first told, but the emotional part—That's why we rotate. If you have any type of feeling, you know. I have a relative with AIDS. I try to think of it like cancer. You gonna love 'em anyway. Some of them know they did some things wrong, and they don't need you to tell them again."

Robin James's small apartment had a downstairs living room and kitchen, two upstairs bedrooms and a bathroom. A clear plastic runner cut diago-nally across the living room to protect the carpet on the most traveled path. Three large goldfish swam in her rectangular aquarium. The filter bubbled softly.

She said she was the first one in her family born at Grady. "Nine-eight-forty-seven. September eight. That was a good year." She chuckled long. "I had my first girl September twenty, nineteen-sixty-two. Her name is Pauline Daniels now, but she was Pauline Louise James then. She was born feet coming out first. So they had to push her back up in and get her to turn around right for her to come out. When I was carrying children I had problems toting them. My grandmama used to would take a white string and tie it around my stomach and pin it. And that kept my baby up. My daughter won't let me do the things to her that my grand-mama-n-'em did. They don't let me doctor her. For arthritis, my grandmama used to tell us to take dishwater and rub down"—she rubbed her own hands and arms—"and rub it out and it works, stuff like that. Like migraine headaches, sniff spirit of ammonia, up under your nose. You don't have to take all those pills.

"Grady is the best place in the world, I feel, for Pauline to be, for help with having a baby, because I would not have had four kids if I—I went to a private doctor once, and he wanted to take my womb out, and my husband liked to have a fit. When I went to Grady's they fixed me right up. I done had two more children since then. I have real bad problems with my menstrual cycles, but I don't want them taking out my—Nobody has really explained to me why is it necessary that we have to have our insides taken out. I just can't accept it. Sometimes I think about when I used to see my mom and my grandmama having pains during that time of month . . . they took it. I feel like I can hurt for most of mine and keep everything intact.

"I'm not just trying to sit up here and tell you that everything has worked out fine at Grady's, but when it comes to knowing what to do and what's wrong with you, they a little slow, but they thorough. I'm telling you, I have friends that won't even go to Grady. When I got into the job world and started working for a living, I'd even continue to go to Grady, even for psychiatric treatment, anything. With me and my family at Grady's, like my brother shooting my baby brother. With a sawed-off shotgun. My oldest brother shot my baby brother. Grady put my brother's arm back on. He don't have all the usage in his hand but with the therapies he went through with them, he's a little handicapped, but he still has his arm."

She recalled the trauma that brought her to the Grady ER. Fourteen years ago, she was riding on the back of a motorcycle. The bike hit a car and skidded down the road. "I said, 'Lord have mercy.' When I said 'mercy,' we was hitting. Death was looking me eyeball to eyeball. I said, 'Lord have mercy,' and he did. I had on leather T-strap shoes. I couldn't get off the bike because my straps had got hooked in the kickstand. It was dragging me. The top of my feet, my knee, and my hip hit the telephone pole. I could only hear the scraping of my helmet. I heard the Lord speaking to me, 'Don't fight the fall. Roll with it.' And every way that bike went, I didn't fight it. When it rolled, I rolled. Kshhhh, that's all I could hear, my helmet dragging the ground. I got taken to Grady. That was worse than having a baby, to have your skin scraped down. It seemed like they used a SOS pad when they scraping you. It be just some soft stuff, but it just feel like it's metal scraping through your flesh. Oh God, when I see a motorcycle, I don't even touch it. My mama took care of me, changed them dressings, oh my God. I used to be ashamed to take my clothes off when I met a man and everything. But now, you know, I look at my scars and: trophies. Where I done been in life, how many times the Lord has brought me out of dangerous situations.

"My mama-n-'em always went to Grady. You learn about yourself, too. When something wrong with you, they going to tell you what's wrong with you. If you go in there and say, uh, 'I just took a overdose of pills,' they going to ask you what time, why, or, you know, everything they gonna ask you. They not just gonna pump your stomach and send you home and give you a bill. They want you to talk to a psychiatrist. That's why it takes so long."

Trying to recall just how many times she had been to Grady, Robin looked at the ceiling and thought a good little while. "I'd say . . . two or three hundred times. Patrick, he was born the seventh month in seventy-one, at seven-seventeen. Then Sheldon, ten-twenty-seven, seventy-seven. I was trying to get Patrick in the Guiness's book of records. He was born in the seventh month, the seventh day, in seventy-one at seven-

seventeen. He was born on the seventh floor, the room number was seven-something, but the only reason we couldn't get him into the Guiness's book of records was because he weighed eight pounds."

"Instead of seven?"

"Uh-huh. Other than that we would have made it.

"When my third sister was eight years old, she got caught on fire, and she got all burned, and the burn unit, they took real good care of my sister. She has three boys now. The scars and things are still there. My mom got hit by a car one time, got knocked up on the telegraph post and the hood got caught in her leg. Grady saved that. She's walking and everything. She's old now, but she still goes to Grady. My mama's sister still goes to Grady. Broke hip. I want to say something. In my life, uh, I want to say something about the psychiatric ward at Grady. I went there for depression. Suicidal tendencies. I have been to the best doctors but not like the ones at Grady. That's why I'm trying to sit here and tell you about when I used to would be depressed. And want to commit suicide or attempted it—I don't know if you can see the scars now, but I had attempted it—"

She gently touched the gray, lumpy scars on her wrists and rubbed her fingers over and over them.

"The people at Grady, they knew me. I don't know if it had to do with the charts they keep on us, but my history was there, my *history* is there. Robin James is in that folder." She made that statement intensely, her high-pitched voice softening yet firming, like she was talking about a dear child rather than her own self. "When the doctor opens up my folder he knows everything about me. They knew how to talk to me. They knew, I guess, everything about me. I felt like if something really seriously got wrong with me, take me to Grady because I know they'll find out. I'm not bragging. It's just that I'm trying to tell you these are people that helped me. Every lady was proud to have her baby at Grady."

She looked intently at the ceiling. "I'm just trying to eliminate some people, like I asked this lady next door, 'You don't go to Grady?' She said 'No, I got cancer,' and I just looked at her. I'm sure a lot of people done died of cancer at Grady, but I just don't know nobody."

Recalling the long waits for a Grady card, she laughed. "That's a

Grady tradition. Waiting for the Grady card and for the prescription. The hurtin' part about it is that the people that was waiting on you was just as po' as you were. And sometimes you even knew the people. They even came from the same neighborhood that you did. But they was treating you bad, and you always hope that somebody in the same predicament get out so they could help somebody else. Understand maybe they don't know how to read and write, not even sign their name good. Don't holler at 'em. Don't do everything but spit in their face. I've seen old folks treated so bad. Sometimes young people don't understand old people's mind dance around. They could be standing up there looking in their billfold for their Grady card and then all of a sudden something else will come to their mind. Their mind dance. Thoughts. They know what they're trying to do, but it's just going to take a few minutes. Sometimes you might flip through your billfold and see something that reminds you of something that happened, and then they go to fussing at them. 'If you can't find it, get out of the line and move to the side because I don't feel like being bothered today.' And then they go and tell the other person over here what a bad night they had, and sometimes we would have to stand in line and let them talk about their personal problems. And they know people be standing there waiting to see the doctor, but they would talk about their men friends or what happened at the club or their children or act like they not at work. I think the people working there didn't feel good about their jobs, when we thought they should be happy that they had a job. Because a lot of times a lot of us didn't have jobs."

Robin stopped talking for a few moments, then said her daughter, Pauline, was eager to have a baby, finally. "She is thirty-something years old, and she been career-minded all the time and now she think the clock ticking. So now she's in this great big hysterical rush to want to have a baby, and she's very fragile, very tiny. She's just not strong so my baby girl, Cheryl, told us that if we had enough money, would you let me carry your baby for you? Cheryl had five.

"I remember holding Pauline's baby. He didn't have no lungs, but they let me hold him. I needed that. Even though my grandson didn't live, I know when I get to heaven I'm going to see him because he was a person.

I told him, I'll see him when I get to heaven. Pauline was just looking there because I was talking to the baby. She said, 'Mama, look at his feet. He was going to have big feet, wasn't he?' I said yep, just like his daddy, you know, stuff like that. He looked like him, too. Dark complexion. They had him with a little hat on, just like they would a baby if it was alive. Pauline said they told her, we could try to keep him alive, but I'm just now finding this out when I was talking to her about you. She said they could try to save the baby, but they couldn't promise he was going to be normal, so she told him she didn't want her baby like that. I was really shocked because, me, I ain't never had to make such a critical decision, and I didn't even know that was on her then. She's kinda strange. I'm just now learning this, look how long it's been. I guess she knew if I had had something to do with it, I would try to fight for the baby life. I woulda. I guess she said I don't want to go through that. It was a cute little baby, though. I got to get to heaven and see."

In the kitchen in her apartment, with her brother Franklin washing dishes, Lisa Dean said her mother suggested she wait three to six months after the baby was born before going to work. "She thinks I need to stay at home. That PEACH program, they'll help you put your children in a nursery 'til you get on your feet. That's pretty good. If you're eligible.

"Go! Get upstairs!" she shouted to Biloxi, her new dog, who didn't obey.

Rob came downstairs and started playing with his X-Men action figures on the kitchen floor. Lisa shouted, "Biloxi, stop!" The dog was chewing on a pair of Rob's shoes. "Get away! Oooh, I ain't never seen such a nosy dog."

She talked about her first pregnancy, when she was only seventeen, fondly recalling her mother's help. She had recently considered having her tubes tied but changed her mind. "I'm not going to," she said. "My mom said, 'You're still young, and you don't know what will happen in your future.' She's right. I'll just be twenty-three. My mom had her tubes tied, but she had five kids." Laughing, she said, "I don't want any more kids any time soon. But I might want another one five years from now, and I won't be able to have one because my tubes will be tied. So I decided not to.

"I've been thinking about the . . . um IUD, but I don't know. I can't take birth control pills. They had this weird effect on my legs and chest. Sometimes I couldn't get up in the morning. I do not want the shot. I'm big enough, and I know everybody that got the shot got big, and I don't need to be any bigger. And the Norplant, you know they have emphasized that. I don't know what it will do to me, and I do not want to be a guinea pig. I know a girl who had to have hers taken out because it was bringing her hair out so bad. Some gain weight, some lose weight. Weird. I know a girl, she had a cycle for a whole month from the Norplant."

She again said she wanted a natural delivery. "I don't want any drugs. I *got* it natural, heh heh. I don't feel I need an epidural or anything. Sometimes it slows down the baby's heartbeat."

"Git!" Rob shouted at Biloxi. The dog remained. Finally, Franklin told him to go upstairs, and he trotted up.

About her new baby, Lisa said, "My mom's gonna spoil him, so everything will be the same. A little spoiled brat just like this one. Now I'm by myself instead of living with my mom, so it's going to be more of my own family. I want our whole family to have a portrait, with my mom in it. Get it blown up and put it right there." She pointed to the wall across from the sink. Biloxi came back downstairs and started chewing and tugging on one of Lisa's shoes. "Biloxi, go on upstairs with your greedy butt," she said. "Go on! But, yeah, it's good. I feel better about being pregnant now, but if I could start all over again I wouldn't have any kids right now. But I *love*, I love my son. But I wouldn't have any more. I would have done better for myself. I would have been financially stable and able to take care of kids. Without a man. But even if I did I would rather have the man around."

The next week Lisa arrived at the OB clinic with her friend, Tameeka Nesbitt. Hoop earrings dangling, Lisa wore denim shorts, Nike running shoes, and a Snoop Doggy Dogg T-shirt. They stood in a long line at the registration desk. Tameeka said, "I'm telling them I'm getting my tubes tied. This is it."

After their weight and blood pressure were taken, they sat in the waiting room, near where several babies were crying and three children crawled on the floor. Two Muslim women sat across from them. Their clothing and veils covered them all over, except for their eyes. One read the Koran.

"Have you got your baby stuff?" Lisa asked. "I done got the bed."

"I'm going to Wal-Mart to lay away some baby stuff."

"I might get the Norplant," Lisa said, "maybe a diaphragm. The pill makes me gain weight."

"I'm not getting no shot," Tameeka insisted, "no Norplant, none of that stuff."

"Lisa Dean, to exam room 8, please," Lauren Foley announced over the intercom. Lisa walked back through the double doors. In five minutes, Walt Robinson, a physician assistant, called Tameeka to exam room 10.

Azi Torres entered the blood pressure room, and Nancy Forrest said, "We don't want no excess weight." She pointed at the large bag Azi still held in her right hand as she stood on the scales. She took Azi's bag and put it on the desk. To the next patient, a large woman holding a McDonald's wrapper, Forrest said, "You got to stop eating that sausage. That's what's doing it."

Azi sat in a row of chairs near the front desk. She looked at a woman holding an infant several weeks old in her arms and said, "I want mine like that, right out." She had already begun moving her belongings, starting with the baby's things, to the apartment of her friend, Kenneth, who said she could stay there for three months, without charge. After that, she would share the rent. "He's funny," Azi said. "He said, 'I'm getting a roommate who is pregnant. It's like, Buy One—Get One Free.'"

A patient walked by wearing a T-shirt with the Tasmanian Devil cartoon character on the front. The beast's mouth was stretched wide by the woman's pregnant belly.

"Yesterday and Wednesday I felt terrible," Azi said. "Yesterday I woke up and threw up all the food from the night before. I felt like I'd explode. I can't explain it. He moved again. Hurts. I wish I could see inside, what he is doing. Weird. I just have to be content and let it move in there. I didn't sleep much last night. I woke up from the baby pressing on my bladder. More and more I'm pregnant, I wake up more. I am thirstier and thirstier, but my bladder is being pressed against.

"I'm a little afraid of the baby being switched. That's why I want friends there so they can see the baby and say that's Azi's baby. I'll probably be a little bit groggy. I told my doctor he better be good because I have friends who will be there. They are from different parts of the world, and they're crazy."

She was called to exam room 2 by a woman's voice. Her doctor was not in the clinic that day; another resident was seeing his patients. Some patients who would normally be seen the next week were scheduled for this day because Resident Research Days had been scheduled for Thursday and Friday of the next week. Azi passed by Ms. Griff, who looked haggard. The clinic was crowded with the extra appointments, and they were short on residents. A woman asked her how much longer until she was called. Politely, Ms. Griff told her things were backed up and to be patient.

"We have two doctors missing," Ms. Griff said. "And each doctor has about twenty patients. I'm about to go crazy."

Two weeks later, on a cool sunny spring morning—another sparkling clear day that made Atlantans think maybe the summer to come might not be so hot and muggy—Ms. Griff and Nancy Forrest entered Grady from the broad cement walkway between Grady and McDonald's. They knew this would be a long day. The residents had been out of clinic the Friday before, so half those patients were scheduled for today. Plus, two doctors were absent.

Ms. Griff went through the patient charts, pulling the ones for her patients. Behind her, on the clinic aides' desk, the Joke-A-Day gag was,

Father: Heather, you'll have to send your boyfriend home earlier from now on.
Heather: Sorry, Dad. Did the noise keep you awake?
Father: No, but the silences did.

The waiting area, the front desk, blood pressure room, exam rooms, and hallway—all were so quiet that air could be heard flowing through the

AC vent; in a while it would not be noticeable at all. Glancing at the printout of a doctor's patients, Ms. Griff fingered down the long stack, arranged numerically by Grady card number. Each patient's records were in a thick manila folder marked CONFIDENTIAL, MEDICO-LEGAL RECORDS in large letters. Most of the folders were worn and smudged. She was in charge of exam rooms 1 and 2. She stacked the folders on the ledge behind the doctor's seat that faced the computer, in the little office between 1 and 2.

Clinic assistant Sarah Lucas arrived and thumbtacked her printout list of patients to a narrow cork band attached to a wall. Physician assistant Walt Robinson entered the clinic, looked at Lucas's list, and crossed out two names.

"These won't be in today," he said. "One came in sick yesterday. This one delivered."

By 8:00 the waiting room began to fill. Conversational buzz increased every few minutes. Azi Torres came into the clinic at about 10:00. Like most everyone else, she came through the door by the front desk, paused, and fished through her purse for her Grady card and her appointment sheet. She handed them over to the clerk, who placed the card in the electric imprinter, a little boxy machine with its plastic jaws open, its purple inky roller clinging to the roof of its plastic mouth. She held a vital signs sheet in the imprinter and clamped it down, which triggered the roller, clicking and whirring, to move over and back across the sheet, the card's raised letters printing Azi's name and number. The paper came out with an identity.

Azi walked to the blood pressure room. She held up the lab sheet and asked what it was.

"That means they're going to test your blood," Forrest replied.

Azi grimaced. "That means they'll stick my finger."

"You can have it taken from your arm if you want, but it's easier from your finger. Just tell them."

"I think I prefer arm."

Returning from the lab a few minutes later, she picked at the Band-Aid on the inside of her elbow. She finally picked it off and looked at the small red blotch in her skin.

"I move everything the baby but no me yet," she said about her new apartment. "I work only once this week, three and a half hours, staying with an elderly lady. And I had baby shower last week. In America they only invite women, they tell me. I no like that. I have many—" she mumbled, thinking of the right word, "—masculine friends, so I invited everybody. I got almost everything that would be expensive to me. We make a little party to welcome everyone. If baby born tomorrow, the baby is ready. Car seat, stroller." She put her hand on her belly. "He's moving. I think he dropped a little. I hope he's ready because I'm ready.

"I drove to South Carolina this week, Tuesday, with my friend. I have a friend moving back to Brazil. They gave me things they did not take back. Kitchen stuff, another stroller. My new roommate, he no have too much stuff. I was scared to have a baby, had no stuff. I got a lot of stuff but not enough for chicken . . . uh, kitchen. I left Tuesday seven a.m. and back Tuesday eight p.m. I told the baby, 'You hang on. I need to get this stuff.' "

A woman Azi had met at Grady walked into the clinic and saw Azi. She said her baby was in ICU with respiratory problems.

"Was labor long?" Azi asked. She looked intently at her, waiting for her answer.

"Twelve hours."

"Was it hard?"

"No, not too bad."

"Was it on your due date?"

"One day over."

"Was it natural?"

"I only had an epidural."

After she left, Azi said, "She from Macon, single mother. She moved here to have the baby. The father doesn't care. Her family is not supportive. I hear some families give the daughter a hard time for getting pregnant. Some say, 'You got pregnant. You're on your own.' I think sad. She doesn't have money for a telephone."

Azi's OB visit was a quick one. Everything was fine. The doctor told her not to drive to South Carolina again. They didn't want the baby born in a car.

Azi walked to the Grady cafeteria for lunch. She had turkey noodle soup, cornbread, and salad. She added ice cream, topped with chocolate syrup and strawberries. She skipped the coffee. "I no drink alcohol, no caffeine while pregnant. I no eat anything bad for me." She turned her nose up at a meat loaf. "I no like American beef," she said, doing the sign of the cross on her chest. "God help me. Come to Brazil and eat beef. You'll see the difference."

Azi sat down to eat and said she was on her way to a job interview to be a babysitter. As had become her practice, although it probably was no longer necessary, she dressed down and wore no makeup. She recalled her job search two years ago. "The women behavior toward me was strange. I work one time with a painter, and I was his model. They were looking for a babysitter, maybe live-in. They said I was too competent. I finish two years of college in Brazil. No say, 'I don't want a girl like you, maybe trouble with my husband.' Sometimes would say I was too pretty and intelligent, not exactly what I want. They probably think, 'She's Latin, and nice, and want a husband.'"

Azi came to the United States for the first time to learn English and to visit friends in Washington, D.C. Before she left Brazil, however, she met Randall, an American from Columbia, South Carolina, who was touring Rio de Janeiro. He convinced her to go to South Carolina—something about a school there being the best place to learn English.

"But he just wanted me near him," Azi said.

She moved into his apartment, and they dated for two and a half months, unable to speak to one another. He spoke no Portuguese; she spoke very little English. She was twenty-seven; he was thirty-eight. She took an English class for foreigners at the University of South Carolina, which Randall paid for, but she did not attend it regularly. The teacher did not speak Portuguese, and Azi became frustrated. When she and Randall wanted to communicate, they wrote each other notes and consulted a dictionary. It was crude but effective. One day he wrote, "Will you marry me?" She flipped through the dictionary and learned she held in her hand a proposal. She wrote to him that she had to think about it.

"I was a little surprised when he proposed, but I had been proposed to three times in Brazil. He was a good guy, very traditional, religious, did nothing before marriage. Very respectful. But he said I must wear long dresses, show no body. My clothes too sexy to him. He say I must go to church every Sunday. His mother said, 'Are you going to marry her? Look at how she dresses.' He pick out the clothes I no allowed to wear. I said, uh-oh. He thought he could change me, like that." She snapped her fingers. "You cannot change someone like that. I was sad because I was starting to like him. He would not let me pay any bills, like Brazilian guys."

She decided to visit her friends in Washington, D.C., and think things over. She flew first to Ohio to stay with a college-age friend whose mother was Brazilian. He was the only person with whom she could speak Portuguese. She wanted his mother to help her learn how an American household works, so she could get a job housekeeping or babysitting. Randall, however, thought she was leaving him.

"He no understand why I stop in Ohio first. Explaining to him was too hard. In Brazil, if too hard to understand, you say, 'No explain.'" She flipped her hand in the air. "Would complicate things more to try, but he thought I was going with someone else. But this guy in Ohio, he was nineteen, like a brother to me."

She flew to Ohio, and the friend met her. They sat in the airport awaiting her luggage, and suddenly Randall appeared. He had flown after her and found her in the airport. He looked at the two of them, said to her, "Now I understand," walked away, and flew back to South Carolina. She turned to her friend and asked what was going on.

"He tell me, and I think this is a dream. I felt deceived. He did not trust me at all. He think I trade him for a nineteen-year-old in college. Ridiculous. If I had been kissing him, OK, but miscommunication. I could not explain every little thing to him. I understand him better later. Living here, relationships are very complicated. They value money over love. People divorce and fight about money. No see this too much where I come from. I didn't understand why he so insecure when I was with him. We used to go to the grocery store, and people would talk to me, and he no like that. I could no explain to him that in Brazil if see someone interesting, stop and talk to them. You have to give someone a chance to be a human. I was shock. I could not run after him and say it no what you think. My English was too little. Too shocked, so frustrated, him thinking a thing like that. My friend said, 'This guy crazy.'

"When Randall was younger, he use a lot of drugs. He get into religion, say he is born again. He thought everyone had to be born again. Everybody have done something bad and need it, but he thought I would switch to his culture, but it would not come natural. His pressure didn't work. It scared me, and I left. I was glad and sad at same time."

She stayed in Ohio a week, reveling in the linguistically uncluttered freedom of speaking Portuguese day and night. She learned how American houses function. Then she went to D.C. and got sick. Her friends worked, so she was often alone. She called Randall in South Carolina and, trading bad English for bad Portuguese, tried to explain that she had not had an affair. He flew to D.C. to visit for a weekend and took her to see a doctor. Azi decided to go back to Brazil, and he bought her ticket. When she arrived home in Brazil, he called her from South Carolina. Her phone system provided translation services for international calls. He had already called the mother in Ohio to ask what was going on between Azi and her son. She had told him she thought they were just friends but did not know for sure. That little hesitation restored his doubts. So he called the son, who was so angry at him that he did not say, "Of course not." He said, "What do you think? You have to listen to her, not to me."

"He call me in Brazil," Azi continued, "and accused me of affair. I wanted to say, 'Go to hell,' but I remember him being nice to me."

"You've done something wrong," he, in South Carolina, told the translator, somewhere in Brazil speaking with both of them, who relayed it to Azi. "So you have to confess to me."

For a few months they repeated the same conversation. "I finally told the translator to ask him if he will be content if I say, 'Yes, I have affair.' I am thinking let's make him happy, say what he want to hear. She ask him, and she said to me that what he want to hear, so I said tell him I did. He said now it's easier because you told me the truth. The truth he wanted to hear. I started to think I was in a movie or a soap opera. I was in Brazil for six months. I became more mature about what I want. I was in no relationship. No one tell me what to do."

She returned to the United States and lived with a friend in Orlando, Florida. Randall called her, and she tried to convince him she could have nothing to do with him. "I was frustrated because I had come to America to learn English, and I had not learned it. Though I did learn about Americans. He was nice and kind, but he still couldn't trust. We got in the crap again from before."

She soon went to Atlanta. A friend went there on business, planning to be there only a week, and she went along. His work kept him there several more months, so he rented an apartment.

"He took me to English as Second Language class three nights a week. The apartment was filthy, and I cleaned it, whole apartment. I cleaned everything. I spent one whole day cleaning and another day to put stuff back. He was very nice, very intelligent. He had been married three times, two times to the same wife. He had one daughter, who did not like him. We had things in common. He had been a race car driver, and I used to race for fun in Brazil. We close an avenue, have illegal races. Everybody get there and have people watching. I didn't race my car. I race my boyfriend's car."

Two months later, she met Jeff, the father of her child. She was riding in a friend's car, stopped at a red light, and Jeff pulled his car up beside theirs. He chatted and invited them to dinner. "You would not catch us if I was driving," Azi shouted. They started dating, and he asked her to move in with him. Her friend returned to Orlando, vacating the apartment, so she moved in with Jeff, hoping to stay until she found a live-in job. Not long after, she returned to Brazil, just before her six-month tourist visa expired. Jeff got a job right around the time Azi went to Brazil. They talked on the phone frequently, and they felt they were falling in love. She returned to Atlanta and moved into his apartment. He quit his job.

"We had problems because he was out of work. And he had family pressures because he was living with me." She learned that Jeff's family was wealthy and that, job or no job, he received a monthly dividend from his family's enormous fortune. But money was still a problem. "He had little control with money. He put bills on top of the dresser and leave them. He buy things he use only one or two times. He put everything in boxes and left them. He buy things he already had in boxes. His phone was cut off, no pay the bill. I decided to pay the phone bill, so I opened a checking account. I have social security card but not one that let me get job here.

"I got driver's license, too. When I get it, they asked if I was white or black or Hispanic. I'm not Hispanic. I am Latin. I live in Latin America. I say, 'I think I'm black; what do you think?' She said, 'I think you're white.' In Brazil, when we say someone is white, we mean they are sick. The clerk was really black, and her last name was White. I thought that was funny. I said in my country you are really black, and I'm *morena*, between white and black."

She returned to Brazil the next year, when she was pregnant, and Jeff arrived five days later. Jeff wanted to tour Brazil, and Azi threw up every day. "But he realized I was not a miserable Brazilian coming to America for money. He see we are comfortable. My sister has money and bought a big house. His family warned him about me, but in reality I am closer to my family in Brazil, while I am here in the U.S., than he is with his family here in Atlanta. He was fifteen days without do anything, sit at home. He accuse me like you should be careful; it was my fault I was pregnant. He start accuse me everything, and he was bored. I didn't expect to be so sick, damn sick, throw up whole day, and night. He was upset because he woke up, and he used to walk alone first around my house, and that is not beautiful like this Atlanta. My city is so poverty and everything. I think that's why he was upset. Then he went to north Brazil and saw a lot of people and made a lot friends. Women is available everywhere, and I think he have a lot of fun. I don't know what he did, but I know he had a lot of fun. And when I try call him once because was couple days he didn't call me and I gave him number to call me collect. He felt like I was spying him, and I got so upset because I said, 'The son of a bitch is in my country, no speak any bullshit Portuguese, and wants no think I will not worry about him.' Thinks I am calling to spy him, the hell with this, why do I have to spy him? I never call anymore, and I said you know something, he can do whatever he wants here.

We have an expression in Brazil, 'Who have mouth go to Roma,' means if you can talk, you can do anything."

Back in the OB clinic, the line outside the blood pressure room was getting long, stretching out into the waiting room. A child scampered through the line, playfully screeching. In the exam room area, a teen patient walked back from the waiting room and asked Ms. Griff how much longer until she could see a doctor. Ms. Griff told her there were five patients in front of her.

"Can I go somewhere? McDonald's?" the patient asked.

"No, dahlin'. We don't know when you'll be back."

Ms. Griff took the charts into room 11. She then walked back to the lab supply room. Coming out she said, "Lord, have mercy." A patient had picked up the staff phone from the desk. Ms. Griff opened her eyes wide, smiled, and said, "Excuse me."

"Excuse me," the patient answered.

Speaking in her soft voice, Ms. Griff said, "Go ahead. Dial 9 first. But you're supposed to ask."

Seeing the OB attending physician walk by, she picked up a chart and said, "Dr. Pell, Dr. Pell, we got a new one." She handed him the chart and said, "Room 9." She picked up the next chart and walked to the waiting room and called a name. In the waiting room, the children were beginning to get impatient and loud. As Ms. Griff returned to the desk, a woman walked to the back and asked, "How much longer for me?" A resident came out of an exam room and asked Ms. Griff for a chart. "I'm going to Medical Records to get some others. I'll get that one, too." Before she could leave, another patient walked back and held out her Grady card. Ms. Griff responded before she could say "How much longer," with, "We can't call you yet. Be patient, and we'll get to you." She went into room 12 to clean it and prepare it for the next patient. She finished and went to the supply room to get a gown for the room. Walking back, she saw a teen with a child angrily chase the child down the hall. Ms. Griff sat the teen down gently.

"Somebody was patient with you when you were little," she told her. "You should be patient with her."

Another teen asked Ms. Griff where to go next.

"Down the hall, to the liaison nurse's office, dahlin'."

Ms. Griff then went to the lab supply room, picked up a gonorrhea culture and form and took them to 12. Leaving room 12, she saw Dr. Pell looking around. He needed a chaperon with him for an exam. "I'm right behind you, Dr. Pell." She followed him into room 9.

At 3:30 a woman from India approached Ms. Griff and asked if she could be seen by a female doctor. She replied, "None are still here. If you had told me earlier, I could have. I'll see if they'll let you see a midwife."

Ms. Griff entered room 9, then exited and went to the nurse's desk. She had a few moments to sit. A patient walked through the double doors and asked Ms. Griff how much longer. The staff were all going about their work, tiredness creeping into the edges of their faces. Ms. Lucas asked Ms. Griff, "Do you think we'll get away by four?" She responded, "It doesn't look hopeful."

Sitting at the clinic assistants' desk, Ms. Griff tapped her heels together and intoned wearily, "There's no place like home. There's no place like home." Next to the computer, the Joke-A-Day calendar had, "My girlfriend's so selfish, she won a trip for two to Paris, and went twice!" She stared at the computer screen, waiting for it to change to the right menu. Her imploring eyes were round and sweet. "It's down," Ms. Lucas said, walking by with an armful of medical charts.

Dr. Holcomb stepped out of his office, and a woman showed him her ultrasound print. She said, "Look at this," and let the meaning sink in. There were Baby A and Baby B. She had twins. "I just found out at ten-thirty this morning. I'm still shocked. What have I got myself into?"

Nancy Forrest walked by carrying a can of disinfectant spray and a blue cloth. She had come from cleaning the lab room. "They had things every whichaway," she said. She walked to the blood pressure room, to clean it.

Finished with all his patients, physician assistant Robinson walked by, his bag slung over his shoulder. "I had a lot of patients today," he said. "I got bombarded." His day had started at 5:00 a.m. when a patient called him at home. She went to Labor and Delivery; they sent her home. Instead, she went to his exam room and wept. He measured her cervix at four centimeters. She had been three in Labor and Delivery. He took her back up, and they admitted her.

Outside the blood pressure room, in the waiting area, the last patient was called to exam room 5. The day at the OB clinic had begun slowly, then become hectic and rushed, and then wound down slowly in the late afternoon, as the number of patients tapered off. The poor waiting room, after a day of too many patients, most of them teenagers, was littered with McDonald's cups, bits of potato chips, straws, napkins, brown bags, torn magazine pages, pamphlets torn to shreds by children, and other assorted bits of paper.

In the exam room area, Ms. Griff removed dirty linen from her rooms and stuffed them in a linen bag that was draped tightly over a wheeled three-legged metal frame. She checked her rooms to make sure all the dirty instruments had been removed. She cleaned her rooms, 1 and 2, and helped clean 9, 10, and 12, rooms she had worked in some during the day. "I'm going home, watch the Braves' game, watch Erkel, and by then I'll be asleep. My granddaughter will punch my arm." She put her head back and closed her eyes, imitating herself sleeping on a couch. "She'll say, 'Bram-mama, Bram-mama, don't be mean.' I'll say, 'I'm not being mean. I just need my nap.' "

Other clinic assistants cleaned their rooms as their last patients left. One cheered softly, "Hooray, hooray," as she cleaned the last midwife exam room. The entire clinic felt somber, after the day's busy clatter had subsided. By this time, they could *hear* the slight click of metal instruments down the hall, the tinny squeak of the linen carrier's wheels on the tile floor, the soft rush of air vents. At precisely 4:57, Forrest finished her last chore and said, "Hooray, I can finally go home."

Seven a.m. on a cool morning, the sky still dark, Diane Williams arrived at Grady's Women's Urgent Care Center. The front of the building was lit by street lights and the horizontal beams of light glowing from each floor of the Grady parking deck. A large man selling newspapers intoned, "Morning paper, morning paper," as if chanting at a temple. "*Morning* paper, *morning* paper. Get your *morning* paper. You know you're going to be waiting two hours. Read the paper while you wait. *Morning paper, morning paper, get your morning paper.*"

Williams put her lunch in the refrigerator in the break room and stepped into the routine of cleaning an exam room, preparing it for the next patient. She put the dirty laundry in the hamper and tossed the used chuck, an absorbent sheet placed across the exam table, in the garbage. She sprayed and wiped the exam bed and spread fresh paper on it. She put out a gown, specimen jar, specimen slides, and sterile equipment. She squeezed a daub of KY Jelly onto a small sheet of gauze. "Sometimes the doctors squeeze the tube with their gunky hands," she explained.

Within a few minutes, two EMT's wheeled in a patient on a gurney and moved her to a bed in the observation room, which they called "obs." She was a small, very thin woman.

"Lord, please help me, please help me," the patient moaned desperately, repeatedly.

"What can I do to help you?" asked Lynn Tronowski, the obs nurse. "Are you pregnant? Have you missed a period?" She did not answer any of the questions. "Let's check your blood pressure."

"It feels like something is pressing down on me."

Tronowski wrapped the cuff around her arm and pushed the "Start" button.

"Oh God, help!" She squirmed until she was half off the bed.

"Lay down, just a minute."

"It feels like something is pushing on my stomach!"

"This is very important. Have you ever used crack cocaine? Today or yesterday?"

"No," she moaned.

"When did this start? When did you last have a normal period?"

"I don't remember."

A nurse came in and asked the triage questions. She stood by the bed, holding a clipboard and pen.

"How many babies have you taken to full term?"

"None. Oh-oh-oh, God!"

"Did you have a period this month?"

"No. Oh, God help me."

"When did this pain start?"

"Last night."

Tronowski slipped a thermometer into her mouth. The patient curled up on her side and shook.

"Sign right here," the triage nurse said.

"Ow, ow! Oh!" She signed her name.

"Sometimes, when somebody uses cocaine, it makes you hurt like that," Tronowski said. She spoke softly and calmly. "You need to tell us if you had drugs today so we can help you and give you something for it. Tell us if you used crack. I can tell when we take this blood."

Cocaine can induce preterm labor, and some women, the WUCC staff had learned, take cocaine to end the pregnancy. Cocaine also closes off blood vessels and can cause heart problems. Such patients were usually given fluids, and magnesium sulfate to slow the painful contractions, although it can make a patient agitated.

"I know you can tell," the patient said. "I haven't used it in a month."

"If you can wait a month, you can quit that stuff," Tronowski said. She urged her to stay still while she drew blood.

Diane Williams pushed in a wheelchair with a miserable-looking pregnant teenager. She told Tronowski the girl was having a sickle-cell crisis. She added, "We've gone over this with her. She's going to tell us if she feels pain or if her water breaks." She spoke with the tone of an instructive mother, yet still the detached professional. She put the girl in a bed at the other end of the room from the patient moaning about the pain in her stomach. She started to leave obs, but when she saw that Tronowski and the triage nurse were busy with the first patient, she said, "I'll take care of this one." She knew it would slow the process for other patients waiting, but she did not want to leave the sickle-cell patient with her treatment not yet started. She brought an IV setup over and muttered, "This is going to be another Monday."

Dr. Donald Fillman came into obs, and Tronowski filled him in about the first patient. He instructed her to do IV fluids and run the usual labs. She asked if she should give her aspirin for pain. "No, not until I examine her," he said.

"Oh, Lord, help me!"

"I'm getting an IV for you," Tronowski said. "It'll give you some fluid. That oughta help."

She got the IV ready, but could not reach the hook over the bed. Williams walked over and hooked it for her. "We're going to have to get you some stilts. If I call you shorty, don't get mad."

"Oh, God, please take the pain away. Please help me." She cried much louder. When Tronowski pushed the IV needle in, she cried, "Ow! That hurts!"

At the desk, Williams said, "If she's abused something, she's going to have fragile veins."

Within a half hour, she began to settle down. She moaned steadily and shivered. Williams finished the IV for the sickle-cell patient and helped Tronowski with her patient. Williams said to the patient, "You're at Grady. We're going to take care of you. Every time you feel pain, take a deep breath, like this." She breathed in deeply and exhaled.

The sickle-cell patient's mother quietly entered obs and sat in a chair next to her daughter, who whimpered softly.

At the obs desk, as both patients quieted, Tronowski whispered, "When you take cocaine, your gut closes real tight, like you're passing a kidney stone. Sometimes tissue dies in there. Usually we fill them with fluid to drain it out. Some kick and scream. We try to keep the blood pressure level. If it goes too high, you can have a stroke." She wrote on a patient record, then pointed back over her shoulder with her pen. "I wish they would put this on TV and tell how much pain it causes. They warn about AIDS, especially for women who prostitute themselves with anybody and don't use a condom, but I wish they'd tell 'em about the pain, too."

The sickle-cell patient began sobbing. Her mother had just left. Tronowski called the residents' office and asked if she could give her something for pain. "She's on an IV and taking oxygen . . . OK." She turned to the patient and said, "We're going to get you something for your pain." The cocaine patient curled up her legs and slept, shaking slightly. Tronowski went to the medication cabinet and returned with the medicine.

"I just want to sleep," the young girl sobbed. "I want my mama."

"I'll go get her when I'm through."

She screamed when the needle entered her arm. "Hurry up!"

"I know it hurts. I'm almost through, and I'll go get your mom."

A nurse came in to replace Tronowski, who left for her lunch break. As she was leaving, two EMTs wheeled in another patient.

The first two patients soon slept peacefully. Williams came in and wheeled the sickle-cell patient into one of the exam rooms to see a doctor. Dr. Fillman returned and asked questions of the patient with the severe gut pain. Her lab results had come in. "How much cocaine did you do yesterday?" No answer. "Did you do any this morning?"

"I didn't—"

"Let's try this. I know that you did it. When did you do it?"

She mumbled that she wasn't sure.

"Have you used alcohol, beer, or other drugs during this pregnancy?"

She said she drank about a six-pack of beer a week. She was calm but quivered slightly. Dr. Fillman tested her sensory responses by touching a foot and asking her which foot he was touching. He turned her foot and asked which direction it pointed. She answered correctly. When an exam room became available, they wheeled her out of obs, around the corner, and into the room.

By this time, three more patients had been taken to obs. One had also used cocaine. Folding the corner of a sheet under a mattress, Tronowski said, "I expect obs to fill up tonight."

The woman whose gut had tightened from cocaine use was admitted to 4B, the antepartum floor. The sickle-cell patient was admitted to Labor and Delivery. Williams called there and reported that the patient was sedated but beginning to feel the pain again. The patient's mother told Williams that her daughter had been molested by a relative, but they had discovered the pregnancy too late for an abortion.

Lisa Dean arrived at the Perinatal Center, where she had an ultrasound scheduled. Lauren Foley had told her her fundal height was a bit low. As the ultrasound date neared, Lisa worried what that meant. She thought Foley seemed calm about it, but then she thought, "But why are they scheduling another ultrasound?" She checked in, sat down to wait, and said, "My mom says this baby's going to be mean. How you are when you're pregnant, that's how the baby's going to be. They think I'm mean."

Walking, she had looked tired. She said she felt tired.

Rob became restless and started running around the room. "I hope I don't have another one like you," Lisa said. He came back to her, and she held his hands. "I'll find out what I'm having today. I think I'm going to have a boy, but I want a girl. Boys are into everything. My mom talks to my stomach, and Rob says, 'Grandmama, that's *my* baby. You can't have my baby. I want a boy baby.'" She said to her son, "I got to take you to the dentist."

"No, they'll take my teeth out."

"No, they're not."

"Yes, they is."

"Are," she corrected him. "I acted like him when I was pregnant. I was crazy."

She mentioned Dwayne, and her face turned sour. "He's getting on my nerves. He doesn't want me to go anywhere. He says it's too close. He says I might have the baby off somewhere else.

"My grandmother had a dream where I had twin girls, and if not twins, it will definitely be a girl. Everybody's been saying I'm going to have twins."

Rob began squirming. Lisa corrected him, and something Rob said caught Lisa's attention. She asked him, "Did you curse?"

"No," he said.

"What did you say?"

"I said, 'Leave me alone.'"

"Come here," Lisa said, and he walked right up to her.

"I didn't curse," he said, beginning to cry.

"Come here then."

"You going to whip me."

"No, I'm not. Come here."

She put her hand on his shoulder. "Did you curse?"

"No."

"Tell me the truth, or I will whip you. Did you curse?"

He nodded his head.

"Why did you curse? That's wrong and not nice. Don't talk like that again."

He nodded and returned to his seat.

She said the previous Saturday she attended a funeral for a man who lived near her apartment. "He called a guy who owed him money and asked if he had the money. The guy said yes. He walked up there to get it, and he was shot before he got there. He was twenty-six and had six kids. Three by one girl, two by FiFi, and one by the girl he was about to marry. The funeral was at the church where he was in the men's choir. He loved quoting the Bible. My mom said, 'You better move, or I'm going to come get my two grandkids.'"

An ultrasound tech pushed through the double doors and called Lisa's name. She walked to the back, undressed, and lay on the exam table. Rob stood by, nervously playing with the yellow curtain the tech pulled around for privacy. The tech spread the ultrasound gel on Lisa's swollen belly and held the transducer against her. She slid it around, holding it to Lisa's skin, watching the shadowy screen.

Moments after the tech started, Lisa said, "Can you tell what it is?"

"It's a girl."

"Yeah, just what I wanted." Lisa grinned widely. All through the exam, she smiled at the screen. The tech pointed out the baby's head, rear end, arms. She stopped every so often, marked and labeled a section of the screen, and punched a button so the machine churned out a picture.

"There's the baby's spine," she said. "These are chambers of the heart. That's normal. See the eyes rolling around? The mouth is wide open, there."

"How could you tell it was a girl so quickly?" Lisa asked.

"Its legs were apart for me to see. There's the baby's little belly."

Rob began wandering around the room. He was noticeably more restless after the tech said the baby would be a girl. "What's that stuff on your stomach?" he asked his mom. "What do they do with that?" The tech explained to him that the gel helped her see the baby better.

"I can't wait to get home and tell my mama," Lisa said to the tech. "She was right."

"She predicted it, huh? What did she go by, the shape?"

"Yeah, and my attitude."

Rob rubbed his own stomach and said, "I got a baby, too."

"You'll be a first," the tech said. "Is it a boy or a girl?"

"Boy."

To Lisa, the tech said, "The baby's a little bit small, about two weeks behind. How much weight have you gained?"

"Twenty-five pounds."

"That much?" The tech finished the exam and told Lisa to wait in the hall. She gave Lisa an ultrasound picture of the baby, a front facial shot, the baby's mouth wide open, much like the solitary figure in Edvard Munch's painting, "The Scream." The tech said she would check the records in the computer and see if Lisa needed to come back for another ultrasound.

Sitting in a chair in the hall, Lisa exulted in the knowledge that her baby would be a girl, yet her demeanor was grim. Her face was a battleground between two emotions. She smiled as she talked about naming her baby, but her face briefly lost its smile as she rehashed what the tech had said. She couldn't remember if she had said the baby's growth was two weeks behind, or two *months*.

"I'm going to name her D'Lisa Marsha." She said she took the "D" from Dwayne and added it to Lisa. She chose Marsha because Dwayne's middle name was Marshall. "I'm getting nervous now." She shifted in her chair. "She said it was growing two months behind." Her face settled into a serious stolid expression. She remembered her mother saying recently, "Where's the belly? You look small." To Rob she said, "Are you going to be nice to your sister?"

"It's a boy."

"It's a girl."

"It's a boy."

They repeated this exchange several times until Lisa looked away and said, "He's really upset about that." She sighed twice and said, "I'm praying there's nothing wrong."

The tech emerged from her office and said, "The baby's doing OK. It's not quite two weeks behind."

"I thought you said *months*," Lisa said, chuckling at herself.

Lisa scooted quickly out of the exam area and danced across the waiting room. "I got to call my mama," she said, and picked up the courtesy phone. "Guess what?" . . . . "Guess." . . . . "Yep, a girl. I got a girl," she squealed into the phone. "And Rob is mad."

"I told you that was my little granddaughter," her mother said. "And she's going to be a little hell-raiser, too."

Lisa hung up the phone and grinned all the way down the hall, on the way down in the elevator, and across the atrium. "I'm having a girl," she beamed. "I got a boy and a girl. I'm not having any more children. I'm having my tubes tied." She thought a moment and added, "My mom said don't do that."

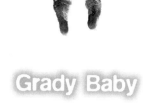

Grady Baby

Azi Torres swept her arm through the air, pointing at a row of vases filled with congratulatory flowers and a clear plastic bag of free sample products from Grady. "Look at all my stuff," she said, in postpartum. She wore a white hospital gown and green foam-rubber slippers. She had had her baby, a boy, two days before. He slept in a wheeled crib next to her bed. She named him Robert. She sat on the edge of the bed and said, "That's a strong name. It's quick and easy to pronounce, here and in Brazil. It is also Jeff's middle name, but I no pick it because of that."

The night before the delivery, she said, she thought it was time, but she was not sure. "I start to feel the pain, strange pain, and stuff. Pain. It comes and goes. I read so much about what is like pain, come and go, come and go. Then I said, 'This is look like the baby is want to come.' But I thought it was very soft pain; it was not hard. But then it getting hard and quick, little space between, and I start to get crazy. I was crying and I said probably can be false, and I did try relaxing, do exercise, breathe, things like that. Then I try sleep and I could not sleep and it was whole night like that. Then six-thirty in the morning I start to feel more and more. I called Jeff and he finally get here at nine. I almost died waiting for him. I was feeling the big pain, and I said I go to hospital and it will be false alarm. Then I went to the bathroom. I see something that look like that what they said about—pink. My water didn't, was not broken. Jeff get here and I get to hospital I was two cili—, centimeters. I was scared because I said gosh, I will die if I feel something more than this. The pain was getting strong and the space between the pain was very short and the stro-o-o-ong and short, and stro-o-o-ong and short, and then in one hour they check and everything, and I was really, really in pain. I start to bite my hand and screaming. Screaming loud, like crazy. I was shamed of myself I screamed so much. Jeff started to get crazy too because he never saw me screaming like that. I hit him because he was hold my hand. I hit him a lot because they start put something to help me breathe, the oxygen mask. I told them before that I wanted epi-, epirudal. The doctor broke my water when I was six centiments, centimeters. And then another doctor, she was supposed to give me the epidural right away, but was busy with somebody else that was deliver time. After they broke the water the pain get worse because, um, the baby, I don't know, the baby's totally there, you know, and ah, gosh, was hell. Probably hell is better than this pain. Jesus Christ and everything like that. I think I get more pain than everybody because, no because I am, I am not different. Everybody can have the same pain, if broke the water and the doctor is not there to give the epidutoral, and I was not prepared. I did not have the dilation. That's why they cut me, to help me, but the pain was so strong that even with the epidural I felt whole pain in the world, and I am very strong to pain. I am not like—" in a high voice, mocking someone exaggerating her pain, "'aaah,' a little bit like some people that just 'aaah.' I am strong. I bit my hand a lot. My hand the next day was bruised. And I hit Jeff a lot. I think that helped me a little bit because I didn't know what to do with the pain and I did that and, 'Oh shit,' with the arm of the bed, I kill—I don't know how to describe this pain. I don't know how some women have another baby. So painful." She whispered, "Jesus Christ."

She smiled a phony syrupy smile and said, "I didn't have 'oooooh' emotional experience I hear about. I was exhausted. I didn't feel nothing. I look and I didn't believe it. I said, 'He's big! Where is he come from?' I thought it was really amazing thing. They put him beside me and I was keeping looking him sometimes, thinking he's huge."

She had similar memories of the episiotomy stitch-up. "They said it was minimum, ten stitches. After a while I ask, 'Are you done?' They said no." She smirked and said flatly, "Minimum ten. I don't think I'll go through this again. Would be better if have husband."

She was surprised by her sister, Luciene, who arrived from Brazil to help her for two weeks. Though she lived thousands of miles away, Luciene had already had an eerie connection with Robert. Luciene practiced spiritism, a religion with elements of Roman Catholicism, African religions, science, philosophy, and Brazilian culture. Or: charismatic evangelicalism, Buddhism, and Brazilian culture. Vibrant and diverse, spiritism is best experienced, rather than summarized. Most spiritists believe in reincarnation guided by the law of karma, the existence of a spiritual otherworld, and psychic communication through mediums. This communication may involve past lives. Spiritists often receive messages or advice from mediums at spiritist sessions. Or they may have healing energy transferred to them through mediums. Many middle-class spiritists, including Azi's sister, who volunteers for an orphanage and adoption organization, do charitable work. Some mediums receive messages while in a trancelike state. Luciene heard her message in a dream.

Before Azi knew her baby would be a boy, Luciene dreamed she was walking along a beach and saw a man's name, Scopius, written in the sand. Scopius, Luciene told Azi, was King Solomon's name in a previous life. A voice spoke to Luciene in the dream, saying, "This will be your sister's son's name."

And it was. "It will be a strong name," Azi said, and chose it for Robert's middle name.

Azi's sister had one more message for Azi. Luciene went to a spiritist medium, who gave her a message from the spirit world. It was an incomplete message, one that would be unclear to Azi until later. For now, her sister said only: "Meet Jeff's grandmother. There will be your support."

Azi pushed her baby's crib down the hall to the nursery. While she was gone, her roommate turned on a TV, a small black-and-white with fuzzy reception. Just as a friend of the roommate entered to visit, Jerry Springer asked one of his guests, "So for three years you had this relationship and you never told your husband you were bisexual?" The roommate's friend asked, "Is it my imagination, or are those women holding hands?"

A tag under a man announced, "Just Found Out Girlfriend is Bisexual."

"They are," the roommate answered. "That woman in the middle is in love with her, and that guy wants to marry her."

On the TV, a tag said, "'Michelle' Says 'Tonya' Is Trying To Seduce Her."

"When we come back," Jerry Springer said, "we'll see if these women will stay with their current lovers or be swept away by the other woman."

A determined woman's voice on TV said, "He may or may not be man enough to take it, but he can *never* be woman enough."

"TV's starting to get boring," the friend said.

The next Wednesday the OB/GYN department gathered for Swan Song, the ceremony honoring the graduation of fourth-year residents. Each resident was given the podium to say final words to the other residents, attending doctors, and staff. Some residents gave elaborate slide presentations; some gave a few spontaneous comments. Some used Swan Song to spew their complaints about the last four years. Some were hilarious; some were serious; some were both. Swan Song was notorious for its candor and cutting wit, as well as heartfelt reflection and occasional schmaltz. The fourth-years were also known to exaggerate a bit. The mood was boisterous and chatty. The chatter quieted when Dr. Goldhill stood and began the ceremony.

One resident received his certificate and said, "I feel like a mosquito in a nudist colony. I know what I'm supposed to do. I just don't know where to start. I'd heard about Grady, about the obstructions in getting something done. It's amazing how many places you have to walk around, how many doors are locked, stairwells are barred, policies you have to get around, but there are some people here who have done remarkable jobs. I'd like to thank them for it. They've helped to work through some of the difficult times. When you can't think of what to do next, they'd say, 'How about this?' One other thing: I'd like to thank the faculty for all I've learned from you."

One resident drew big laughs with his sarcastic comments about physician assistant Walt Robinson considering himself the equal of a third-year resident. Two residents merely thanked everyone, said the last four years were great, and sat down.

The next resident got a nice laugh with, "I know you're hoping I'd get up and say some really nasty stuff. But my boss is in the audience, and I do want to get paid next year. So I can't really burn any bridges. But I do have a few things to say. My first call day at Grady I was the only intern because there was some sort of screwup. Dr. Denson came to help. He was more of a hindrance than a help." The residents laughed at that, some glancing at the director of the obstetrics department. "They set up the bed, then the thirty people came that are always there for a delivery. It has to be a big spectacle. The patient had already had like six babies so she didn't have to push very long. She gave a little grunt and the baby came shooting out about thirty miles per hour." More laughter. "I went to grab the baby and I turned to the table for the instruments to clamp the cord and I slipped in that slimy water. I just went flat on my back." They roared with laughter. "I looked up a few seconds later and I was thinking, 'Where's the baby?'" She was on a roll; they laughed even harder. "I heard Dr. Denson yelling, 'Are you OK?' There was the baby in the bucket, blood spurting out of the umbilical cord, and of course there were thirty people there to see it. The baby did OK, and one of the nurses said, 'Don't worry, it's still moving all its arms and legs.'" They roared; she was slaying them. "Dr. Denson, after a couple of beers, likes to remind me of that story.

"Also, I wanted to say hi to a whole bunch of people. And a few special people: First, Dr. Baker, my advisor. Dr. Neel, I admired his sense of humor. He taught me to try to not take myself so seriously. It didn't work. Dr. Holcomb, whose calm and common-sense approach to obstetrics I've always admired. I've learned a lot from him. Dr. Jennings, he taught me everything I know about diabetes and pregnancy. I hope I remember some of it. Dr. Cawthon taught me how to dissect, and he's been a good friend. He's the biggest resident advocate I know. You can go to him any time and he'll give you good advice. I do appreciate his love of teaching. He goes to great lengths to give a conference every Monday that hardly anybody goes to. That's been a pet peeve of mine. Dr. Bishop taught me to take pride in my work and taught me that if you pay attention to details you can hopefully stay out of trouble and take good care of your patients. And a surprise person: he takes a lot of flak from the residents. Ninety-nine percent of it is well-deserved. Dr. Denson has the hardest job in this program. He taught me how to stretch a six-centimeter cervix to complete." Big laughter.

She showed slides with quotations on them and asked the audience to guess who said them. "Some are private jokes," she alerted them. "Here's a blast from the past: 'If you had kept your legs shut, this would never have happened.' She named a former resident as the speaker of the line. In a soft voice she read, 'You don't have to *touch* AIDS patients, do you?' She paused and said, 'That was my mom,' which got a big laugh. "Here is what I hear when I get a phone call from patients at night, who go to a private doctor but wait until midnight to call." She whined, " 'I'm having severe pain, the worst pain I've ever had, and this is worse than the pain I had last night, which was also the worst pain I'd ever had. I need some pain medicine right now, at three in the morning. By the way, I am allergic to codeine, morphine and Tylenol." She concluded with a chipper, "I'll miss everybody in my class. Especially the people who helped me out, who laid off the criticism and just gave advice." She thanked Ms. Griff and said, "I know they made her quit saying, 'Come on in, take everything off but your skin.' It wasn't professional but it set the patients at ease."

On the phone, Azi Torres sounded very sleepy. She spoke slowly, her deep voice creeping through her words.

"I am on the speak phone because I don't know where the phone is. Robert is doing good. He's zleeping right now. I am so tired. I can't sleep at night. Oh, he just woke and make a lot of noise. Robert is so cute. He eat a lot. I am breastfeeding him. And I have a lot milk, very full. My breasts is too sore. It hurts a lot. But now it's getting better. I cannot walk too much. I think I have to go back before the date that they told me because sometimes I am still bleeding. I don't know if it is normal."

Then she mentioned her roommate. "Kenneth sounds like he's jealous, said, 'some guy' when you called. He's kinda funny, but he's nice guy."

The next week, Azi and her friends were watching the televised final match of soccer's World Cup. Brazil's last title was in 1970, when, led by the great Pelé, they had defeated Italy—today's foe. It had been twenty-four long years since they had celebrated a World Cup championship. Brazilians, during this tournament, placed their national pride on the shoulders and feet of their revered soccer team. During each game over the last month, national energy consumption in Brazil dropped by one-third as schools, factories, and shopping centers emptied. All day before the championship match Catholic churches in Rio de Janeiro echoed with prayers for a title.

Azi held a grudge against Italy for past victories over Brazil. "I *hate* Italia," she snarled as she settled into a chair.

The Brazilians created a crescendo of noise in anticipation of each shot, the noise shattering into groans with each miss. They chattered through every moment of the match. Every pass or block or shot was treated as the turning point in the game. Two men angrily shouted obscenities in Portuguese at a player who kicked too high.

"¡Oh carralho!" one muttered.

Several people wore T-shirts with Brazilian symbols. One shirt's design combined an American flag with Brazilian colors, green and yellow. Another announced, "We are coming to invade America." The walls and ceiling of the living room were decorated with green and yellow paper. Junk food was everywhere: Lays Barbecue Potato Chips, Wheat Thins, Santita's Tortilla Chips, Royal Gold Pretzels, Budweiser beer, regular Lays Potato Chips, Heineken beer.

Azi paced the room, stepping over people, breastfeeding Robert. "I can't watch," she said. "I'll die. I'm so nervous!" She placed Robert in a baby pen in an adjoining bedroom and quickly returned. She sat next to her roommate, Kenneth. They touched each other affectionately and called each other, "Dear." With her thick Portuguese accent, with the Latin way of giving each vowel its own syllable, Azi's "dear" came out, "dee-oh." Azi heard the front door open; always the first to welcome someone at the door, she hopped up and dashed to the door to welcome two Brazilian women. Exuberantly, they exchanged hugs and kisses.

Brazil almost scored from the left side as the shooter received a well-timed pass and kicked the ball toward the goal. But the Italian goalkeeper blocked it. The cheers in the packed room sank into a loud groan. Within a minute and a half, Italy nearly scored.

"Oh no!" someone shouted just before the shot.

"¡*Para ele!*"

"¡*Segura ele!*"

The shot missed, and dread filled the room again as they saw another Italian play come together, but the goalkeeper blocked the shot.

Azi stood watching the game, again breastfeeding Robert. She wore a chain necklace that featured a large gold "A" surrounded by a square frame. When she fed Robert, she tossed the "A" back over her shoulder so that it hung down her back.

At 25:15 in the match, Italy almost scored again on a shot kicked at a tough angle, but the Brazilian goalkeeper deflected it at the last moment. Within a minute and a half, Brazil again moved into a scoring position. "Kick it! Kick it!" someone screamed. Miss! Azi finished feeding Robert, turned him around on her shoulder, and patted his back until he burped.

"¡*Para ele!*"

"Cut it off! Cut it off!" someone echoed in English as the Italian star, Roberto Baggio, deftly moved with the ball into a good scoring spot but missed.

Azi put Robert into the car seat on the floor and rocked it. A group of four people Azi did not know came into the room. "Is anyone Brazilian?" Azi asked. A woman said, "I'm Italian." A mournful "Aaaagh!" arose from the group. The first half ended with no score. The group broke up into several chattering groups. Some went outside to smoke. Some retreated to the kitchen, where food was spread around the table. The nervous tension was manifest in eating, chatting, drinking, smoking.

During halftime Azi sat in a corner and talked privately, quietly. She was worried about Jeff. His car had been repossessed. His family had stopped sending money. "He feel alienated from his family. They no accept me when we were together." She wondered if he would be able to send the child support he had promised for Robert. "If he can't pay for his car—" she said, not finishing. "I need to be strong with him, say give support or will take to court." She was not sure about her relationship with Kenneth, either. He was in another room as she spoke. He had a set of rules for them if they got married. They would tell his family that Robert was his child, and they would not tell Robert about Jeff. "Lie to him and family," Azi said. "And he say I don't do enough for him. I no want to lie to son. No want my life to be any harder."

At 52:45 in the match, a Brazilian player nearly knocked a header through, but the Italian goalkeeper blocked it. "Aaaah!" they groaned. The weather outside the house joined them. Thunder rumbled across the dark sky. At 55 minutes played, the television showed the two announcers for twenty seconds while the game was still being played. The crowd in the room was furious. "Get off there!" someone shouted. Someone snarled something in Portuguese about American television.

Azi turned to Kenneth and said, "I'm glad you don't know Portuguese. A lot of bad words are said here." At 67 minutes played, heavy rain began. Outside, a sheet of water overflowed out of a gutter full of leaves. The crowd became reverently quiet when the television showed an interview with Brazilian soccer great Pelé on the importance of soccer to Brazil. A Brazilian shot bounced off the Italian goalkeeper's chest, to the ground, and *just* caromed off the goal post and out of bounds. The Italian goalkeeper kissed the pole. The crowd in the room heckled him.

"That guy lucky!" Azi shouted "Lucky guy!"

With 10 minutes to play, the group in the room was almost hysterical. They rose and shouted at every close play. Azi paced around, again breastfeeding Robert. The game ended with no score, and they went into overtime. Azi continued to breastfeed Robert. Two of Azi's close friends, Isabel and Lina, hugged each other tightly and stomped the floor. Azi paced, holding Robert. No one scored in the first overtime, and they moved to the second. At 17 minutes, Brazil nearly scored, and the group screamed their agony. They were louder, more anxious than ever. Another shot just missed! Several people leapt to their feet and shouted. "Shit!" one yelled, amid all the frantic Portuguese that surely expressed the same sentiment. At 26 minutes Azi lit a candle and walked around the room touching people with her free hand and snapping her fingers. "For good luck," she said. Everyone eagerly touched her. The second overtime ended with no score, and, for the first time in World Cup history, the match would be settled by penalty kicks. One kicker versus one goalkeeper. Each team got five kicks. Italy kicked first.

Italy's Franco Baresi reached the ball, kicked right-footed, and—

horrors!—the Brazilian goalkeeper guessed the wrong way, leaving a wide open net. But the shot missed! It sailed over the crossbar. Baresi fell to his knees and grabbed the back of his head in despair. The Brazilians in the room sank in relief, disaster just averted. Brazil kicked, but the Italian goalkeeper guessed correctly and dived to block his shot. In the second round, the Brazilian goalkeeper again guessed wrong. This time the ball flew into the upper left corner of the net for the first score of the long match. The room became dead quiet. But the Brazilian hero, Romario, strode forward and placed the ball for his kick. His shot struck the inside of the left post and ricocheted into the net. A score! Azi and her friends shouted in relief. The score was 1–1. The Brazilian defender moved to his right, and Italy's Albergio Evani kicked it down the middle, at the place the defender had vacated. Silence again. But they shouted when Brazil scored on their third kick, too. Isabel and Lina held hands tightly, quaking, their eyes riveted to the screen. Italy kicked again, and Raffarel blocked Daniele Massaro's right-footed shot. Another chance to take the lead. The Brazilians in the room leapt up and down, hugged and shouted. Dunga swung his foot right as if to shoot to the left, but he turned his foot at the last second, fooling the Italian defender. He scored! At last, Brazil had the lead, with one final round of kicks to go. A miss gave the World Cup championship to Brazil. A goal tied the score. The great Baggio, Italy's last kicker, approached the ball confidently. Baggio had already dramatically saved Italy in the opening game of the second round, when they were one minute from elimination against Nigeria. A Turin, Italy, newspaper had announced, "Baggianism is the only faith which unites Italians." Italians everywhere believed Baggio would always deliver them from defeat. Baggio kicked high, past the goalkeeper, but the ball barely skimmed over the crossbar. Brazil won!

The room exploded. Azi hugged and kissed all her friends and jumped up and down, over and over. Several women kissed the TV screen when it showed Brazil's players, holding aloft the World Cup trophy. The TV showed an outdoor scene in São Paulo, Brazil. A mob celebrated in the streets. A TV reporter holding a microphone casually, looking around, apparently could not hear that he was on the air. The Brazilians in the room cheered, proud that their country's celebration disrupted mighty

American television. Azi and her friends sang Brazilian songs. They danced around the room, cheering and laughing. The stunned Roberto Baggio stood in the penalty area, hands on hips, hanging his head, inconsolable. The most celebrated player in the world missed a free shot into the net from twelve yards, one he could make in his sleep.

Far from their wildly celebrating home country, Azi and her friends partied into the yard and the street. They waved Brazilian flags and danced exuberantly. And before the night was over, Azi met a new man.

A DeKalb County policeman drove by the celebration on his way to a call. Thinking the rowdy scene was too close to the street, he decided to return after his call. When he pulled into the driveway, Azi immediately walked over to the police car and met James. He found out why they were celebrating, said he wished he could have watched the game, Azi said she had a friend who taped it on a VCR, he said he had a VCR, and she gave James Isabel's phone number. Then she said Isabel's not home much, so she gave him her own phone number.

A young Hispanic woman approached the OB desk, a little girl with her. Speaking for the woman, the girl said she was not sure if she was in the right place. A clerk asked if she had already had the baby. The girl shook her head and started crying. The woman cried, too. All the clerks became quiet. One whispered, "She must have lost the baby. Where's the interpreter?" A clerk offered to take them to a room where they could sit in private. The girl said no. They all stood quietly for a few moments, not sure what to say. The woman and girl, apparently familiar with the routine, walked into the blood pressure room, where Forrest was waiting. In a few minutes, she had them chuckling.

Lisa Dean entered the OB clinic, accompanied by her son Rob. She sat and said she had been with her friend Tameeka the night before she delivered. "I am so mad at her. She already had hers, and I got to wait until August twenty-nine." She added, "I'm thinking about getting my tubes tied."

Rob put his hands on Lisa's belly. "Mom, let me kiss my pooky-pooky."

Lisa reported that Dwayne was in jail, arrested for driving without a license and, for the second time, without insurance. "I tried to visit him Sunday, but they said he was in church. I started crying. Later, he told me he wasn't in church. I'm gonna try to see him on Friday." She said she rode to Grady with a man who was a good friend.

Lisa was called to the desk to check in, then was sent to the blood pressure room. She got in line behind three women, and eyed the scales. "Do we got to do that?" she said. "I don't want to know."

A thin woman—thin except for her bulging belly—stood on the scale and shook her head, grimacing.

"This is not a quick-weight-loss program," Nancy Forrest said.

"I'm not going to gain any more weight."

"Yes, you will," Forrest said.

"I'm one thirty-two now."

"And more to go."

"No, I'm not."

"Yes, you will."

The next patient, a postpartum, sat next to Forrest. She squealed, "It's over! You don't remember me, do you?"

"Oh yes, I do. How are your dermatology treatments going?"

"Just fine. What do they do at postpartum?"

"Pap smear, breast check, see if your uterus is back to size, pregnancy test."

"Pregnancy test?! How can somebody do that? My thing was, 'After nine months of pregnancy? No way.' "

"The average person feels just like that," Forrest said, "but not everybody."

Lisa had gained two pounds over the last two weeks. She returned to her seat, then decided to get lunch at McDonald's before her exam. She ordered a Quarter Pounder with cheese, a Super Size order of French fries, and a Super Size Coke. "And give me a chocolate sundae with nuts," she said. After she ate, she visited her friend Tameeka in post-partum.

"I told you, that night," Tameeka said, laughing, as Lisa walked in her room. Tameeka wore two hospital gowns and flimsy hospital-issue green foam-rubber slippers. "He's got my big nose." She gave Lisa an account of what happened after Lisa left that night. "I was sitting out on that cement wall, and everybody was saying to go rest. But I walked and walked. My sister said you need to sit down. I sat down and said oh well the pain done stopped. And as soon as I stood up they started. I said I was going to have the baby, and they said nah. My mama said you're not going to have that baby. You'll know when you see that pink discharge. This other girl told me when you get ready to lay down you're going to know you're going to be in labor for real because it's going to be really painful. Boy, when I laid down, boy, they really came, but I just made myself sleep through it. Then they just got so bad where I couldn't stand it. It hurt so bad I woke up before six o'clock. When I went to the bathroom I didn't see the pink discharge. I seen a brown discharge. Everybody kept saying no, no that's not it. My mama was the only one saying you may need to go now. When I got in the ambulance, they believed I wasn't in labor because my back wasn't hurting. I was just hurting down in here. I saw that discharge, but it was brown. And when I got here I had dilated six centimeters. That fast."

"Girl!" Lisa cried.

"After they put in that epidural, I felt some pressure and I wondered if that was it. Tammy looked and said, 'The head is showing, and it doesn't have any hair.' But it was that water bucket. It went back in and came out again. Then it busted. Pow! Yellow stuff went everywhere."

"When did they put in the epidural?"

"About ten-forty. Boy, them pains was killing me. I said will you hurry up? What in the world is you *doing*? I say you supposed to be trying to *beat* the contractions. And I had about four before he got the epiderman in. I had one right when he was doing the epiderman. He started massaging my back, to calm me down. But them pains was hurting. I told him if he would hurry up we wouldn't have to go through this. I said, oooh wooooh. Don't want no more children. That pains, ooh God. I couldn't stand it. It's amazing how your body will hurt like that. Amazing." Gingerly, she shifted herself in the bed. "Girl, these tubes got me hurting so bad. This is the first time I've been up since I got here."

"I might get my tubes tied, too," Lisa said. "Or maybe in five years. I asked my midwife if they come untied after five years. She said they shouldn't. She said do that only if I'm sure I'm not going to have more kids."

"My mom said I was too young," Tameeka said, "but I don't want no more. That pain was killing me." She leaned over and looked at her son, Felton. "Look at his hands. They going to be *black*. He's gonna have a lot of hair, and his little balls are jet black. His daddy's real black. Look at that little black wee-wee."

"He's got big feet, girl," Lisa said, laughing.

Tameeka got up from the bed to stretch and walk around carefully. "He's got big feet because I used to talk about Ni Ni's feet. Every day I used to talk about how big her feet were."

"Girl, I can't wait," Lisa said. "Has he been circumcised yet?"

"No, they do that today," Tameeka said.

"That's mean. They should do that first thing. You're walking like you're sore."

"Girl, I'm real sore. I was so sore yesterday I couldn't move."

Felton started sucking on his top lip, emitting a gentle 'smack smack.'

"You're greedy," Tameeka said. "My sister couldn't get my layaway out from a baby shop downtown yesterday. It was some blankets and stuff like that. She went down there and paid the money, and they wouldn't let her take the layaway because she didn't have no ID. She told 'em my sister had just had a baby. They told her they required it because if I had come down there and tried to get my layaway and it wasn't there it would be their fault. They said some people's stuff was stolen like that last Christmas. I gave her my picture ID and then they let her get it."

The conversation paused, and they stared at Felton. Tameeka said, "The doctor said he's light, but he's gonna be dark. When I saw that wee-wee. . . ."

They began talking about a man they knew who had fathered several children by three women. "She's pregnant again?" Lisa said, of one of the three.

"Twins," Tameeka said.

"Lord God have mercy."

"They're talking about getting her tubes tied. They need to tie something on *him*." She stroked Gregory's hair and said, "I missed him so much I got him out of the nursery as soon as I finished my class."

"They cut my phone off at home," Lisa said, "but it's not due 'til the twenty-seventh."

"My labor pains was totally different this time," Tameeka said. "My contractions came every ten minutes, but I was dilating like that." She snapped her fingers. "It's amazing to see that water bag hanging out of you. I felt down there and felt it go back in. Then all of a sudden, pow! When I got that epidural I felt so weak."

"I don't want that," Lisa said. "It can slow the baby's heartbeat."

"I know that discharge is supposed to be pink not brown. So I kept it. I put it in a bag. I told Tammy I kept it to show them. She said, 'I don't want to see that.' "

Tameeka said that Walt Robinson, the physician assistant she saw for her prenatal care, came by to visit her yesterday. "I said I really thank you for coming, but I won't be seeing you downstairs again. He was good to me. He always joked around about whatever you said. You could ask just anything. He took his time. That's the reason I didn't want no 'nother doctor. Some of them just whisk you right on through. I just want everything to be done right, and I don't want to be too scared to ask anything. I had always said I would never like a man to check me no way, you know what I'm saying? But he always had somebody with him, you know what I'm saying?"

Lisa called the phone company and said to the clerk, "My phone was cut off, and it's not supposed to be 'til the twenty-seventh. . . . This Friday I'll be able to pay that amount. . . . Probably that next Friday or Saturday." She hung up and said, "I forgot that I had worked out an arrangement. I owed three hundred dollars and I was supposed to pay a hundred and eighty on the fifteenth. I forgot. I'll pay some this Friday and some the next." Lisa said the bill was high because Dwayne called collect from jail repeatedly.

"When they go to jail," Tameeka said, "they want to talk to you all night. When they're on the streets they don't give you five minutes."

"Next time I'm going to tell him, 'I pay this bill, not you.' "

"Lisa will not go the hospital!" Tameeka Nesbitt said worriedly. "She's got marks all on her neck, and her stomach got tight and small. I was mad at her because she did NOT go to the hospital, and she was hurting so bad yesterday. Her neck was all bruised. She say, 'Well, my stomach isn't hurting.' I said regardless . . . but she didn't go."

Calmly, looking at her kitchen floor, Lisa explained that it really was not so bad. A black bruise spread across the brown skin on the side of her neck. "We were on our way home, at Lakewood. All of a sudden we couldn't stop, the brakes went out, and we spun all around. We hit a pole. Other than that, everything's fine. It didn't do nothing to the baby, just the seatbelt, it just did that right there." She pointed at the bruise. "The baby was moving OK. I had called Lauren Foley and told her about it. She asked if the baby was fine, if I was OK. I said everything was fine. She said if there were any abnormal changes, to come in. You know how you feel like you just got in a fight, and your body feel sore? That's how I felt yesterday."

"My grandmother worked for thirty years in a Rhode Island hospital," Ms. Griff said, sitting at Thursday night New OB Clinic, when pregnant women had their first general exam. "My father was a medic in a hospital and in the service. I stayed across the street from Grady. I had a nice experience here having a baby, and I wanted to make a difference. I kept coming over and applying and finally got a job, at first in the nursery and postpartum. I've been in the OB clinic for fifteen years. At first, every day I said I wasn't coming back. I was eighteen. Some had abortions before they were legal, and I saw how sick they got. Women who had gone to someone to do the abortion and got infected from it. I felt sorry for 'em, though they didn't want pity. They were in a tough situation and made that choice. One of my friends died from an illegal abortion. We went to school together, and she was very popular."

She said even though she sees many patients each day, she becomes attached to some. "I do those that I see a lot. You can't help but do that. One woman just lost her baby, and I remembered her here from two previous babies. The majority don't wait 'til they're seven, eight months. Most come like they're supposed to, but the myth is that they come at the last minute. Sometimes they speak when you see them in the store. If I see 'em there, I wait and let them speak first because some don't want others to know they've been to Grady, so I let them speak. And most do. Some call me at home and ask advice, or they just need someone to talk to. Some had children when I first got here, and their kids are fourteen and fifteen, so I'm starting to see my grandchildren."

"How many patients, Ms. Griff?" yet another resident asked. During the day, she heard a stream of questions from patients: "Am I next?" "How much longer?" At New OB, it was the residents. She reigned over the stack of patient charts, which were numbered according to when the patient arrived. Each resident took the next one and looked wearily at the rest of the stack.

"Let's keep it moving tonight, Ms. Griff," the next resident said.

A fourth-year resident walked to the stack, and Ms. Griff handed her a folder. The resident looked skeptically at the number, apparently noticing it was out of order. "This is a real sweet lady," Ms. Griff said. "I wanted her to see someone nice." After the resident left, Ms. Griff said, "This patient weighs nearly four hundred pounds. She brought her sheet back here, so I knew she didn't want people to see, so I wanted her to see someone nice and someone who's a fourth-year and knows what they're doing. I'm not as thin as I'd like to be. I have friends who are fat, and they get discriminated against."

A resident picked up the next folder and counted the folders under it.

"When I was a child," Ms. Griff said, "I wanted to be a nun. They lived a nice simple, peaceful life, and they praised the Lord all the time. In the pictures and movies their lives were quiet and simple and they were always helping people. My house was peaceful, but a lot of those around me weren't."

A resident walked by, carrying a tote bag, on its side was the logo, "MetroGel—metranidozole vaginal gel." He looked at the pile of folders and grimaced.

"We usually have a doctor in every room," Ms. McGriff said, "but not tonight, so we're really having to push it."

A young woman walked to the back and asked Ms. Griff if she had been called. "Anybody call a Ms. Terry?" Ms. Griff boomed down halls. No one answered, so she told the woman she would be called soon.

Another patient walked by, and Ms. Griff said, "Tell Tracie I'm mad." The patient nodded and walked to an exam room. "Tracie's dealing with drugs, and that's what she's running from."

Later in the evening, a resident picked up a folder, counted the number left, considered how many doctors there were and said, "Will I only have to see one more patient, maybe?" Ms. Griff shrugged.

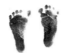

Like Grady Forty Years Ago

Before flying to Mexico on a medical mercy trip, Grady OB physician assistant Walt Robinson said he planned to set his computer so that when his teenage son booted it up, Robinson's voice said to him, "Don't forget to make up your bed. Mow the lawn. Surprised you, didn't I?" Robinson told this story, snickering, sitting in the small computer room next to his exam room.

Robinson was a PA in the OB clinic. Around twenty years ago, he took an Emergency Medical Technician course. At Grady's ER, he observed these medical people who seemed to be physicians but somehow were not. They were not nurses, so what were they? He asked. "We're physician assistants," they replied. Robinson applied to Emory University's PA training school, and was accepted. His clinical learning took place at Grady.

"I'm looking for my babies now," he said, explaining his work. "I look at the date of birth for my patients to see if they were born here when I was training here."

He loved to talk about being a PA. His face crinkled in a cutesy smile—which some people around Grady found irritating—and his eyes twinkled. "A PA is a highly-trained person who practices medicine with the supervision of a doctor," he explained. "We receive broad training, including the different specialties. Our authority comes from the fact that we assist a licensed physician. Mostly, we work alone, though some problems require a doctor."

His patients, seeing his white coat and stethoscope, usually assumed he was a doctor. The OB resident doctors *hated* it when patients called him "Dr. Robinson." What they detested even more was that Robinson, when called 'Doctor,' often said nothing.

"The nurse-midwives," he continued, "work under a protocol that says what to do in X circumstance. PAs can use more flexibility and judgment." [Ooh, *that* would irk the midwives.] "The training is based on a medical model, rather than a nursing model. You are trained by doctors."

Before Grady's prenatal patients began seeing the same medical care provider at each visit throughout their pregnancy, Robinson's specialty had been vaginal warts. "I saw all of those. They became 'my patients' and saw me every time. It was unfortunate that they had to have warts to get continuity of care."

Robinson bounded down the hall to the waiting room to call his next patient, which he often did, rather than page her over the intercom. He pushed one of the double doors open, stepped halfway into the waiting room, and called her name. She stood; he gave that crinkly smile. He walked with her to room 10. He asked her how things were going, and she said fine except she had thrown up that morning.

The only procedure scheduled was a belly exam. Robinson moved his hands across and stopped and felt.

"This is the head," he said. "Do you feel your baby moving yet?"

"It started last week."

He measured her fundus, the bulging belly's curvature. He squeezed ultrasound gel on her belly and smeared it around. He placed the transducer against her belly and moved it until the baby's heartbeat was distinct. The thump-thump of the heart, magnified by the monitor, sounded watery, as if it beat amidst slowly swirling ocean waves.

"When are you due?" Robinson asked.

"July."

"Is that this year or next year?"

She laughed, shook her head, and rolled her eyes.

The next three patients also only needed belly exams. He used his "this year or next year" joke with two of them. They laughed and shook their heads, too. After the last patient left, Robinson said about his trip, "A lot of my patients are Mexican, and I want to understand their culture.

I can also practice my Spanish. One patient told me, 'I understand you, but your Spanish is terrible.' "

The day before, he had asked the interpreter how to ask his patients, "Has your water broken?" He told her he has been asking them, "*¿Se quebró tu agua?*" She said that was not right. He should ask, "*¿Se le rompió la fuente?*" He carefully wrote down the correct translation. He then asked her how to ask if a patient had any abnormal discharge. He told her how he had been asking, which she said was not correct, either, and she told him the correct way.

"They don't understand 'vagina,' " she added. She told him they use a phrase which means "that part."

"But I'm in a professional setting," he objected, "and I'm used to speaking accurately about a person's body."

"But it's important that you speak in a way that they understand. You may be professional and correct but may not communicate well."

Then Robinson got funny. "In English we say, 'that part.' " Saying the last two words, he waggled his eyebrows up and down.

She did not laugh. She had said flatly, "Don't do that with them."

He began installing a program on his computer. "Computers is my hobby," he said, twinkling his eyes. Six pens and pencils filled his plastic pocket protector. He proudly said he had assisted the company that installed the software that computerized OB patient records. He punched keys on his laptop computer, and a record of deliveries came on the screen. He kept a log of every delivery of his patients. "I used to work labor and delivery, and I loved it." The log included each patient's name, Grady number, age, number of pregnancies, delivery date and time, infant weight, infant sex, procedures done during delivery, any notable incidents, who assisted, and which doctor supervised the delivery. He punched more keys and a statistical breakdown of his deliveries appeared on the screen. He had delivered exactly the same number of girl and boy infants.

"You can do all kinds of things," he said, pecking keys. "You can do a bar graph of the number of boys and girls. You can determine the difference in weight of boys and girls. See—"peck, peck—"fifty-one percent of the weight to boys, forty-nine to girls." He looked down the list of

"Assisted by." "That's usually a medical student, sometimes their first delivery, my hands over theirs." Though PAs perform no surgeries, he added, "When they assist on a C-section, they usually hold the forceps. Ah, this one I helped do her first. One resident was angry with me for doing a delivery when he was going to teach a first-year how to do a forceps delivery. They learn how to do forceps on an easy one, so if a difficult one comes along, they'll be confident. I see the importance of them doing it, but I don't want them to do it on *my* patients."

He said about once a month he had to tell someone her baby died. "I recently had to tell two patients in a row. That was a bad day. One was thirteen or fourteen weeks pregnant, spoke no English. I tried to pick up the fetal heart tone, tried and tried, moving it around. I couldn't pick it up, so I sent her to ultrasound. She came back with a report written in English. But she knew. I have to be forthright when I tell them." Using a bland professional tone, he removed his smile and imitated himself: " 'The test shows the baby has died.' They usually know already. They usually start screaming and crying. Yeah, that was a bad day. I think about it while I'm here, but I separate it from my home life. I strongly believe in that prayer: God, give me the serenity to accept the things I cannot change, the courage to change the things I can, and the wisdom to know the difference."

Robinson walked up to the fourth floor to see if any of his patients were in labor. Just outside the entrance, a woman using the payphone in the hall, and a young woman standing next to her, sobbed. Robinson looked down the list on the board in the residents' room and saw one Hispanic patient of his, fifteen years old. He walked to her room and spoke with her and her boyfriend.

"*¿Contracciones?*"

She nodded.

"*¿Mucho?*"

"*Si.*"

He checked her cervix and walked out to the nurse's station. He told the nurse, "She's only fingertip."

"You get out of here! With *those* contractions?"

"She needs to walk and be checked in an hour. The baby's head's down."

"Did you write it in the chart? And did you tell *her?* I tried to triage her earlier, but they don't speak any English."

"I did. Just take the monitor straps off, and she knows what to do."

At the end of Robinson's work day, he rode the MARTA train home. The train ran rhythmically along its tracks, emitting an electric clickety-clack. The cars jerked, squeaked, and popped when the train stopped at each station. Commuters sat and stared blankly ahead or out the windows, their faces, like those in Robin James's dream, masking who-knows-what thoughts. Robinson took out his Spanish dictionary and learned two more Spanish words, a daily ritual.

Robinson taught himself Spanish when he worked New OB Clinic every week for a while. With the help of an interpreter, he first learned to say a few simple requests, like "Open your mouth, please." The first time he tried that request on a patient he said, *"Abre su vaca, por favor,"* which means, "Open your cow, please."

"This is my first time to leave the country," Robinson said in Atlanta's Hartsfield International Airport. "So I have a virgin passport," he snickered. He traipsed through the airport like a flower-hopping bumblebee. He looked at magazines at the newsstand and purchased none of them. He bought a bag of popcorn and ate it from bag to mouth, tilting it a little higher each time. At the metal detectors, he paused a while to watch luggage pass through the X-ray. "I like to see what other people bring," he said.

Robinson had told all his patients about his trip. With his Mexican patients, he brought out a map and asked where they were from so he could see how close they lived to his destination, the Sierra Madre Mountains, near the city of Atoyac, in the state of Guerrero.

The trip was coordinated by Flying Doctors of America, a volunteer medical mission group that provided the services of American medical professionals to people in poor countries. Each team member was warned: things that should work, do not; schedules on paper may turn to pulp. This team—one physician, one physician assistant (Robinson), one veterinarian, two registered nurses, one dental hygienist, and three non-medical volunteers—flew to the Acapulco airport and piled into a large Chevrolet Suburban. Outside of Acapulco, the rough, narrow road curved among hills then valleys. Every so often, cars slowed to a crawl to jostle over huge speed bumps called *topes*, which suddenly appeared on a highway. Rusted signs sometimes warned of *topes*, but they gave the driver hardly a moment to slow the vehicle and save its suspension.

On the way, the team got acquainted. They told about their families and jobs. Dewayne Biddle, the veterinarian, worked in an animal emergency center. Jostling in the back seat, he said he often had to tell owners it was best to put their pet to sleep.

"It's hard," he said, "when the family is pushing the owner to have the pet put to sleep to save money, or because it's inconvenient not to, but I'm not sure the owner is ready. Some rich people want to put them to sleep just so they won't have to spend the money or just so they won't have to put pills in a dog's mouth for seven days. Then you have some poor people with terrible shoes on, and they bring in their pet and pay to have it treated."

In a couple of hours the team arrived in Atoyac, an agricultural town in the foothills of the Sierra Madres known for coffee and coconut industries. A prominent family that owned a coffee processing plant hosted the team the first day. The third-floor balcony offered a rooftop view of Atoyac, the hazy mountains in the eastern background. Palm trees appeared in the skyline here and there, like green fireworks frozen in the air.

The family served a huge dinner of rice, chiles rellenos, tacos with hot green sauce, chicken, beans, and tortillas. And they kept bringing it. The director of Flying Doctors, Allan Gathercoal, asked each person to name one thing he or she was thankful for. "Most groups," he said, "change their mind about what they're thankful for the more they're around poverty." Robinson said, "I'm thankful for the opportunity to have this fascinating experience, and I look forward to having it with everyone."

After dinner, they organized what would be called "the pharmacy," a dozen cardboard boxes filled with the donated medicine. Each box was labeled by hand, with a black felt-tip pen, "Antihistamine," "Antibiotics,"

"Analgesics," "Worms," "GYN," "Emergency Med," or "Prenatal." The medications were tossed into the boxes, which, though labeled, were piled randomly with little cartons and plastic bottles of medicine, like a child's toy box after a hasty cleanup before mom's inspection. Robinson contributed a large supply of birth control pills from Grady. They had a box of toys to give to children and a box of sample toothpaste and toothbrushes.

Robinson asked one of the interpreters, Marguerite, whether the Catholic church discouraged women from using birth control. She said she was not sure what church leaders told the women in this area, but she was skeptical that the women would use birth control anyway. Robinson gave Marguerite his speech about the many benefits of the pill, hoping she would similarly convince the women they would meet in the clinics.

The next morning, they had their last hot shower for a few days, then left for San Vicente de Benitez, a remote, tiny mountain town where another translator, Javier, lived and where his father was the mayor. Standing, the team rode in the back of a pickup truck, hanging onto ropes or each other or the metal rods that framed the cargo area. Dust filled the air and covered the wide green palm fronds along the side of the road. The driver careened from side to side to avoid the rough mountain road's enormous potholes. They passed an American couple standing by the side of the road, each of them holding binoculars, peering into the trees, apparently looking for birds. They stopped briefly at Javier's house to unload luggage, then drove on to the small town of Paraiso.

The team set up the clinic in a medical building inside a large courtyard surrounded by a white brick wall. The building was plain and flat, with a broad entrance that was already full of people waiting. All the rooms were small and stuffy. Small windows allowed for little movement of the hot air inside and outside the clinic building. Team members carried plastic bottles of water they had poured from a huge glass jug. The clinic was staffed by a woman still in medical training, fulfilling her one-year requirement in a clinic as repayment to the government for educating her. She had completed her MD, but she would receive her diploma only after her year practicing in Paraiso. Javier said many medical students served such a year in such a town far from any sophisticated medical equipment. Students whose families have money and political connections would likely be assigned to a more desirable place, such as Mexico City or Monterrey.

Cindy Edwards, a dental hygienist, and Diana Graves, an employment assistance director, set up the pharmacy in a small room, the walls lined with three tables for the boxes of medicine. "Let's put the antibiotics here, and the analgesics there," Edwards said. They arranged the boxes on tables and set out a pile of plastic sandwich bags, into which they would drop pills. They kept the most commonly used medicines—Tylenol, Motrin, Vermox—on top of the piles, but for other prescriptions they would be digging around in the boxes. Gathercoal reminded them that the medicine had to last three days. "So keep that in mind when you are giving them out," he said. When the first prescriptions began arriving, they did not always match what was in the boxes. One asked for four-hundred-milligram tablets of Motrin, and they only had six-hundred-milligram tablets. Another asked for Vermox tablets, and they only had it in liquid.

Early in the day, Rebecca Damiani, the RN who treated minor problems, spoke to David Freeman, a pediatric cardiologist who was the team's one MD, about a man with arthritic pain and parasites. She had in mind the laws governing who can give prescriptions in the United States. "I'll give him Tylenol for the aches and pains," she said, "but he also has parasites. I'm not comfortable prescribing anything for parasites. So maybe we could practice together on this one." By the end of the day, she would be prescribing, on her own and constantly, the parasite medicine Vermox.

In front of the building, a long line formed outside in the heat and humidity. Biddle, the veterinarian, stood to the side of the building treating his first wave of animals, mostly dogs with worms. His stethoscope draped across his neck and shoulders, sweat pouring from his brow, he wiped and wiped his face with his handkerchief, which he unfolded and refolded. He finished treating the animals, including a goat that had caught its penis on a barbed-wire fence, and went to help in the pharmacy. He told Lorenzo and Graves, "The pets all have parasites. That's why the people do." He treated dogs with a banana-flavored parasite medicine that they lapped up quickly. "In a few weeks, the parasites will return," Biddle said. "And the dogs are not neutered, so they're biting me." Soon Gathercoal peered in the pharmacy and asked him, "Dewayne, are you ready?" Another bunch of about twenty-five children with dogs had arrived.

One boy, looking very tired and miserable, with blisters on his face, was given Advil and sent to the hospital. They told his mother he probably had chicken pox. He would have a long, bumpy, unhappy ride to Atoyac.

Biddle brought a letter into the pharmacy. A young man had given it to him, on behalf of the young man's friend, who was too embarrassed to explain his problem in person. The very polite letter, written in English, began, "Good day my friend. What a good work you are doing." It then said the letter writer, because he had lost an apparently unusual bet, had had to push a peeled mango into his own rectum. The poor fellow's rectum was swollen and painful, according to the letter. He was also having diarrhea. They prescribed Preparation-H and Imodium A-D.

In the exam room he shared with Freeman, Robinson had tied a rope across a corner of the room and hung a blanket from it. He put his exam table behind it, to give his OB/GYN patients some privacy. The electrical outlet on his side did not work, so he used his flashlight. His pocket protector filled with pens, normally tucked in his shirt pocket, he had pushed into a pants pocket. He slung his camera pouch across his shoulder. He rotated six speculums, soaking two in soap for a half hour and rinsing them and letting them dry. Two at a time, they went through this cycle all day. Damiani's room had a desk and medicine cabinet with glass doors. On the wall above the desk hung a calendar with a picture of Jesus.

Over lunch they talked about the morning. Team Leader Tom Reckersdrees said the local doctor was feeling ignored, as if the bigshot Americans had strutted into town and invaded her clinic in front of her own people. He said he had tried to include her in their work, but with little success.

Nurse Damiani said she was feeling inadequate. "If I was at my work,

I wouldn't be seeing half these people. A doctor would. I wasn't quite prepared for the number of people and how quickly I was supposed to get people moved in and out." She also said she would like a list of what and how much to prescribe for certain conditions, since she was playing doctor all day.

"David?" Gathercoal asked.

"It's going reasonably well, considering I haven't done general med in a while. We're more triage than a clinic. And we don't have time to do a lot of things I'd usually do."

Damiani wanted to know how the worm meds were holding up. They thought it would last the day, but Gathercoal said he would get more from Atoyac. Robinson said he needed urine specimen cups and urine dipsticks. (He would not get those luxuries.)

Gathercoal, cheering the team on, acknowledged that a lot of the patients they saw simply had aches and pains. "Out of five hundred we see, we'll truly help two hundred. And without us, what would they do? You're doing the best you can under the circumstances. Keep up the good work."

Reckersdrees said he wanted things to move faster. "If someone has worms, give them a prescription for that, and move on to the next one."

Freeman countered, "But some people you can't diagnose that fast, and there might be some other problems. Unless you're willing to ignore them."

They left it at that, each having made his point.

After the meeting, Robinson said the conditions were not sanitary. "Everyone sits on the same place. I wonder what kind of prenatal care they get. They don't keep up with their menstrual cycle, and they probably deliver their babies at home. I'm giving birth control pills to those it's appropriate for. I was afraid at first they wouldn't want it, but they do."

Damiani and Freeman huddled to rehash the unusual mix of symptoms that one patient had. Like residents at Grady who saw the same things over and over, they were excited to talk about something new. They could not arrive at a diagnosis without a lab, though. She might be a diabetic, and there were other possibilities, but they could not know, so they prescribed something they thought might help her. But they did not know.

After lunch, they resumed seeing patients. The clinic ran more smoothly, though the whole day was rushed and hectic. The crowd never diminished, and everyone felt pressured to move things along. Sweating, breathing hot stale air, they saw patient after patient. The medical people and the pharmacy worked together better as Damiani and Robinson and Freeman learned what the pharmacy had and did not have.

When the clinic closed at 5:00, they began cleaning up. Robinson was still seeing his last patient as brooms whisked across the concrete floors. Some people still had not been seen. "This is like Grady, forty years ago," Robinson thought.

As they were driving away from town, the translator Javier laughed and said, "I didn't want to tell you this before we got here, but Paraiso is well known for having members of organized crime." He laughed again.

They returned to San Vicente de Benitez for dinner at Javier's home. Over dinner, Damiani said by afternoon she felt more comfortable coming up with a quick diagnosis and treatment. She mentioned a badly malnourished child she was almost certain was going to die. They tried to reassure the parents, and encouraged them to feed the child as best as they could. "But I feel very sure it is going to die," she said.

The side of the home facing the street was the family's small store, which was fronted by a covered porch. After dinner the team talked, sitting on the porch. Some purchased beer or soft drinks from the store. "Don't forget to wipe off the top before you drink," Gathercoal warned them. The sun sank behind the mountain, and the hot day became a pleasant evening, blessed with cool mountain air. Half the village extended up the mountain behind the house, and the rest of the village spread out on a small plain across the street from the house. Rutted dirt roads snaked among the houses.

Javier explained that the people come thinking the American doctors and equipment are superior to that of Mexico. "They want to see the American doctor and sometimes they expect a miracle," he said. "Even if it's the same medicine but they changed the name. Sometimes they're not really sick, just aches and pains, but they want to see the American doctor. They've heard great things about America and its health training and equipment and system."

Robinson spoke with his usual eagerness. "It was frustrating for me," he said, "because of all the things that I check in patients in my clinic at Grady, blood type, ultrasound, blood counts, checking for infection and checking for Pap smear—I could do none of those things here. I was amazed at how many babies most of our patients today have had. It was not unusual to find out that a patient was pregnant and she was having her sixth, seventh, eighth, ninth, or tenth baby, and I think the oldest patient pregnant was in her late twenties or early thirties. Can you imagine being thirty years old and having your tenth child? Many of them have had a fair amount of fetal mortality. One lady was having her third baby, but both of her first two babies died within her. All these patients would be considered to have a high-risk pregnancy in America, and we would do all kinds of major manipulations and checks. Here all I can do is give them a month's supply of prenatal vitamins.

"Every patient had to be convinced to take her clothes off for the examination. It was not easy, and—it was fascinating to note—every one of them was dressed in her Sunday best. Every one of them had a dress and slip on. Everyone had clean underwear. Everyone had a bra and a tight frilly dress. It was hard to get their clothes off, and most of them would just lift up the dress which meant I could examine either their lower abdomen or upper abdomen but not the whole abdomen at one time."

He said he spoke with the local doctor, and the exchange began like that of Reckersdrees's but ended well. "She brought a patient, and she seemed a little put out that we were there using her space. She kinda pushed in and pulled this pregnant lady in. I said, 'Hello, how are you?' While the patient was getting undressed I said this is my specialty, *'especialidad obstetricos,'* and she took an interest in me and answered my questions and asked me some questions. She asked me if I wanted to help her examine the patient, and we listened to the baby's heartbeat together, and she seemed very happy about that. She invited me to spend the night and help her deliver the baby, but I declined. I'm amazed that she works here every day with these facilities which are so limited."

Robinson said his self-taught Spanish served him well, but he often relied on his interpreter, Nancy. He added, "Most of the patients looked very anemic. Of course I had no way of confirming that. All their conjunctiva and mucosa of their mouth were very pale. You could look at the vagina and you can tell by the pallor if a patient is anemic, and most were very white. They probably have hematocrits that would floor you or I. We wouldn't get up in the morning. We wouldn't have the strength."

The three nights in San Vicente de Benitez, the women slept in Javier's home, and the men slept on cots across the street in a barn, which had a small bathroom where the toilet and shower shared the same space, the shower head protruding from the wall above and just in front of the commode.

"Yee-aah!" came a shout from within the barn, as the team prepared for sleep, and everyone knew it was a man on the team taking a cold shower. The barn had no hot water—and no water at all from 7:00 p.m. to 7:00 a.m. During the night, the pipes to the mountain villages were shut off to allow water to flow down to Atoyac. Every day, each family filled buckets and tubs with water before the evening shut-off.

The men sleeping in the barn were awakened throughout the night by horses and donkeys chased by dogs. The dogs barked; the horses and donkeys clopped their hooves frantically. Then roosters crowed before the sun rose over the mountaintop. San Vicente de Benitez came to life slowly in the early morning. A worn blue pickup truck crept down a rough road toward the main highway that bisected the village. A girl walked down to the road wearing a backpack full of books. She would ride a bus to school. A small group of boys holding machetes waited for a truck to take them to work in the coffee or corn fields for the day. They teased each other and tossed rocks back and forth, laughing. Some women swept the dirt in front of their homes. Smoke from burning trash piles rose slowly here and there, blending with the morning mountain haze. Robinson, who had risen early and walked across the highway, across the plain and up a rise, looked out over this scene and took pictures.

The mountain was lush with thick tropical greenery and brilliant red, yellow, and white flowers. Huge banana flower spikes, shaped like hearts, hung beneath clusters of bananas that grew outward from a central stem. Banana bunches ripen from the bottom of the stem to the top, so that when most of the bananas had been picked and only a few green ones remained at the top of the long bare stem, the lone flower spike at the bottom of the stem was a purple pendulum.

Robinson walked back down the rise, by the town's outdoor basketball court, which was never used while the medical team was there. The metal rim of one goal was bent down almost parallel to the pole. Robinson stopped at one home and took a picture of Rosaura, a six-year-old girl who preened for the camera, grinning widely. She held the post supporting the roof over a porch and tilted her head just right. She would charm every man in the team by trip's end. Reckersdrees, who had met her on a previous mission, called her "my little girl." Throughout the town, residents welcomed him and others, showing the guests around their homes and courtyards, always offering a bunch of bananas or a handful of sweet mangoes.

A group of women and girls gathered at the little building that housed the village's small mill. They held small pails filled with soft corn kernels that had soaked overnight in lime water. The kernels formed yellow and white mounds, filling the pails like ice cream cones. They were waiting to have their corn ground into *masa*, the soft moist dough they would form into balls, flatten, and cook on a flat pan to make the day's tortillas. The women and girls formed a line and placed their pails on a counter. The owner poured the first bucket of corn into the slot and turned a large metal wheel attached to the side of the mill, which set the grinder in motion. She flipped the switch that filled the little building with an electric roar as the mill came to life. Ground corn came out of the bottom of the mill and collected on a metal shelf. A slight burning smell filled the room. The first woman in line knelt and, using her whole arm, scooped the *masa* into a bucket. She scooped a few buckets, then stood, and someone took her place. Without any signals or words, they took turns kneeling and scooping, and filling a few buckets, which were not necessarily their own. They just filled their pails to the same level that they had brought. Each brushed white flecks of *masa* off her bare arm.

The girls and women, talking and laughing over the undulating noise, moved down the line, pushing their pails along the wooden counter, working together in a routine that had become habit. The owner would occasionally shout for the next person to put her corn in quickly; she didn't want the mill to grind away at air. When someone's buckets were filled, she would show them to the owner, who would eye them and name a price, which would be paid. Little Rosaura took her turn; the white flecks collected in her long black hair like fresh snowflakes. When she finished, she pulled the white handle of her blue pail over her arm into the crook of her elbow and carried it home. The whole process, a dance of women and machine, lasted about twenty-five minutes.

The clinic for the day would be there in San Vicente de Benitez, up the hill in an open-air school, where the town's kindergarten met. Standing in the big main room watching boxes of supplies being carried into the school, Javier said, "Most of the kids go to this school and to our elementary school, but we don't have like a middle school or high school. The childs that finish the elementary school, they have to go to another town to study middle school or high school, if they want to continue their education. Most of the people don't send the kids to school. They spend money on the bus every day, and it's kind of hard. Most of the parents take the kids to the field that they're going to work. I would say that 40 percent of kids in this town go to school. The others, the parents say we don't have the money for materials they use in school. There are so many reasons why, you know."

The three spaces for Robinson, Damiani, and Freeman were arranged out on the patio that extended from the main room all along one side of the building. The balcony was separated from the main room only by columns and a waist-high brick wall. Perched on the rim of a sharp drop, the patio featured a view of the mountains spreading out to the west and a refreshing breeze that blew away memories of yesterday's tiny, stuffy rooms. But it offered no privacy. Using ropes and clothespins, they hung white sheets between the patio and the main room, and between sections of the patio, so that they each had their own "room." Robinson was at one end, Freeman at the other, Damiani between. Damiani had become an almost equal member of the medical triumvirate.

Robinson arranged his supplies and equipment on a small wooden table. The only exam surface he had was a large wooden table that he knew would be uncomfortable. He imagined himself trying to do a speculum exam on that flat hard table, without the patient's hips elevated, and he knew it would not work. A speculum exam can be painful anyway, but without the proper angle, it would be worse. He saw a round blue plastic bowl and remembered an old trick from Grady: on a few occasions when a woman needed to be examined right away, and an exam bed was not handy, they would slide a bedpan under her hips. So all that day, when a speculum exam was required, he brought out the plastic bowl. He told his interpreter Nancy, "It's uncomfortable, but it's not near as bad as that table would have been."

The clinic was less hectic than the day before. The town, and thus the crowd, was smaller. Rosaura and her friends came by the clinic and amused whomever they could distract for a few moments with their giggles. As on the day before, the team saw women, children, and older men. Few young male adults appeared. Much of the team's work would be treating everyday problems that Javier explained would usually not get treated at all.

"If they get sick," he said, "they have to go to Atoyac or a clinic at another village. They usually wait until they're very sick because it's so much trouble to go to Atoyac. It takes a lot of time, and the roads are bad. If it's an emergency, they usually die."

The schoolroom was by the town square, *el zócalo*, which was rarely used anymore. The concrete tile surface was cracked and overgrown with weeds. Broken concrete benches had fallen in pieces to the ground. There was one little-used store at the corner of the square.

Javier said, "That's the story of this town. Twenty years ago, it was very important for this region. All the business from the coffee was in this town. So the boards of societies of coffee workers was here. There was a lot of people that had money right here in this town. But when the price of coffee changed businesses started going down. The people started moving out. We had a lot of things to do in this town, but now the square is not used too much. They use it, the donkeys and dogs, the animals right there, you know."

Reckersdrees kept things running, and he translated in the pharmacy.

Each of the three primary medical people had a translator, as did the triage desk. Damiani, Freeman, and Robinson worked all day, seeing patient after patient, except for a lunch break. In the afternoon, Damiani peeked around the sheet separating her from Freeman and asked him when was the last time he had seen diphtheria.

"I've never seen diphtheria," he said.

One small old woman with a face crowded with wrinkles came to the clinic complaining of a pain in her forearm she had had for three weeks. They determined she had a broken arm, but they had no casting materials or splints. They found someone to whittle a piece of wood into a makeshift splint, and Damiani and Biddle wrapped it tightly in white gauze, to hold the bone in place so it could heal.

One shy young woman came to see Robinson, complaining of vague discomfort in her abdomen. On a hunch, he decided to listen to heart and lungs. He heard a murmur in the bottom part of her interior chest. Not proficient in diagnosing murmurs but aware of what a normal heart sounds like, he asked Freeman to check her. Finally, Freeman was in his field, cardiology. He diagnosed her as having mitral valve regurgitation, a damage to the mitral valve that allows for reverse flow of blood into the chamber of the heart—leakage of the heart valves with each pump of her heart. Freeman said he wanted to order an X-ray, which was impossible there. "So there really isn't much we can do for her," he told Robinson. Freeman gave her a diuretic to reduce the amount of fluid in her veins. "That might help her heart work a little better," he said. He wanted to give her Dijoxin, which enhances the function and strength of the heart muscle. He wrote her a prescription for it in case she ever got to a pharmacy.

Biddle was gone from the clinic much of the day. He visited several farms, where most of the animals' bones could be seen through their skins. At the first place, the farmer cut a dead chicken open, and Biddle could see from its lungs that it had pneumonia. He gave the farmer antibiotics to put in the chickens' drinking water. At the next farm he showed them a new medicine that had just been introduced, a liquid parasite medicine that Biddle poured on the cows' backs. The medicine was absorbed and killed most common intestinal worms, lung worms, and skin parasites—grubs, lice, mites, ticks—for three days. At one farm, he saw children swimming and adults washing clothes in the same pond where cows waded to cool off and to urinate.

That evening before dinner, Reckersdrees and Gathercoal said they were going to see the building where they would hold the next day's clinic, and Robinson jumped into the truck with them. Later, after dinner at Javier's house, Rosaura asked Robinson about a bump on her neck, and he recommended she put a hot wet cloth on it. She went home and told her mother, who came to see him with a complaint of her own. Freeman and Damiani also saw people who dropped by the house with complaints. Freeman was up until late at night seeing people.

After Robinson finished eating and treating Rosaura's mother, he returned to the rocking chair and talked about the second day. "A lot of patients, especially the older patients, had complaints with their vagina, such as irritation, pain with intercourse and discomfort in general in the lower abdomen. Some had post-menopausal symptoms like hot flashes. It would have been good for them to take estrogen and progesterone, and, of course, we had none of that. Or to use estrogen vaginal cream, which is a good local treatment for that problem, but we didn't have that, either. So I wrote prescriptions in case they can get the drug somewhere. A lot of patients had dysmenorrhea, or painful periods. Of course, birth control pills are wonderful for that. I feel real good about having those."

Robinson was also mulling over a decision he had made. "I regret what I did. This is a patient about four or five months postpartum who is breastfeeding and came to me, asking about something poking her uterus. Come to find out, she had an IUD, but she didn't know it was there. I asked her if she wanted it in there and she said, 'I don't know what it is.' So I decided to pull it out. Without really thinking anymore, in order to relieve her discomfort I removed the IUD and then I realized what a dummy I was, because here's a lady four months post-partum. She's breastfeeding now, but she may not be after a few more months. And then she's going to be—if she's sexually active—at risk for getting pregnant. And here she had a perfect form of—almost perfect form of—contraception already in there. I regret pulling it out. I hope that maybe she'll find a way to get another one, wherever she got that one. IUDs are an ideal form of contraception because it's easy to put in, you can leave it there for many years, it needs no attention, there's no hormones, which means you can give it to people who cannot take oral contraceptives. There's no active participation required. You can just ignore it. There are a couple of potential problems with it. One is that women with IUDs tend to bleed a little bit more when they have a period, with more cramps. And they're more likely to have intermenstrual spotting or bleeding. But besides that, the other big risk is—which my patient did not have, I don't think—is that if you have many partners, you are much more likely to have a pelvic infection, which could be very serious, if not fatal, with an IUD. But primarily if you can prescribe it to a patient who's going to be monogamous and not have multiple partners—for someone who is married and monogamous and whose partner does not have multiple partners—it's an ideal form of contraception. Anyway, I regret having pulled it without having talked. . . . She may have decided she didn't want it after discussing it, but I pulled it without really discussing it with her. I wish I had not done that."

After this conversation, Robinson walked outside to visit with folks, and his interpreter, Nancy, sat down in the rocking chair and talked about working with him. Nancy and her husband, Manuel, an amorous young couple in their early twenties, often cuddled and smooched. She grew up in California, but she moved with Manuel to Acapulco, his home. She raved about Robinson.

"He wanted them to trust him. He always tried to explain everything to the patient. They understand him clearly. And he understands *so much.* He always taught them that you need to check yourself on your breast and stuff like that. Some of the women were scared, and he would always say it's not going to hurt. 'I'm not going to do nothing that you don't want. If you want me to stop, please tell me.' And he let them know what he was doing at all times. 'I'm going to do this and this.' If they had a daughter, he would say, 'Can you bring her here so I can check her?' When he wasn't with a patient he was always outside with the next one, talking to her and getting information from her. He said, 'If I had to, I would stay up twenty-four hours with them. I would work through all my lunch hours if I had the chance, if some woman needed me.' There was one patient eight months pregnant, and the head was all the way up here, and he let her feel the head, and there was a father that had never felt the head before, and he felt the head."

She said she learned a lot about her own health from Robinson. "As he was teaching them he was letting me learn. If she had a lump or something in her breast he would let me feel it so I would know what it feels like. He taught me basically what I need to know about being a woman myself, things that I didn't know I had to do, so I kinda feel more comfortable now. He would let me listen to the heartbeat of the lady that he was working with and he would also let the patient hear the heartbeat of their baby. There was one couple that had five kids, and this was their sixth, and they had never heard the heartbeat, and it made them so happy. They were smiling so big. And he always walked them out after the exam as far as he could. 'Take care. Go to a doctor. Maybe I'll see you next time.' "

The next day the team drove up the mountain past the school where they had held the clinic the day before, out of the town, and on to San Vicente de Jesus, another tiny town. They bumped along the dusty road, coughing and jostling, again standing in the back of a pickup. The young doctor there was also completing his year of medical service. As they had the first two days, they prescribed Vermox for worms all day.

Over lunch, Freeman said he thought a surgeon could be more helpful than himself on a trip like this. "For a surgeon, a one-shot fix does a lot of good. But if I give someone blood pressure medicine for one week, I've helped them only one week. I could sometimes see the disappointment in their eyes when I say we can't help you. Some of them expect a miracle. Or we say there's medicine for you, but we don't have it here." He paused a moment and said, "In reality, this is what's normal, and we live in an unreal world."

One woman brought her son to the clinic near the end of the day and said he had *parásitos*, and as proof she produced a bag of worms that her son had passed. She plopped them on the floor, a good little mound, and the team members gathered around, gawking. The three primary medical people, trained to look at human sickness with a scientist's steady eye, were fascinated by the revolting sight. Robinson took a snapshot.

After dinner at Javier's, some of the team drifted out to the porch, some stayed inside sitting in chairs. Robinson's translator, Nancy, sat in one of the chairs. The day before, Robinson had asked Nancy if she used birth control, and she had said no. Aghast, Robinson had said, "You didn't learn from everything I said to the women!" On this night, Robinson came into the house from the porch and plopped into Nancy's lap a year's supply of birth control pills.

The next morning, before the team rode back to Atoyac, Robinson rose early again, to walk around the town, this time walking up the hill toward the school. He walked through the square and to the town church. Outside the church stood a wooden crucifix decorated with pink streamers and a chain made of red and white paper loops. A white arch set in the ground rose just behind the crucifix. A man who lived across the road saw him and unlocked the front door for him. He let people in to pray; if a family needed a priest, for a wedding or funeral, they sent for one from Atoyac. The crucifix inside the church had a dying Jesus on it, an almost life-size figure with red blood dripping from his wrists, ankles, and side. The ceramic figure was shaded a pale white color, accenting the bright red blood and Christ's jet black hair. A crimson shawl with white tassels was draped around his neck, like a stethoscope, and a skirt of the same colors and pattern covered his loins.

After Robinson left the church, the man asked him to come look at his mother's leg. They walked to the porch where pots and pans hung from the ceiling, above the wood stove. The house had electric power, but it was built in pre-electricity days when the outside of a house and the inside were not very distinct from one another. Like many other houses in the town, some of its windows had no glass, and some entrances had no doors; they were simply open places in the wall.

The man's mother emerged from the house and showed Robinson an open sore on her ankle. It was likely she had scraped it on something, and it had not healed. Here, he struggled with his self-taught Spanish, trying to explain that she could provide her own treatment. He said, "*Es posible tener con, con usted. Necesito lavarse y* I don't know the word for 'keep it clean,' *lavarse,* wet to dry. . . ." This translates, "It is possible to have one with you. You need to wash it, and I don't know the word for 'keep it clean,' wash, wet to dry. . . ." He told her to elevate her leg often, but he said it in more English than Spanish: "Elevate *su* leg."

The team packed their luggage and rode back to Atoyac. At their hosts' home, the men took their first hot shower in three days, then they all had another sumptuous lunch and a nap. Some walked around Atoyac, shopping at the community market, *el mercado*. The market covered a large city block, but from the street they could only see a few entrances that appeared to lead into dark alleys. Inside, however, the market opened into a maze of crooked narrow aisles crowded with tables and shelves filled with merchandise. The merchants sold fresh meat, vegetables, fruit, hardware, farm implements, clothing, household supplies, and a wide range of odds and ends. Some items—hats, shirts, sausages—hung from ropes draped from pole to pole. Shiny metal scales sat on counters ready to weigh a few tomatoes or a slab of beef. Wide straw baskets were filled with bread for sale. Shoppers ducked or pushed hanging items aside to pass through narrow aisles. A patchwork of colored cloth sheets formed the market's roof. Sunshine slanted through narrow slits between sheets. Each booth was run by one or two people, who dickered on their prices according to the savvy of their customers. They sold some tourist items, even though Atoyac was not a tourist town. Mostly, local folk shopped there. To the Americans, they spoke their prices, *"Cinco pesos,"* and signaled with their hands—in this case, spreading out five fingers.

In the afternoon, the team rode back to Acapulco for the evening. The city was hopping, with thousands of visitors in town for the annual city festival. The ocean air, unlike evenings in the mountains, was thickly humid. Streets were jammed with cars. A six-lane thoroughfare with a narrow grassy median was blocked off on one side for the parade. The team crept through the traffic until they finally reached their hotel, a Days Inn. Next to the hotel was the "Rodeo Roundup" restaurant, which was decked out in American Western movie decor: wagon wheels, saddles, pictures of cacti and horses. On the sidewalk in front of the restaurant two young women beckoned people inside. They wore frilly shorts, dime-store red cowboy hats, bandannas, boots with tassels, and holsters armed with toy guns. A short walk from the hotel, the parade was in full swing. Floats sponsored by hotels, corporations, and various associations rumbled past the cheering, predominantly Mexican crowd. Except for a few self-contained resorts where foreigners rarely left the grounds, Acapulco had become a vacation stop for middle-class Mexicans. A Pepsi-Cola float advertised the soft drink and the "Flintstones" movie. A Hollywood-theme float included a Marilyn Monroe impersonator standing over a grate; intermittent gusts of air from a concealed fan blew her white dress up around her head. She acted surprised and thrilled at each gust. On the same Hollywood float posed a woman wearing a black-leather-and-chains dominatrix costume. Many floats had large speakers booming rock-and-roll music. Dancing men and women on floats waved to the crowd, who waved back and danced to the music, then waited, and, a few moments later, danced to the music on the next float. Most floats, regardless of their theme, had contingents of young women in tiny bikinis. One float with a Middle Eastern theme featured a belly dancer gyrating provocatively at the back. Twenty leering men walked behind this float throughout the parade route.

The team ate at a restaurant with an outdoor patio and panoramic view of the horseshoe-shaped Acapulco Harbor. In San Vicente de Benitez, where they were fed by local people and where there was little to purchase, no one had spent more than a few pesos a day for beer or sodas. Suddenly, they were spending thirty to sixty pesos for one meal. After dinner, most of the team, including Robinson, returned to the hotel to sleep. Some went to a disco next to the restaurant for a night of dancing. They boogied on a dance floor with two walls of floor-to-ceiling glass, looking across the harbor at the glittering, sloping hillside reflected in the calm water.

Saturday morning Robinson made a little mistake before returning to the purified water of the United States. The relative luxury of a hotel clouding his thinking, he rinsed his toothbrush in faucet water. He had diarrhea for a week.

Sitting in his seat on the airplane flying back to the United States, Robinson mused, "I didn't enjoy Acapulco half as much as the other. That last night was unsatisfying." He wrote on his evaluation form that he thought they should conduct two clinics instead of three and hold them for two days each. He noted that they were gone six days and conducted clinics only half those days. Some people, he wrote, traveled a long way and had to be turned away at the end of the first day. Before the plane landed, Gathercoal asked Robinson to make a return trip, next time as assistant team leader.

Tired and Swollen

On a cloudy August morning, Azi returned for her six-week checkup. James, the policeman she met after the World Cup, helped her with Robert. They sat near where a tape that explained an episiotomy was playing on the VCR/TV. Breastfeeding Robert, Azi said, "I hope they don't call me now." In a few minutes, they called her to the lab. She rolled her eyes and told James, "I think I can do it with him." She carried Robert, still breastfeeding, to the lab, as she had done pacing while watching the World Cup the month before. Waiting for the tech to draw blood, Azi said, "I now able to hold him and do anything with one arm, even cook. In Brazil, when I saw my sister doing that, I thought, that not me."

After her blood was drawn, she gave Robert to James, who moved to the OB waiting room. In the Family Planning office, the counselor asked about her period. Azi said it would start, then stop, start, stop. "Now it stop for two, three days." The counselor asked her about birth control. She said she had taken the pill in Brazil and it made her sick.

The counselor gave her a form and said, "The doctor will give you a pill compatible with your body, and one you can take while breastfeeding, so check if you've had any of these conditions."

The form had a list of diseases and conditions, some of which Azi did not recognize in English. She asked what a gall bladder was, what sickle cell anemia and stroke were. She finished the form and returned to the waiting room, where she resumed breastfeeding. James put his arm around her. A tape about C-sections played on the TV. A calm woman's voice from off-camera said, "I was in labor for several hours, and my cervix wasn't changing." A male doctor's voice told about the decision to do a section. The woman said, "Mike and I wanted a natural delivery. . . ." James stroked Azi's hair. "A C-section may be necessary if you have had one before, or if you have high blood pressure. . . ." Across from Azi a husband and wife sat together, the husband holding his hand to her belly. Next to them, a mother and three enthralled children watched the tape of the delivery.

Ms. Griff walked to Azi and glared, pretending to be angry. Azi's name had been called twice for her exam, but she had not heard it over the TV. "I had to put somebody in front of you." Ms. Griff said. "Come to the back in five minutes."

After her exam, Azi went to see discharge nurse Robbie Dimler. "Look at my baby," Azi said proudly.

"Ooh, look at the baby," Dimler said. She cuddled the tiny boy in her large arms. "How's the mom?"

"No sleep. I wish he had two mothers. One to get dressed, one to feed him."

Azi removed a camera from her purse and took a picture of Dimler holding her baby, who quickly fell asleep on her broad shoulder. The two chatted for a while about breastfeeding, laughing and shaking their heads. Dimler gave Azi information about her next WIC appointment, and Azi wrote it down on a bag labeled, "Disposable Bag for Sanitary Napkins."

That afternoon, Azi held Robert in her lap, at Kenneth's apartment. It was typical of low-cost apartment complexes scattered all over the northern suburbs. Young couples or singles lived inexpensively while they were in school, in their first jobs, or until they could afford a house. The two-bedroom apartment had a small square kitchen and ample living room. Between the television and sofa in the living room, several layers of blankets formed a pallet on the floor, where Kenneth enjoyed playing with Robert. Azi flipped through a pile of photographs on the small dining table between the living room and kitchen. A pile of English/Portuguese flashcards were scattered near her elbow. In one picture, she stood next to a pickup truck. Perched in the back was a motorcycle.

"It was mine," Azi said. "Last year. I sold it before I left to Brazil. I bought a motorcycle and I get pregnant—I no bought. Jeff bought the motorcycle. Who is I am to buy a motorcycle? He always wanted to give me a present, something because I used to pay his bills when I used to work. I said I bought because in reality the money that he expend buying motorcycle was nothing in comparison to the money that I spent, almost a year with him."

She said that when she first brought Robert home, she felt overwhelmed. In a high-pitched voice, she cried, "Ach! Hell. You have a pain and you walk and you feel a pain, and your milk, your breasts are painful. . . . The whole pain you feel in the first week and the second, because too much pain. And the pain when breastfeed him, because my nipples is so sore, so painful, and then one pain help you forgot another, like that. Something crazy. I can't describe. After the baby born I was constipated completely. Is worse than have the baby is go to the bathroom after because everything that I can't make any, do that, because the pain is—you have stitches. They cut me like that, what is they call, episomi—"

"Episiotomy."

"Yeah. I was walking funny, very slow in the hospital. Because they stitch. I remember something funny. When Kenneth get there, I could not open my eyes because I was too tired. I didn't sleep the day before and went two nights pain and everything. I was dead tired. I can't describe how I was tired. I saw he come and I didn't see he left. Is like I couldn't see anything. Like say to me, 'You win the lottery,' and have no reaction if I win the lottery. I just ah! Just never say anything."

She said James, the policeman, had called her soon after the day they met. He still had not seen the tape of the game. Gentlemanly and kind, he was a solid man with a steady job. "Kenneth was jealous at first, but he has his life, and I have mine. And I'm not in love with him. James helps with the baby. He never lets me pay anything. He's really funny about that. He like a lot of men in Brazil. And I like it. No because that. But he means some stuff that he have in common with me. I don't know what to do because he is really interesting guy, but I know he is expecting that I date him. I said that I no want to think about men for so long because I am so disappointed. Even I am disappointed with Kenneth. He work a lot and now James give me so much attention, with the little time he have in his life off work. My friends call me, "Doña Flor," from a movie in Brazil where a woman have two husbands, but I have three. They have to make a movie with me, 'Three Husbands and a Baby.' "

She walked to the kitchen, carrying Robert on her hip, and served herself lunch. She brought the plate back to the table and sat down to eat.

Robert let go with a loud "Wah!"

Azi jostled him gently with one arm, while she ate with the other. "I eat all the time like that. Never have time to eat alone."

"Wah!"

"Is complaining about something. What you upset about, eh? Heh? Heh?" She imitated his squeaky cry. "Sometimes I eat with left hand. He is still hungry. He is tired too.

"Also, he pull me, the nipples, and it just hurts." She took a bite and realized her food was cooling. "Been a long time since I've had hot food. But you know I find out something, a lot of men just stop on the street and look at the baby, say, 'Oh, how old?' and everything. Same thing that the women do in Brazil, the men do here. I thought it was very interesting. James said probably they was not stopping the baby but stop to flirt. Like the baby was an excuse. I don't think so really. Because I was still fat."

"Wah! Wah!" Robert cried.

Lisa Dean was getting ready to go with Dwayne, who was out of jail and on probation, to a family reunion—not Dwayne's family but a family he grew up with. Lisa knew all the family, too.

She asked her brother, "Franklin, are you gonna cut lil' Rob's hair?"

"Is he going with you?"

"Yeah." To her romping puppy, Lisa snapped, "Biloxi!" then added, "She know how to get out the door. She tried to get out this morning." Rob came downstairs to the kitchen, and Lisa told him, "Bring me a peach, and wash your hands first."

"No."

"Yes!" He washed his hands and opened a cabinet drawer. "No, lil'

Rob, in the refrigerator drawer! My mom says this little girl is going to be my payback. She said the way she acted when she was younger, that's the way I acted. Sit down, Biloxi!"

Rob asked if he should wash the peaches.

"I already washed them before I put them in the drawer. Go and get Jerry an apple, please."

"Thank you."

"Say, 'You're welcome.' "

"You're welcome."

"My mom said I was a little girl. Talked a lot. She said I even cursed."

Rob took one bite out of his peach and said, "I don't like this."

"What's wrong with it?"

"It has a spot right here."

"Let me see it. Bring me a knife, and be careful."

Lisa said she was pleased with Lauren Foley. "She's a great midwife. She just so down to earth. You know how some people be mean and don't want to answer your questions."

Sitting on the floor, eating his peach, Rob said, "I like your hair."

"Thank you, honey. She's not like that. She'll answer all your questions. I like the way they have it now. Before, I had a doctor. I had started having contractions and I was at the hospital by myself and I wanted the nurse to check me out and see if I had dilated."

"Mama, get me some more stuff for my book ba-a-ag."

"Be quiet!"

"I want it."

"Lisa!" came a shout through the screen door.

"Come in."

"Is Franklin here?"

"Upstairs. She wouldn't do it. She didn't want to do it. So I told the head nurse, and she made her do it anyway."

"What you gonna cut, Mama?"

"Your hair."

"With your clippers?"

"Yes. He weighed six pounds. I was bigger with him than I am now."

"You were big when you had Biloxi," Rob said.

Lisa laughed heartily. Her deep, almost masculine laugh filled a room. "Baby dog."

A slight rain drizzled the front of the clinic building. The thick warm air seemed eager to release a torrent of moisture, as if this pitiful rain merely hinted at what might come. Tropical Storm Beryl churned toward the Georgia and Florida coasts, bringing who knew what kind of weather the next day. Lisa emerged from a car that stopped on Butler Street. Hurrying, she walked between two vans parked along the road, through the crowd of transportation hawkers, and into Grady. Getting out of the car, she and Dwayne accidently bumped each other and exchanged glares.

Her hair was up in an intricate finger wave. A thin S-shaped band of hair snaked down each side of her face, just in front of her ears, where a man's sideburns might be. She weighed in at two hundred forty-four pounds in the blood pressure room, then sat in the waiting room with Dwayne. He leaned toward her and whispered something. She slapped his knee and snapped, "Get away!" Lisa said she was beginning to buy things for the baby: a few outfits, T-shirts, bibs.

"I need to get more socks. My mom said, 'I got it all covered. Most of it's in layaway, and I'll bring it down.' That's the way she was with my son." She yawned and said, "I'm sleepy. I don't know what time I went to sleep. I was up watching movies."

Dwayne whispered something to her and snickered. She stared at him, looking irritated. He said he was going to find his friends, and he left.

"He makes me sick. He's aggravating. Or maybe it's just me. They say when you get pregnant you get mean. He's why I'm tired. I thought he would leave me after my friend dropped us off. I said, 'Go on.'" She pointed at a little girl with a round head. "She's pretty. That one, too. She's cute." The second girl was an Indian girl with dark features, big eyes, a pretty smile.

The tape about C-sections came on the TV.

"I don't think I could take a C-section," Lisa said. "I had a friend who had one, and she said it about killed her."

"Lisa Dean, to exam room 6, please."

Just before the door shut to 6, Lauren Foley said, "Howya doing? Still pregnant."

The visit lasted ten minutes. Lisa had told her she felt dizzy and that her feet were swollen. Foley told her to lay on her side often and drink more fluids. She added, "See you next week. And don't go wreckin' no more." Dwayne walked in while she was waiting to check out.

"Are you ready?" he asked mischievously. "Is it about to drop?"

She scowled at him and smacked his arm. They walked down to the atrium, where two friends were waiting on them. They scampered through the rain to McDonald's.

It was a shockingly cool August morning in downtown Atlanta. The air was not humid. The breeze felt right; it wasn't merely hot air moving. Lisa got out of a car driven by a young man and entered the clinic building. She wore soft slip-on shoes on her swollen feet. She said it felt like she was walking on cushions. She wore a large, billowy dress. She still moved well, despite being so largely pregnant, despite her waddle.

"I couldn't get up today," she said sitting in the waiting room. "I forgot to call transportation yesterday, so I had to get a ride this morning with a friend." She filled out a green Medicaid-funded-transportation form, preparing for her ride back home. "I didn't want Dwayne to come in this morning. He makes me sick." Her nose running, she sniffled.

She said, "I'm ready to get over this sinus. I can't sleep because I can't breathe. I can't take anything for it. I'm not going to be late next week, if I make it. I'll probably go over."

Lauren Foley called her to room 6. "I guess you're getting tired of this," Foley said before she closed the door. Exiting in ten minutes, Lisa said, "There is something I can take for my cold."

"I'm going to give her some sniffle medicine," Foley said. "You get a gold star for waiting and asking." She handed Lisa a small plastic cup. "Here's your cup for your monthly cup-oh-pee. I guess you wonder what we do with all that."

As Lisa passed the front nurse's station, Ms. Griff eyed her and said, "She'll be back next week. She doesn't look uncomfortable enough."

At the lab, a tech asked her, "Do you know how to do a clean-catch?"

"Oh, yeah."

A clean-catch urine specimen was obtained by wiping the vagina with toilet paper from front to back, then pulling the labia apart to allow the urine to flow cleanly through without, the staff hoped, picking up any extra substances from labia, hair, whatever. The more hugely pregnant a woman became, the more acrobatic this task became.

Lisa left the lab and took a seat in the pharmacy. She pointed down at a hole torn in the front of a shoe. "Look at what the dog did. Look, the left foot is swollen more than the other one. It looks funny, don't it?" Her feet swelled beyond the limits of the slip-ons. She chuckled low. "They look like bear claws."

As the line advanced, the row of people sitting hopped up, moved down a seat, and plopped back down, like sheep slowly bounding over a row of fences, then waited standing in line a while. She advanced until she reached two lines of red tape on the floor. Between the lines, in faded, scuffed red paint, it said, "WAIT HERE." A sign on the wall by the sign-in window said, "Wait behind the red line for the next available typist." At her turn, Lisa handed over her forms. The clerk gave her a bottle of Actifed and pointed to the row of windows at the pharmacy on the next wall, where she would get the Robitussin. As Lisa walked to a row of chairs facing the pharmacy windows, a smiling woman handed her a Christian pamphlet. She accepted it, and the woman continued smiling, holding out a pamphlet for the next person walking by. On the TV bolted to the ceiling, Maury Povich ended his show on how to be a model, and the Channel Two news anchor announced a story about two policemen who accidentally shot at each other in a New York subway. Lisa hopped down this row of chairs until her turn came, then stood, and the line hopped along behind her.

"Kenneth knows, but Jeff doesn't know," Azi said about an upcoming vacation she was planning to take with James. "Jeff is jealous. He start accuse me since the baby born. I no care more about him. I said 'Jeff, you are the only one no work in this city and if I spend time with you, I not spend time with anybody almost. I spend some times with James but is too short. Jeff doesn't know if I see James or not. I think he's pretty jealous."

Azi's relationship with Jeff, which would have ended the year before if she had not become pregnant, held on tenuously only because they shared a child. They had recently spent a weekend at the exclusive Sea Island, on the Georgia coast, where his wealthy family owned a condominium. She agreed to go with him because she thought this would be the last time he would invite her there, and she wanted to take advantage of the opportunity. But it reminded her of the frustration she had always had with him. "He spend, spend his whole money and when his money finish, he say 'Azi, my money finish,' the morning of the last day, and then I start to spend my money. He go to the more expensive restaurant; he is impossible; if he have money he go to the nice restaurant, all the time, everything, is impossible."

She said she paid Kenneth half the expenses for the weeks she had shared the apartment with him, though he had said she could stay there the first two months for free. "Jeff give me some money before we go to the beach, and then I pay a lot of things that I was owing to Kenneth. He's too nice, and I feel he was expecting we would be together and I feel like I got to pay him every little thing that he expended with me and every little thing I wrote on a paper. He didn't know. Then I show him and I say that's the money and you better take it. If you no take, I call you burro, means not intelligent.

"Jeff says, 'I'm in love with you.' Three years together, and now we find out he is in love with me just because I am going out with somebody else. The hell with his love. Is very funny, his love, is very convenient. I think after the baby born, he realize. . . . If he really cares about, I want him care about the baby, no about me. I really wish that he didn't like me anymore, understand? Just help me take care the baby. He's so messy. And he cannot get over me. I think he have been try, but he could not. I think I get him jealous when I say to him, 'I have a lot in common with James.' I didn't think I'd meet someone I'd have so much in common like him. It just kill him."

"Wah! Wah!" She picked Robert up and began breastfeeding.

She looked down at his face and said, "The nursery was looking him, said, he no look like you. He look like the father probably. I said yeah, look just like the father."

Life with a baby was still a baffling experience for Azi. "He no have any routine! Different every day. I have to educate myself. After three months I start do that because he will sleep more. Now he sleep more through night, not through but four hours straight. And that's good to me. Any two hours straight, I get rest."

At the McDonald's next to Grady, a tragic affair came to an odd close. Police arrested a man who had walked into the men's bathroom and shot himself in the shoulder. Atlanta detectives doubted suicide. "Shooting yourself in the shoulder is not what I would call a legitimate suicide attempt," one police lieutenant said to a reporter, "considering all the better targets if you really want to kill yourself." The man was charged not with shooting himself, but with murder. Five hours earlier, it was alleged, he had calmly walked into his estranged wife's workplace and shot her once in the chest. Moments before the shot, when his wife first saw him approaching, she had leaned toward a coworker and whispered, "Call 911." Then she screamed, "No, Ike, no!" Her husband, who that day had told his sister he was going to kill his wife and himself, was taken to Grady, where he was shortly pronounced in stable condition, awaiting arrest.

Lisa stepped out of the car of the same male friend who had given her a ride before, and walked between two vans, toward Grady. Waddling through the atrium, she lightly rubbed her fingers together on one hand and said, "Last night my hands were so swollen I couldn't do this. I feel like, today—maybe. Last night I had a headache and a toothache. I felt like I was falling apart. I'm so tired." She exited the elevator on the second floor and walked toward the OB clinic.

Someone announced over the intercom, "We have a lost little boy in the OB waiting area, wearing blue overalls, red shirt, and white shoes." The boy was standing by the front desk, sniffling and breathing hard. A woman walked in, picked him up, and dashed out.

"I can't believe she left him," the clerk said.

"She could have said thanks," Lisa said.

A patient standing next to Lisa said, "If that was my boy, I'd be so scared if I lost him."

The clerk said to her, "You wouldn't have lost him."

"Slip off your shoes and step up on the scale," Nancy Forrest said to Lisa in the blood pressure room. "Keep that Grady card." Lisa put it in her purse and stood on the scales. "Put down your purse, please." She weighed two forty-eight.

As Lisa left, Forrest said, "Maybe she won't be back next week."

Lisa plopped into a chair in the waiting room. "I feel nauseated, like that headache's ready to come back. I put vanilla extract on my toothache. It numbed it. My little boy daddy used to put it on there. This old lady told me about it. It works. I wonder who would leave their kids. He was so scared."

She said she had noticed how swollen her face was when she scratched the outside of her nose using the two fingers that form a peace sign. She had to spread them more than normal, to scratch. "That's weird, isn't it?" she said. She said she was going to call Rob's aunt and ask her to take him home because she had a feeling she was going to have the baby soon.

On the TV, a tape about breastfeeding began playing. Lisa said, "That girl looks like the weather woman on Channel Two. My mom didn't discourage me from breastfeeding, like they're saying. She encouraged me. She breastfed all her five children."

"Lisa Dean, to exam room 6, please."

"Hi there, this is gettin' old, isn't it?"

Lisa told Lauren Foley that her mucous plug had come out the day before, and Foley told her she would probably start having regular contractions soon. Lisa asked about her swelling. Foley checked the form and said her blood pressure was OK. She checked Lisa's reflexes, which were normal, and told her not to worry about the swelling. Her blood chemistry, according to last week's lab report, was normal, so the circulation to her liver was fine. "Everything slows down when you're pregnant," Foley said. "Circulation, and so forth, so you're constipated, you have swelling, you're tired." She told her to drink plenty of fluids, rest, eat less salt, and prop her feet up. As Lisa was leaving, Foley said, "Call me. I'll be listening out for you."

At the desk, the clerk asked Lisa, "What time do you want to come back, Miss Dean?"

"Same time, ten." She rested her head in her hands on the counter. "I hope I don't come back."

The clerk handed Lisa the appointment sheet. "I hope not to see you."

Lisa got on the elevator beside a woman in a wheelchair. The woman had a long railroad-track-shaped scar on the stump just above where her right knee once was. In front of the clinic building, waiting for her ride home, Lisa said, "Did you hear about that man who shot himself in McDonald's after he killed his wife?" She narrowed her eyes and said, "They say most women that are killed are killed by someone who said he loved her."

The Perinatal Mortality and Morbidity Conference, in a fourth-floor classroom, included residents, nurses, attending physicians, medical students, and Walt Robinson, a physician assistant. Dr. Melissa Avery, the resident presenting the cases, sat in a desk in front of the room. Before the conference started, she explained its purpose. "The second-year high-risk antepartum resident presents cases from the month before, so she had no role in them. It's easier to hear general criticism than personal criticism. They want placenta information, blood studies, pathology report. Peds is there if the infant lived long enough. Sometimes we find something that should have been done, but usually it's just academic, to raise the level of suspicion in prenatal care, what to look for earlier. But it's mainly for academic discussion."

She began by rattling off information about the first case quickly, numbingly, clinically. Sixteen weeks pregnant, no prenatal care. Complained of abdominal pain. Drug screen was negative; said she was a former IV drug user. She had lost one child before, in an automobile accident. Vital signs were stable. An echocardiogram revealed severe aortic deficiency. The woman elected termination of pregnancy due to likely poor outcome of pregnancy. Patient was transferred to surgery, where she was given an aortic valve replacement. Due to other problems the doctors discovered, a splenectomy was performed.

Dr. Scott Jennings orchestrated the discussion. He asked one resident if the therapy had been appropriate. The resident named several other possibilities and concluded with, "It depends." Everyone seemed to agree that with the woman's severe heart problems and serious risks of continuing the pregnancy, the woman's decision to terminate the pregnancy was a good one. Dr. Jennings turned to the pathologist, who, in addition to giving his report on the fetus, said he was not happy that the placenta had not been delivered to pathology. They like to see everything. Dr. Jennings agreed it should have been sent.

"It might not have made any difference," the pathologist said.

"But it could have."

The next case involved a midwife patient, thirty-seven weeks pregnant. The fetus had shown normal movement, and the pregnancy was uncomplicated. But the patient sensed no fetal movement for a full day. The fundal height measurements over several weeks were given, and Dr. Jennings asked if that should have been investigated. Avery said it seemed to be normal growth. Dr. Jennings asked how far off the expected fundal height would a measurement have to be for it to be checked out.

"I use three centimeters or more," one person said.

"I use two," another said.

"A four-centimeter difference at that point is impressive," Dr. Jennings said. "At forty weeks it's not impressive."

"Would you recommend urgent ultrasound?" someone asked.

"That's a good question. This one was three centimeters from the month before. We were pretty close on gestational age." He asked, "How much did she weigh?"

Avery flipped through the records. "One-oh-four."

"So the fundal height should have been accurate."

"She was admitted for induction," Dr. Avery continued.

"What could have been the cause of this?" Dr. Jennings asked.

"It could have been cocaine, but that's rarely the case with our Hispanic patients."

"Any other congenital problems that could cause it? Especially at Grady Hospital?"

"We could be headed toward syphilis," a doctor said.

"So what happened?"

"She had dilated seven centimeters, RPR active."

"Was the membrane ruptured?"

"No. And she denied feeling contractions, only decreased movement."

"A lot of women wish they didn't feel contractions at seven centimeters." A few people chuckled softly.

A short discussion ensued about using a needle to draw fluid from inside the membrane. Someone pointed out that sometimes the sac is like a balloon, and it pops when a needle is used, and you get no sample. Then a discussion followed on a number of procedures that are done, which may not be cost-effective or necessary but which doctors at some hospitals perform routinely.

At the end of the discussion, Dr. Jennings said, "So, aside from being very depressed, she went home OK the next day?"

"Yes."

Looking at the pathologist and chuckling, Dr. Jennings said, "We did get a placenta on this."

The pathologist responded by showing slides made from analysis of the placenta and fetus. A discussion followed about possible reasons a fetus can die when there is no obvious reason. Dr. Jennings concluded with, "Some die from mechanisms we hardly understand. It's a mystery. This deserves some kind of study project. Any other comments?" There were none so they moved on to the third case.

It involved a pregnancy estimated at twenty-three weeks. Fetal anomaly was suspected, and the patient was admitted for elected termination. A four-and-a-half-centimeter by four-and-a-half-centimeter mass of tissue was detected attached to the fetus's neck. Patient had received counseling and elected termination. Medical history did not contribute. A six-hundred-four-gram female infant was delivered, dead at birth.

"What did it look like?" Dr. Jennings asked.

"There was no description," Avery said, "but a pathologist described it to me on the phone as a partially cystic mass."

Pathology slides were shown of side and front shots of the fetus. A huge red mass bulged from the neck. The pathologist said this type was rare. He gave the Greek etymology of the complex medical term for it. He said it may have arisen from a primitive thyroid, but research says that's unlikely. A close-up slide revealed an aggregation of immature cells, which had no diagnostic significance.

"If she had not elected termination, could this be removed?"

A host of likely complications were identified around the room.

"I saw two in a week with cystic masses," a doctor volunteered. "One had a mass bigger than the head. Another patient refused termination. She was fascinated by it." He paused a moment and said, "I guess we'll see that one in here before too long."

The next case had been one of Robinson's patients. Twenty-three years old, thirty-nine and two-sevenths weeks pregnant. She arrived with irregular contractions, and she reported decreased fetal movement. Her cervix was at two centimeters and was fifty percent effaced—about halfway to being thinned out enough for delivery. Heart tones had been normal the day before when she saw Robinson for her prenatal visit. But this day the ultrasound revealed no movement or heartbeat. Social and family history was negative. She took vitamins and iron. She tested negative for gonorrhea, lupus, syphilis, and everything else they tested for. It was in every way a normal pregnancy, but the baby was dead. The doctors gave her Pitocin until she delivered a dead little girl. The second-year reported the placenta was intact, and the patient had an uncomplicated postpartum.

The fetal lungs tested positive for bacteria, but it was a slight amount that many healthy babies have. Dr. Jennings noted that since the membrane had not ruptured, there was no clue, obstetrically, as to what happened. "Let's look at the pathology slides," he said. Robinson reached behind his head and dimmed the lights. He rattled the ice in the bottom of his cup and drank some down, the plastic top removed now. He waggled his foot—a nervous habit.

The magnified placenta membrane on the screen, the pathologist said there was no severe infection. Dr. Jennings asked if there was more from the fetal or maternal side. "There's not much from either side," she answered.

"So the baby was responding to something inflammatory?"

"The baby was responding to something. The usual organisms we look for were not there. There is some inflammatory reaction here."

Someone asked, "Can those be post-mortem?"

"No. It had to come from a live baby. Well, some studies show otherwise. I don't know. But it was probably a pre-mortem phenomenon."

Dr. Jennings clicked a button, and a slide of the fetal kidney shifted onto the screen. It confirmed there was no body abnormality. Slides of the lungs revealed probable slight asphyxiation, but nothing severe enough to be fatal, and slight evidence of meconium contamination, which was also too minor to be harmful. Meconium is fecal material from the baby, which if inhaled at delivery, can cause infection in the lungs and major health problems. Dr. Jennings concluded, "I guess we're tempted to blame all this on infection, but it's not the most beautifully illustrative case."

Robinson volunteered that this couple really wanted a baby. "It was hard to explain to them. They were model patients, never missed a visit."

Someone asked about the umbilical cord. The second-year flipped through the chart and said there was no description of it. The pathologist said the section of the cord they got revealed nothing significant.

Dr. Jennings said, "Sometimes life is not fair at all, is it? Some patients who abuse everything are great breeders, if you will. And sometimes those who do the best can't pull it off. I wish we were smarter." He paused, and the room was quiet. Robinson turned the lights back up. "Any other questions or comments?" There were none, so he said, "Let's go to the next case."

Robinson whispered, "We have no clue whatsoever what happened, flat out."

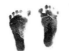

Get It Out of Me

Sipping coffee from a large Convenience Food Mart mug, Jodi Reeve listened to the morning report. Attached to her Grady nametag was a button that said, "Trust in Births Trust in Midwives." She sat in the midwife office with the third-shift midwife, who was ready to go home. Behind Reeve was a locker labeled "Dolls and Pelvis."

"In 19, you got a thirty-seven plus weeks by ultrasound," the outgoing midwife said. "She said she had a gush from her vagina yesterday. She was booming out contractions. Requested an epidural and received one. I was busy with other deliveries, and the doc examined her. She had an amnio infusion. No meconium. Contractions now every three minutes. Her Pit's on 4.

"Then there's the fourteen-year-old, in room 21. Tall and skinny, she has a needle phobia. She's been treated for STD's. Big variables. I thought she had a couple lates. Her contractions are six or seven minutes apart. They were going to start Pit, but they didn't. She wanted no epidural either. Fear of needles. And she's by herself. She does OK if you hold her hand."

Reeve first went to room 19 and looked at the strip coming out of the fetal heartbeat monitor. She sipped coffee. "We don't like this, but it shows movement, and that's good." She glanced at the monitor and said, "This machine hasn't done as much good as everybody thought. With it, we think we know all about what's going on in there. Sometimes it shows something, and the baby's doing fine. Sometimes the strip is normal, and something's wrong. It hasn't done much for OB/GYN. Except increase the C-section rate."

She walked to 21 to see the fourteen-year-old. She introduced herself and said, "You look a little spaced out." An oxygen mask on her face, she extended her hand toward Reeve, who gently held it. Reeve looked at the strip, then asked, "Can I have my hand for just a second?" She used both hands to tear off the end of the strip, then held her hand again. A contraction started. "Nice and easy," Reeve said. "All the way through. Don't tighten up. Breathe all the way through, nice and easy." She looked at the doctor's order for Pitocin and said, "This is ridiculous. I'm going to talk to his wife."

She released her hand and walked down the hall. Walking briskly, commenting on the inherent tensions between the approaches midwives take toward delivery and that of MDs, she said, "A lot of what we do is cover our ass. We take plenty of notes to show we've consulted correctly." She sat at the nurse's desk and wrote in charts. "Especially as midwives. We've had more experience than the docs, but some docs don't understand midwifery. They don't learn about normal delivery and rarely get to watch a normal delivery develop without medical intervention. I'd prefer to have a woman in a warm bath and walking around. But this is a medical delivery here, the monitors and needles. This third-year group of residents, in their first year spent a month with us to learn about normal delivery. Most were frustrated. After the first few residents it didn't work at all. This one here today, Timothy Crews, was one of the few who really learned from it. He married a midwife."

"Heyo, midwife," a nurse walking by said.

"Hey, baby."

"Whatchoo know?"

Reeve wrote progress notes for fifteen minutes, glancing occasionally at the strip torn from the monitor in 21.

She returned to 19; the patient said, "I wish I'd get it over with."

"The first one is unpredictable. You've kicked in to active labor, so maybe the baby will respond, and the cervix will dilate. You may have a big baby, and you're not real tall, so we're going to keep an eye on it."

To her friend, the patient said, "You shocked me, coming here."

"I heard you were in labor, and I drove like I was flying across town."

"Ain't nothing happened."

"Yes, it has," Reeve said. "A lot's going on in there."

Reeve walked to the residents' room and showed the strip from 19 to Dr. Crews. Happy to be on the same shift, they exchanged big hugs. "Whatever you want to do is fine," he said.

Magical words, to a midwife.

Returning to 21, still carrying her large mug, Reeve said, "As midwives, you learn who your allies are. There's a level of trust with some docs who understand what we're doing and trust what we do. Like, doctors tend to use Pitocin to induce labor, or artificially break their water, but I'd rather give an enema or something else."

She checked on the fourteen-year-old. "I think she's going to deliver."

Another midwife patient was brought up from the ultrasound clinic. She was put in 20. Reeve had patients in three consecutive rooms, 19, 20, and 21. The tech attached the new patient to the monitor. The shifting monitor strap, already connected with the speaker, made a rough scratchy noise like a hand brushing a live microphone.

"She had a decel," Reeve said, thinking aloud, looking at the strip. "The baby's heart slowed down during a contraction. It decelerated. Now, why would this baby do that? Is it trying to say, 'I'm ready to come out?' "

Back with the fourteen-year-old, Reeve held her hand with both her own hands. "Nice and easy. Stay with it." The patient moaned, uncomfortable during a contraction. "Is it still in the lower part of your stomach?" Reeve asked. "Do you want to get on a bedpan and pee?"

"I already did," she said, muffled, through the oxygen mask.

Still holding her hand, Reeve looked at the strip and wrote on a yellow progress sheet. The strip showed occasional contractions closer together than the others. "This is not a good pattern. We like them consistent. The fetal monitor is technology we've brought into the birthing process, and now we can't get rid of it. We have to monitor them all the time, so I can't have her get up and walk. Even ultrasound, we don't really know its effect. We think it does no harm, but we're not completely sure."

Back in 19 with the patient ready to get it over with, Reeve looked at the strip. "It looks good." She showed the strip to the patient's friend. "Each of these vertical lines is a minute, see? This squiggly horizontal red line is the baby's heartbeat. This black one shows the contractions. This means the contractions are every two, three minutes. I'll show this to the doc and say this is the contraction pattern and this is how far she's dilated, and decide from there."

The red heartbeat line moved along in little scribbles that barely edged up or down, until a contraction hit. Doctors and midwives liked this "reactive strip," a band where the heartbeat jumped up a bit during a contraction. The contraction line scribbled along in more dramatic up-and-down shifts, climbed sharply when a contraction began, and descended sharply as it ended, creating a little black-lined, craggy mountain range on the screen.

The patient said something Reeve did not want to hear. "When you talk to the doctor, will you go ahead and take the baby out?"

"No, we'll do everything we can to have a vaginal delivery. It's the best way and safest. You don't have to recover from major surgery and with a vaginal delivery, you're a new woman, the hormonal and all that. But if you do need a C-section, we do them safely here, and Grady has a very reasonable C-section rate. Some places, you may have a C-section because it's five o'clock, and the doc is ready to go home, but not here."

"My mom and sister both had C-sections."

"That makes me pessimistic. You're all probably built the same, so you might. You probably already have it in your mind, to—"

"Take it out."

"—have a baby. It depends on the baby's head."

Reeve walked to 20, to see the new patient, who was two weeks past due. A nurse was asking her triage questions, a clerk getting her signature. A nurse putting in the IV said, "Little stick. Sorry, darling." Reeve wrote on a progress sheet and said, "I'll be back."

She returned to 19 to check the cervical dilation. "She's about four, five," Reeve said. "The head seems down further."

"Four to five? I've been that for a while."

"Yeah, baby. Roll back on your side. I think your baby liked it better."

Down at the doctor's room, she said to Crews and the attending doctor, "I think it's inevitable she's headed for the operating room. Her mother and sister did. That's depressing."

The attending said, "I'd grit my teeth and give her a little more time."

"OK. I'll check her in two hours." Walking down the hall to 19, she said, "Sometimes we don't cut even if it seems inevitable." To the patient she said, "The doc says don't throw in the towel yet. The baby has come down some. There's some change in the pelvis. There's molding on the head, so the baby's trying to get through the pelvis. That's why the baby's head's so soft. Have you seen a newborn's pointy head?"

"Yes."

Reeve wrote on the progress sheet. The monitor echoed its watery thump, thump, thump.

"Prepare the OR for a C-section," came over the intercom, from some room.

She walked to 21. "Howya doing, baby? That medicine helping any?" Drowsily, the fourteen-year-old nodded. Moaning through a contraction, she extended her hand, and Reeve held it. "Do you want something more for pain?"

"I want something to ease the pain."

"That's what I mean. I'm going to examine you."

"Don't. It hurts."

"I won't do it during a contraction." Reaching to check the dilation, Reeve said softly, "I'm just going to touch you a little, right here."

"My stomach hurts, for real. Can I walk? It'll stop it from hurting."

"It won't stop it from hurting because you're in labor. Here's what's going on in there. The top of your uterus is pulling the bottom up, pulling the cervix over the baby, like pulling a turtleneck sweater over your head." Reeve wrote on the progress sheet and said, "We can give you more pain medicine through the IV in your arm, or the best is an epidural."

"What's that?"

"It's medicine we put in through your back. It makes you numb from the waist down. Which do you want?"

"IV."

"Well, it'll take the edge off a little."

She walked to 20, where the nurse was having trouble finding an arm vein for the IV. Reeve felt her arm near where a rubber strap was tied around. "You have some tough skin, you know that?" She felt, then slowly pushed the needle in. The patient grimaced. "Sorry, sweetie." Reeve removed the rubber strap. No vein. The nurse felt the other arm, rubbing and tapping softly with her fingertips. Reeve held a small black wand to the patient's belly, pressed a button, and it buzzed. "This is a noxious noise for the baby," Reeve said, "to wake it up. We used to drop a bedpan."

She returned to the nurse's desk and looked at the large computer screen, where four patient strips trudged across in red and black jagged lines. Watching three patients' strips, Reeve called her house. To her daughter she said, "I want you to do some laundry, clean your room, and get the trash out before they come. And the boys need to feed the dog." Her son got on the phone. "I want you to take out the trash and feed the dog. Rebecca is going to do the wash. Who won't help you? Put him on the phone. Whoops, I'm buzzing. Talk to you later." She hung up and said, "I have three children in my family: a son, a daughter, and a husband." She looked at her beeper. "I don't know that number." She punched the number. "This is Jodi Reeve, one of the nurse midwives. What's up?" She listened a minute and said, "Try that Hurricane spray."

Back in 19, she asked, "Are you still comfortable?"

"A little. I'm starting contractions."

"Where are they?"

"Down here."

"Have you peed in a while?"

"Two and a half hours."

"It may be your bladder."

Reeve quickly checked in on 20, then told the fourth-year anesthesiologist that 20 needed an IV.

"I'll send someone in training."

"No, this is not for someone in training. This one's really tough. We've had some good nurses try."

Back to 21, where a medical student was looking at the strip and holding the fourteen-year-old's hand.

"I want to walk," the still-alone, grimacing girl said.

"I'm sorry. Walking is not an option." Reeve spoke firmly this time. "I wish it was." Reeve massaged the patient's right hip and thigh. The monitor's soft thump filled the room.

The patient's sister entered the room. She wore a T-shirt that said, "Luke In the Nude." Reeve said, "Good, we need a hand-holder and massager." The student and sister exchanged seats; the sisters held hands.

"I had to take mama to work and pay my rent," she explained.

Reeve walked to the nurse's desk, where nurse Marie Costley said, "They have an induction in 9. It's yours, but the docs did it. And you have a new patient in room 4."

Two new midwife patients. She had five patients now, in 4, 9, 19, 20, and 21. "OK, I'll go see her. Right when I'm planning to eat something."

She went to 20, where the nurse said, "We got an IV." Reeve pushed a needle into the arm without the IV, to draw blood.

"Sorry, honey." She drew out the blood and removed the needle. "All right baby, we're done with you. I think."

She walked to room 4, to see one of the two new patients, then wrote the patient information on the board in the residents' room, then checked on the patient in room 9.

After 9, she dashed to the midwife office for a quick bite. "Keeps my blood sugar from bottoming out," she said, eating quickly.

She went to the residents' room and wrote the updated information about 9 on the board in orange ink. Emory Medical School patients were written in blue, Morehouse School of Medicine patients in black.

She walked to 21 and checked the fourteen-year-old. Reeve announced, "This baby's ready to come," then told the student, "Shut that door please; there's no curtain in here." Reeve raised one of the patient's legs, the knee bent, and, standing by the side of the bed, leaned against the bottom of the patient's foot, to hold the leg up. "Breathe, push, easy, easy," Reeve instructed. She repeated this several times, the sister sometimes saying it with her. Between pushes, the patient looked down between her legs, her eyes wide. "Go ahead, push again, sweetie. It's almost out. Go ahead and push again, push for me. Come on, sweetie, the baby's ready."

The patient moaned and exhaled hard and fast. As she pushed again, the baby partially emerging, she screamed loudly, freely, fiercely, twice.

"There it is, there it is," Reeve said, leaning hard against the foot.

The patient let out a loud, long scream, this one spiced with terror, as the baby came on out. The baby cried, and Reeve said, "It's a boy. Well, you little troublemaker." To the new fourteen-year-old mother, she said, "Did you want a boy?"

"No."

Her sister said, "You did good." The patient began sobbing.

Reeve handed the sister a pair of scissors. "Set this little boy free."

The sister looked frightened, holding the scissors in the air.

"Right here, between there and there."

She clipped through the umbilical cord, then hugged her sister, both crying.

Reeve told the patient, "Pull your shirt up." She complied, and Reeve placed the baby at her breast. Reeve covered her breasts and the baby with a cloth. The patient saw Reeve pick up a needle, and she grimaced.

"This isn't for you. It's only for the umbilical cord." Reeve drew some cord blood and handed the needle to the nurse. "Sorry, it's the best I could do." To the patient, she said, "Your placenta is ready to come out. You pushed beautifully, so it probably stretched perfectly." She checked for a tear. "Well, maybe one stitch. Your placenta's ready. Go ahead and push it out."

Nurse Costley came in and asked, "Jodi, do you want me to up the Pit next door?"

"No, I'll do it. All right, push down. Hard, like you did with the baby."

The sister asked, "What is it?" after the placenta slid out.

"The placenta. I'll show you." The fourteen-year-old looked, too. "This was attached to your uterus. This is what the baby was in. This nourished your baby. Cool, huh? You got a tiny tear, and I'm going to put in a couple of stitches. I'm going to give you some numbing medicine. You did so good." The youngster grimaced again at the sight of the needle.

"I don't want that," she insisted. "Nuh uh."

"I have to do some stitches. It'll be more comfortable if it's numb. I'll talk you through it. I won't surprise you."

The nurse picked up the baby and took him to the warmer. The girl still grimaced.

"This is just a couple of stitches, darling. I can give you numbing medicine or just stitches, straight. What do you prefer?" Reeve spoke with a tinge of grit in her voice but remained calm and jovial.

"Just stitches."

At the first pain from the suture needle, the girl screamed.

"Do you want numbing medicine? It'll just be one stick."

She nodded.

Reeve looked around for the sister, who was out of the room. She asked a nursing student who had come in to hold the girl's hand. "You can squeeze as hard as you want," Reeve said to the girl. But before she could inject, the girl changed her mind and said no, eyeing the needle. Reeve backed down.

"You only have a tiny tear. Sit in a tub three times a day. It will burn when you pee, and when you have a bowel movement wipe it clean from front to back." To the sister, who had returned, she said, "She's got to keep her bottom real, real clean, or it won't heal right." She turned back to the patient. "I want you to rub your uterus until it's hard." Cleaning her up, Reeve said, "You did great."

"She's got to get over that fear of needles," the nurse said.

In the hall, on the way to room 20, Reeve said the uterus should be massaged to loosen it; it clamps down the veins so a woman does not bleed to death when she has a baby. "It's really an incredible system," she said. She quickly checked on the patient in 20, then walked next door to 19, where she said, "It looks inevitable that you'll have a C-section, which doesn't sound like the end of the world to you."

"It's not. I'm ready to get it over with."

"It looks like we've come to a dead end."

Timothy Crews came in the room. He greeted the patient politely and pulled the curtain for privacy. He checked her cervix. "She doesn't appear to be contracting. What did you say, five?"

"Five and complete," Reeve answered.

"She's had adequate pattern?"

"Yes, and I've been here since seven-thirty."

"It looks like we gave it our best shot. Miss Burgess, as Jodi explained—"

"Yeah, she did."

While Crews explained the C-section, Reeve returned a phone page, checked on 18, where another midwife patient had been brought, and returned another phone page. She returned to 21 to check on the teenager and baby.

"So, how much did that little peanut weigh?"

"Twenty-nine ten," the nurse said.

"Are you going to breastfeed?"

"No."

"You should. This is the middle of National Breastfeeding Week. We would love for you to breastfeed. You wake up in the middle of the night, you just roll over and put him on the tit. It's the best thing for him, but don't do it if you don't want to. It's your choice. You had this baby."

Her sister encouraging her, she began breastfeeding the tiny baby. Her sister said, "I'm happy now. When I get home I'm going to hand out cigars."

The fourteen-year-old watched closely as the baby suckled at her breast. Reeve, the nurse, and the student all wrote on forms. Collectively covering their asses. As the baby ate its first meal, the only other sound was the scratching of three pens on paper.

"You'll make yourself a healthy baby," Reeve said. "All the antibodies you have, you'll pass through your milk."

Reeve walked to the midwife office and pulled a notebook from her locker. "Most of us keep logs of our deliveries." She wrote for several minutes, this time for herself. She walked to the residents' room and wrote in orange, "Delivered," on the board by the patient's name.

In the hall, she saw the patient from 4 walking the halls, rolling an IV pole with her. "Has it been two hours yet?" Reeve asked her.

"Almost."

She went to 21, where the fourteen-year-old was feeding the baby with her other breast. Reeve said, "You did great. Congratulations. I got to do the baby exam soon. Be back."

She quickly checked with 20, then 18, then looked in on 19 and wished her well with the C-section. "I'll be checking with you."

Her pager buzzed. She darted to the nurse's station to answer it. Behind her, the patient from 19 was wheeled into the OR. She walked to the residents' room, erased 19 from the board, and updated the information on 18, using the orange pen. Crews was explaining the board to Dr. Mildred Hankins, who had taken over as attending physician. Crews spoke in a bland, professional monotone, going down the board line by line, from the lowest room number to the highest.

"Eleven wants a female doctor," Crews said about one patient.

"We should make no promises," Hankins said. "We should say we'll do our best but can't guarantee it. If they demand it, they can go somewhere else and pay for it."

Reeve went to 20. The patient lay on her side, an oxygen mask on. Reeve looked at the strip and wrote in the chart. The patient from 18 walked by in the hall, her husband pushing the IV pole beside her. The loose wheels clacked as they turned. "Feel a contraction?" Reeve asked the patient in 20. She said she wasn't sure. When the patient moaned, Reeve asked, "Feel anything?"

"Yes."

She also said she wanted to make a phone call, so Reeve said she would get a phone and bring it to her. In the hall, she saw the husband of the patient from 19, who was in the OR having a C-section. He asked where she was.

"In the OR. We tried to wait on you, but once they make the decision, you have to move." She escorted him down to the door leading to the OR. He stood across the hall, waiting, fidgeting, leaning against the wall, a plastic bag of his wife's belongings by his feet. She retrieved the phone, a one-piece that hung up when it was laid flat, and took it to 20. When the new Labor and Delivery floor was first opened, all the rooms had phones, but one by one they were stolen. The staff kept this one phone at the nurse's station to pass around, as needed. "There's a contraction," Reeve said, looking at the strip. "Can you feel it now?"

She nodded. Reeve left to take a quick break. She finally made it to the break room. On the table were brochures advertising candy and jewelry. Next to them was an order form. A handwritten note at the top of the form said, "It's school time! You know what that means!!? SALES!!! Please look through and if you feel the urge(!) to order something— great! If not, I hope this has afforded you some pleasurable visual delights!" It was signed by "Joan," who drew a smiley face under her name.

"She's screaming again," one of the nurses in the room said flatly, responding to a woman's agonized, long shout from down the hall. It was part scream, part moan, a deep desperate wail; perhaps only a new word can describe the unique sound of a delivering woman who simultaneously screams in pain and moans in extended agony: she was scroaning.

Reeve said she had her first child in Boston, where she had a midwife she adored. "She was a great midwife; it was a great birth, and I decided I wanted to do that. I thought I would get my experience here and go somewhere else, but I stayed. I love Grady." She saw an ultrasound nurse walk by and called out her name. "Would you get your docs under control? Everyone you send up here is deceling. It's out of control!" The nurse laughed at her and walked by. "There is no birthing center in Atlanta," Reeve said. "It's hard to get doctors to back you up. It's hard to get malpractice insurance. Even though it's safe, no one wants to back you up. Obstetricians are too unsure about their ability to make a living at a birthing center."

She was paged from home. "What's up there?" she said into the phone. "Did Bec do laundry? . . . Did she fold it all?"

"Would the midwife call 4247, please," came over the intercom. She finished talking with her family, returned the page, and walked to 21 for the baby exam. "Howya doing?" she asked the fourteen-year-old. "I heard you had a shower. Do you feel like a new woman? There's nothing like having a baby to make you feel like a new woman, huh?"

She nodded meekly.

"Look at this baby," Reeve beamed, standing over the baby warmer. She put on gloves and turned the baby over, and he cried. "I'm sorry. I know you don't like it." She listened to his heartbeat, gently probed his mouth with her finger, and felt his head. "Your baby has a little bit of a conehead, from fitting through your birth canal. You don't need to shape it. It'll round out all by itself." She flipped the baby over and checked his anus. Reeve noticed a young man sitting on the upholstered couch against the wall. "Is this your baby?" He nodded. "Have you held him?" He shook his head. "Do you want to?" He shook again, but that did not deter Reeve. She carried the baby to him. He held his child in the crook of his arm, staring down at him.

Later that day, the floor became hectic. Sitting at the nurse's station, Reeve heard agonizing scroans from 14 during each contraction. The faint cry of a baby drifted from room 17. From 11 she heard the rhythmic thump thump thump of the heart/contraction monitor. Moans from 14 were joined by occasional screams, sometimes merging into a scroan. From 14 could also be heard, simultaneously, a female voice saying, "Push push push push push push" and a male voice counting to ten. "Take a breath," the female voice said. "Push push push wonderful."

The doctors were going in and out of two rooms. Reeve was in and out of two rooms. It was just announced two more patients were being sent.

Over the intercom came, "Please clear out the OR for a C-section."

A resident stopped by the desk and told Reeve he delivered one of her patients in the admitting office. "She came on MARTA," he said. "I felt her and said, 'This is the head.' Me and the nurse ripped off her shorts; the patient was on her hands and knees. We wrapped the baby in a sheet, and it was OK. That baby was vigorous from the beginning."

"Let me ask you this," a nurse said. "Did she tear?"

"No."

"See, you should try that hands-and-knees position more often." She glanced at Reeve and nodded.

Reeve said that patient had been in before and was sent home.

"So it's your fault," the resident kidded.

"Most of our patients ride an ambulance, and the one that rides MARTA. . . ."

She wrote on progress sheets, then added, "Sometimes very with-it women are with men that don't stay with them. It makes you think not-so-good thoughts about men. When they're here, I try to get the men involved in the delivery." Speaking in a mock dreamy voice, knowing she was being idealistic, she said, "I imagine their being involved will change their attitude about cherishing life and about the woman they're involved with. I wish it was a lasting thing. For my husband, it was an incredible experience. I usually try to get them involved somehow. Sometimes it's easier than other times. I try to stress what a miracle it is, how fantastic it is."

She continued writing and said, "I have a hard time dealing with teens, especially those close to my daughter's age. So many patients today have been teens. Fifteen, fifteen, fourteen. One was one year older than my daughter. Here's my cure for the woes of the world: reversibly sterilize all babies, across the board. Then after parenting classes—"

"Yesterday, we had one who was fourteen," a nurse said, "who wouldn't let 'em take her blood."

"We had one who was fifteen," another nurse said, "her second baby."

"We had one who was fourteen with two miscarriages."

Reeve's pager beeped, and she returned the call, from a fifteen-year-old. "What does the discharge look like? . . . Does it burn when you pee?" She told the teen it might be a miscarriage. She recommended she go to the Women's Urgent Care Clinic.

At the back of Grady, an ambulance pulled into the WUCC emergency entrance. They wheeled in Lisa Dean and rode the elevator to the fourth floor. Dwayne walked beside her. That morning, her friend Leslie had come by to see if Lisa was all right. Lisa had gotten up early; the pain in her belly had kept her awake much of the night. In the bedroom, Leslie timed Lisa's contractions. Dwayne was there, drawing Lisa's ire. "Move! Get out of the way!" Lisa had shouted. Leslie told Dwayne he should talk to her, calm her down. "Let her know you're there," she told him. Dwayne reached over to touch Lisa, and she dived on the bed. "It hurts! It hurts!" Lisa said, groaning. Leslie said, "It's coming," then called the ambulance. They went for a walk, and when the ambulance arrived, Lisa said, "I'm not ready to go." She wanted to be sure. Thirty minutes later, she was sure. Leslie called the ambulance again, and rode with Lisa.

In room 17, Jodi Reeve checked Lisa's cervix. Four centimeters. She asked Lisa to give her a urine sample. Wearing brown house slippers, Dwayne went in the bathroom with her, holding the IV bag. Lisa emerged holding a plastic cup of yellow liquid. RN Holly Eberhart attached her to the monitor. She lay on her left side, moaning, breathing hard and steady. Dwayne sat in the upholstered chair by the window.

"Is this your miserable tiny amount of pee?" Reeve shook her head at the specimen cup.

"It's all I could do."

Reeve dipped a strip of paper into the urine and watched it change colors. "She's got a little bit of ketone; she's dehydrated. When did your contractions start?"

"Eight-thirty."

"When did they get close?"

"About eleven."

Reeve held off asking questions during contractions.

After she finished her questions, Lisa said, "Oh God, here comes another one." Then she said a word that she had scolded her son for saying a few months earlier in the OB clinic. "Oh, shit. I don't know if I can take this."

"When this one ends, roll over," Reeve said, "and I'll measure your tummy." She measured her fundal height and asked, "Where do you feel it?"

"Down here."

"Not in your back?"

"No."

Reeve listened to her back through a stethoscope. "How did you deal with your first delivery?"

"I didn't hurt this bad."

"It was longer, wasn't it?"

"Nope."

"Are you sure? Or do you not remember?"

"When I got here, I was dilated."

"Oh, really? That's good."

"I feel like I got to vomit."

"OK." Reeve held a plastic kidney-shaped emesis basin to her. "It just means things are moving along." She did not vomit, but Reeve handed her the basin to keep, in case she did. Reeve asked Dwayne, "Are you ready to catch this baby?"

"Yep."

Lisa fanned herself with the basin. "I might not have to vomit."

Reeve handed Dwayne some blank progress sheets. "Here, give her a fan." The papers crackled as he waved them in the air. Lisa continued moaning.

"Ooooh, this pain. Oh, damn." She held her head and writhed. The contraction subsided. "I feel so much pressure down there." Dwayne sat on the bed and massaged her belly. "Tell 'em the IV is leaking. I feel water leaking down my arm."

"Jeez," Reeve said, "they're coming frequently, aren't they? Has it been this intense all along, or did it just start kicking in high power here?"

"Oh, worse!" Lisa cried. The door squeaked as Eberhart entered the room. The monitor emitted its watery thump thump thump. "Oh, ooooh."

"Let me check you." Reeve reached and said gently, "I'm gonna touch you right there. Eight centimeters, darling. I'm going to break your water, OK?" To Eberhart, Reeve said, "We need to set up. Tell one of the nurses down there." She got a chuck from the supply cart and said, "OK, lift your buns up, darling. She's clear, water is broken. You can go back on your side now." She removed the chuck and threw it away.

Thump thump thump. "Oh, oh, oh, oh." Lisa gave several quick breaths. "Ooooh." More quick breaths, then a louder moan.

"Are you OK?" Dwayne asked.

"No."

Reeve and Eberhart laughed. Eberhart clanked instruments into place, tore open sterile packages.

Reeve asked Dwayne, "Are you OK? You scared?"

"I'm OK." He held Lisa's hand.

"Oh, shit. I feel like I got to push."

Reeve put on a scrub cloak that covered her below the neck. She turned on the spotlights that shone down where the baby would soon emerge. "You got a little bit of cervix around the baby's head."

"What does that mean?" Lisa asked.

"It means it needs to go away."

"I wish it would hurry. I need to pee."

"Do you want to get on one side or the other, or do you want to go on your hands and knees?"

"I don't want to get on my hands and knees."

"OK."

The clerk from the front desk came in and said, "Miss Dean, can I get you to sign this consent form?"

"Wait until after this contraction, OK?"

"Slow your breathing down," Reeve said. "Don't breathe too fast."

The contraction subsided, and she signed the form.

"What do you have at home?" Reeve asked.

"A boy."

"Do you know what this one is?"

"A girl." In a voice that sounded too weak to be Lisa Dean, she said, "They told me." She let out a big moan. "Ooooh, ooooh," she said in up and down rhythm. She moaned long, then let out a "Whew! I feel it come. This is about to kill me."

"Do you have the name picked out? If not, you can have mine."

"What's your name?"

"Jodi. If you don't like that one and you need a more exotic name, you can have my middle one. It's Eleanora."

"I feel it, ooooooh, ooooooh." She added a little whimper. "I feel something, whatever it is. Ooooooh, ooooooh. I can't push. Oh, it hurts too bad." Louder, she said, "Oh, that hurt."

"Push down for me," Reeve instructed.

"I can't. It hurts," she cried, anguished, her voice trembling. "Oh, I feel it. Oh oh oh oh oh. OOOOOH." She let out a scroan. She stretched it out and panted, "Oh oh oh oh. Aaaagh! Oh, it's hurting. Aaagh! Oh oh oh oh." She grunted. "Oh, I want to see the head."

Reeve said, "It feels like pushing a bowling ball out your butt. It's terrible, but I don't want you to freak out. You still got a little bit of cervix there."

Dwayne held Lisa's hand. Reeve stroked her belly and her leg.

"Breathe through the contraction. Are you still hot?"

She nodded. She lay on her back, her legs spread. She moaned, scroaned, and squirmed.

Reeve continued her chat, passing the time until the lip of the cervix moved off the baby's head. Noticing something in Lisa's chart, Reeve asked, "Did you sign the papers to get your tubes tied?"

"I should have." She whispered a chant: "I can't take it. I can't take it. I can't. I can't."

"This isn't a good time for me to ask that." Reeve wet a washcloth in cold water and pressed it to Lisa's forehead. The monitor steadily fed out the paper strip. "I would go ahead and push with the contraction. Give me a little push now. Get on your side now. It's coming down."

Dwayne said, "Push. Just push."

"Oooh," Lisa grunted. She screamed, "Oohoohoohooh," and ended with an abrupt grunt. She sobbed a little. "Oh, God, I can feel it."

"Go ahead and push," Reeve said.

Lisa let go a loud scream.

"Push a little harder, a little harder, against the pain. Hold your breath and push. Use all that energy to push. A little bit of cervix but I think you're gonna push it away. You don't want to get on your hands and knees, huh?"

Lisa grunted softly and exhaled slowly. Dwayne sat safely in the chair, where he could not see.

"Are you planning to breastfeed or bottle feed?"

"Breastfeed."

"Very good. Did you breastfeed your boy?"

"Yes. Ooh." She let out a big breath. Her face was red, her arms splayed out to the sides.

"You're OK. Give it time. It's coming."

"No, it's not."

Reeve joked, "Let's call the National Enquirer, tell 'em we got a baby that's gonna stay in there forever."

Lisa grunted, then released loudly. "Ooooh! I want to close my legs so bad, and I can't."

A nurse peered in and said Lauren Foley called and said she got Lisa's page and that she's sending good vibes, hoping her labor goes well.

Lisa said a breathless, quick, "Thanks," but with little conviction. She grunted. "Oh! I can't."

"You're pushing hard," Reeve reassured her. "You're doing great."

"Oooooh, ooh." Big "Whew!"

"I want you to do something for me. Roll over that way."

"I can't."

"I know you don't want to move. I want you to move."

"I feel something coming out, what is that?"

"Water. Or pee."

"Roll over that way."

Groaning, Lisa lumbered over. "Oh, oh. I can't close my legs."

"You don't have to close them."

"Oooooh."

"What I really want you to do is get on your knees just for two contractions. Let me lean up against you. What can I do to help you?"

"Oh oh, cover up my behind." Smiling, she looked sideways and gave her deep chuckle, as if she was back in her little apartment laughing at her son.

"OK." Reeve draped a gown across Lisa's behind.

"Oh! Oh, I can't do this! Grrrrnnnt, aaah!"

"You are such a trouper. All right!"

Eberhart reentered the room. "That's a stylish position," she said.

"She likes it." Reeve massaged Lisa's behind.

"Aaah, oh. Oooooooooooh. Wah! It hurts so bad. I can't do this. I can't stay like this." She sounded urgent.

"OK. I just wanted you to move a little." Reeve helped Lisa get on her back. She put one knee on the bed and checked her cervix. "I just want to see if that cervix is gone."

"Is it?"

"Uh huh." She turned to Dwayne, who was sitting silently in the chair, and said, in a cheery voice, "Do you want to put some gloves on, help me?" He did not answer but did not say no, so Reeve said, "Wash your hands first."

"Sterile or regular?" Eberhart asked.

"Sterile."

"Oh, he's gonna really do something."

"Yeah."

Reeve placed her finger where the baby would emerge. "I want you to concentrate on this finger. Pull your knees back."

"Help me hold my legs!"

"Push now, dear."

"Hold my leg! I can't do it no more!" Lightning quick, the thought flashed through her mind, "They said the SECOND one would be EASIER!"

"It hurts more because it's a girl," Reeve said. "She's doing her hair in there." Reeve leaned against the bottom of Lisa's left foot. Dwayne stood woodenly next to Reeve, staring blankly.

Terrified, Lisa shouted, "It's tearing! It's tearing!"

"Here she comes," Reeve said.

"GET IT OUT OF ME!" Lisa shouted desperately, her face flushed, the baby on the verge of emerging from the birth canal but still seemingly forever stuck in a place far, far too small.

The top of the little bluish gray head appeared, featuring a patch of matted dark hair. It pushed forward. Using a rubber bulb with a slender conical tip, Reeve suctioned liquid away from the baby's face. She placed Dwayne's gloved hands on the head, right next to hers, and they gently helped D'Lisa enter the world, face down. For a brief moment, with her ashen skin and blank face, she did not look animate, more like a doll, but she came to life quickly, moving her tiny legs and arms. She cried immediately when she was placed on the bed, the blue, gray, and white umbilical cord still attached. She quickly opened her eyes, which were topped with dark eyebrows.

Reeve coaxed Dwayne to cut the cord. Silently, he stood by and clipped it through. She handed the baby to Lisa, who cuddled her and smiled. Reeve drew blood from the cord. She looked at Dwayne and said, "Pretty cool, huh?" He nodded. She pushed down on Lisa's stomach and pulled out the rest of the cord. She told Lisa to push the placenta out. After it slid out, she showed Lisa and Dwayne where it was attached and where the baby had lived for all those months. Eberhart took the baby to the warmer. She weighed the baby and announced, "Twenty-nine seventy."

"What's that?" Lisa asked.

"Six pounds, eight ounces."

"My boy was just six-three."

Lisa's brother Franklin came in. Eberhart told him, "We have a girl."

"Hey, Dwayne," he said in his low, gruff voice.

"What?" Dwayne answered.

Reeve felt Lisa's belly and said, "All right, I want you to feel right here. It's your uterus. You need to massage it."

"I hate this part."

"And it will be worse this time because you're not in shape. It needs to be hard like a rock. You need to keep your bladder empty, and you need to drink lots of fluids. OK?"

"OK."

"You didn't tear; you just have a little skidmark."

Lisa looked over at the baby, who was wearing a tiny beige knit cap, lying in the warmer. She said, "Dwayne, her bottom lip is just like yours." Eberhart wrapped the baby in a little blanket. The baby lay on her side, quaking, grasping the air with her fingers. "Can I feed her now?" Lisa asked.

Reeve said she needed to do the baby exam first. "Look at how cute she is. Hey, darling!" Reeve sang. "She has long fingers. She's going to be a famous jazz pianist." She examined little D'Lisa all over, then Eberhart inked on a form a black set of baby footprints.

"She's quiet," Lisa said.

"Any medicine?" Eberhart asked, writing on another form.

"Nope," answered Reeve. "We did this cold turkey. OK, dearest, you did great. Are you ready to feed her?"

"Yes."

"Wah! Wah!" D'Lisa cried as Reeve picked her up.

Reeve spoke on behalf of the baby. "OK, Mama, I'm hungry."

Lisa held her baby and eased her large brown breast to the child's mouth. It was clear she had done this before. "She's trying, trying."

"Can you feel it cramping in your uterus?"

"Yes."

Dwayne, still silent, watched. Lisa's hair was thoroughly mussed in the back, the top pushed over to one side, rays of black hair randomly stabbing the air. The finger wave on her forehead, however, was still neatly curled—a pretty flower amid brambles.

"She's got a good suck," Eberhart said.

"She sure do." Lisa laughed, delighted, higher pitched than normal, watching D'Lisa. "Yeah, that's it," she cooed.

Dwayne mumbled something only Lisa understood.

"Yeah, girl, going to town," Reeve said. "She was sucking her thumb in there."

"She got it from her uncle," Lisa said, staring down.

Reeve asked Franklin, "Did you suck your thumb?"

Lisa answered, "He was born with his thumb in his mouth."

Reeve scribbled away on forms for Lisa's chart. "What's her name?"

"D'Lisa."

"And your name is?"

"Lisa Dean."

"How much weight did you gain?"

"I don't know. Two-forty-eight on Tuesday."

"What were you when you started?"

"I don't remember." Lisa's voice was soft and tender.

"Did you come to the clinic more than seven times?"

"I came every time."

"Good for you. Is she doing it, Mom? All right, she's got the bug now." Still scribbling, Reeve added, "We got a twenty-five-minute labor. You can eat if you want to."

"I'm ready to eat." She gave her sly look, moving her eyes to the side.

Reeve said, "When I had my second baby, I could have eaten anything you put in front of me. I ate stuff I never would have touched." She picked up the form. "Let me take this to log her in. She's doing good."

"She sure is."

"I'm out of here," Reeve said. "You did great."

"Thank you." After Reeve left, Lisa said, "They were great with me, weren't they?"

Franklin asked, "Do you want me to go get you some McDonald's?"

"Get me a Quarter Pounder combo meal." To Eberhart she said, "Is that IV empty yet? It's about to kill my hand."

Eberhart finished her questions, then said, "All right," in that tone of finality, the last syllable rising high.

Lisa said, "This IV is about to drive me crazy." She looked inside the baby's blanket. "She made a little stink-stink."

Franklin asked Eberhart, "Where're you from?"

"England."

Lisa said, "I like the accent."

"Where's Dwayne?" Franklin asked, noticing he wasn't in the room.

"Probably calling everybody."

"I heard you screaming, 'Get it out!'"

"You did? Heh heh heh." Franklin walked out, headed to McDonald's. Holding D'Lisa in her arms, Lisa lay her head back, and rested until Dwayne returned. She handed the baby to him. "Here's your daddy."

Dwayne held D'Lisa and stared at her, his expression blank. Franklin returned with food. Lisa munched first on the fries. Watching Dwayne hold the baby, she snorted a quick laugh and shook her head. "She knows who that is." The baby cried, and Lisa said, "She wants to eat again." Dwayne handed her back. She positioned her and said, "I oughta call Tameeka."

"She probably already knows," Franklin said.

"Hey," Dwayne said, looking at his newborn. He sat in the chair, leaned back, put his head in his hand, and slept. Franklin sat in a rocking chair.

"That's cute," Lisa said, watching the baby suck. "She tried to push it back in her mouth with her hand." She watched a moment and said, "That placenta is gross."

A few minutes after D'Lisa finished eating, a nurse came to take her to the nursery. Being carried to the crib, she gurgled softly.

"Look at the little greedy butt," Lisa said. "She just pooped all over the place." After the baby was gone, she lay back again. "I want to get rid of this IV. I'm going to lay down. I'm tired."

Another nurse came in to draw blood. Dwayne still slept. Lisa and

Franklin stared, watching the blood go through the tube. After the nurse finished, she removed the IV.

Lisa rubbed her arm. "Finally, that damn IV's out. It's sore." On the love seat, Franklin leaned forward, resting his head in his hands, a small pile of Lisa's belongings next to him. She said, "Franklin, sit back in that sofa. Relax. Move that stuff."

He moved it to the floor and lay down. In a few minutes—Lisa lying on the bed, Dwayne reclining awkwardly in the chair, Franklin curled up on the small sofa—all three were asleep. Their heavy breathing was the only sound in the room, which a short time ago had been frantic.

Later, Eberhart placed a plastic bag of free samples on the floor in Lisa's room then helped her to the shower. Lisa emerged from the bathroom fully recharged. She wore a blue housecoat with pink ribbons and roses scattered across it. Hands on her hips, she pranced to the bed and sat on the side. "I'm ready to go home now," she sang. She extended her legs straight out. "The swelling has gone down already. Look."

"I'm going to ring transport," Eberhart said. "Look at these men."

They still slept soundly, on opposite sides of the room.

In the midwife office, Reeve waited for her replacement, Kathleen Coleman. Coleman arrived, and the phone rang. She listened, put the caller on hold, and said to Reeve, "She had all her prenatal care here, but didn't want to deliver at Grady, so she went somewhere else, and now she wants to come here for postpartum check-up. Can she?"

"It's up to you. You can tell her to go there."

"I'm afraid she won't get any follow-up if I say that." Coleman punched the flashing button and arranged the woman's appointment. She hung up. "I hate it when they do that."

In postpartum, Lisa wore the same ugly green hospital slippers that she had teased Tameeka about two months before. "You better not get 'em wet," she had smirked. "They'll blow up."

"She's got some long feet," she said now, of D'Lisa. "Heh heh heh. My mom told Dwayne, 'You gave her your long feet.' " She held the baby to her face, and the baby sucked on her cheek. Lisa laughed. "She's hungry." The baby started crying. "OK, OK, I'll feed you." She cried louder. Lisa held D'Lisa to her breast. "I'm sorry. I'll never do that again, make her wait so long."

It had been about a minute.

A nurse came in and asked her to sign a form. Lisa signed it with her right hand while holding D'Lisa in her left arm, settled into the crook.

"What kind of birth control do you want to use?"

"I don't know. For now, foam and condoms."

The nurse gave her an injection. Lisa turned away.

"I'm finished."

"I didn't feel it."

"When you're good, you're good," the nurse said proudly.

Lisa yawned. "All night, they were coming in for the baby or me. Blood pressure, weight, something. Then when I was ready to sleep, it was time to breastfeed or change her diaper. Why don't they have a phone in here?"

A woman's voice from the other side of the curtain said, "I think it's because they're still remodeling. They're supposed to have phones, TVs, music, and stuff."

"Lauren Foley came by to see me." Lisa smiled widely. "She said she'd see me at the six-week visit." She peeked under the blanket covering the breastfeeding baby. "She's hungry. She's sleeping and still eating." Lisa closed her eyes and imitated her baby's face. D'Lisa finished eating, and Lisa put her on her shoulder and patted gently. Within seconds a little hic-squeak popped out.

The voice said, "My other roommate before you didn't know how to burp. That baby was crying and crying. I said to burp him, and she did, and it stopped."

The nurse brought in their lunches. Lisa sniffed the tuna salad sandwich and picked out the red pimentos with a plastic fork. D'Lisa cried, and Lisa fed her again. Watching, laughing, she said, "That's a shame. Eating and sleeping at the same time." When D'Lisa finished, Lisa said, "Maybe she'll sleep, because I'm tired. I'm going to try this tuna fish sandwich." Before she could get it to her mouth, the baby started crying. She picked D'Lisa up, cuddled her and kissed her. "Sssh." She fed her again, grimacing. "It hurts. They're still tender." Lisa peeked. "She didn't want it. She just wanted to lay on it. My mom said there would be times like these, when I won't be able to eat." Cuddling the baby, she picked some tuna salad from the side of the sandwich with a fork.

Two women friends came by to visit, soon followed by two more women, four children herded with them. The children, enthralled by the scene, were quiet, for a while. Dwayne came in, and the women teased him.

"Look at those lips on D'Lisa!"

Dwayne picked up D'Lisa and looked at her.

"Talk to her, Dwayne!"

So he did: "Open your eyes. You've been eating too much." He walked around with her. "Hey hey hey. Whatchu crying for?"

"Lisa done spoiled her already," a friend said.

D'Lisa continued crying; Dwayne handed her to Lisa and left the room.

One of Lisa's friends, a giggly near-teen, looked at Lisa and laughed.

"Are you laughing at me?" Lisa said.

"Are you going to breastfeed?"

"Yeah."

"Your titties are going to be big forever."

"You're so stupid." Lisa began breastfeeding D'Lisa.

"Does it hurt?"

"They're tender."

"I don't want no big ol' titties."

"Girl, get out of my room."

"I got stuck in Grady and had to sleep here one time," a friend said.

"Grady doesn't close," Lisa insisted. "You couldn't get stuck."

"The elevator stopped."

Lisa shook her head. "See what I have to put up with."

Dwayne returned with a sack from McDonald's. Lisa lay D'Lisa across her lap. She picked up a pair of tiny socks. Laughing, eyeing Dwayne, Lisa said, "I don't know if these are big enough for her feet." She ate Chicken McNuggets dipped in mustard sauce. The tuna fish sandwich remained uneaten.

"She's dreaming," Lisa said.

"How can you tell?"

"Because she's sleeping and doing this." She closed her eyes and wriggled her face. She looked at Dwayne and imitated him from the day before, in the delivery room. "'Just push.' Heh heh."

"Can Franklin cut my hair?" someone shouted through the window at Lisa's apartment. Lisa sat in a worn, padded upholstered chair in her kitchen. She wore slippers and a housecoat. Airplanes roared above every few minutes. Outside her window, two boys played basketball one-on-one. The "hoop" was the crossbar of a clothesline pole, which they delighted in dunking over. Dwayne was upstairs—Lisa had just told him, "Get out of here!"

"Franklin's not here," Lisa answered. "So many people came by Saturday I can't remember who all came. Dwayne's sister came by. Robin James. Tameeka came by. 'Look at auntie's baby. That's my niece.' Just like I call her baby my nephew. I told her, 'It about killed me, but it was worth it.' That first night was OK, except for everybody coming by. Later, Dwayne would say that she needed to rest. She slept good. She woke up three or four times to eat, but she slept a good while before she woke back up. I try to get my naps in when she gets hers." She patted at her hair. "I want to get my hair cut."

Dwayne came in the kitchen, picked up D'Lisa, snuggled and kissed her. Lisa asked him to change her diaper. He handed her back and said, "She's too little for me to change." He left to join a group of guys.

Lisa said Rob was still staying with an aunt, his daddy's sister. She raised her tone, imitating her son, "'I'm ready to go see my baby.'" She said about Rob's daddy, "We speak. We're cordial. The only thing I dislike is he doesn't do for Rob like he should. His family does it but not him. Since he found out I was pregnant again, he stopped seeing Rob. His sister told me she's going to get onto him. He used to pick him up on Friday after work and keep him through Sunday. I don't try to be mean to him. He's supposed to start paying child support again, but because he's got so many debts, he hasn't. He has gotten real sorry about taking care of his son."

Someone knocked on the door.

"Who *is* it?"

"Auntie Dina. I need to use your bathroom."

Looking annoyed, Lisa said OK. Dina came in and went upstairs. "She's not my real aunt. I've just known her since I was a little girl."

Dina came back downstairs and sang to D'Lisa, "She got Auntie Dina's nose. She's gonna be nosy like me." She sang, walking out the door.

"I'm so tired," Lisa said. "I haven't had enough sleep. I just feel so sore still. When I'm breastfeeding I'm sore. Cramps! I can feel the uterus shrinking back to normal size." She looked down at D'Lisa, in her lap, "You're gonna be greedy."

Her dog Biloxi, she said, was protective of the baby. "She was laying between the bed and the door when somebody came in. She got up real fast and moved over there and was just looking at her. Dogs can sense things. I said, 'What's wrong, Biloxi?' She's like, 'I'm going to make sure.'"

She noticed a girl walking by, outside her kitchen window. "She's twelve, and pregnant. She has no business having sex at that age. Her mother uses drugs, but she's home. A lot of kids around here come talk to me. I notice. I'll ask, 'Are you pregnant?' 'No.' 'Tell me the truth.' 'OK, I'm pregnant.' I say be careful; take care of yourself. Twelve, thirteen. What can they do? So much ahead of 'em." She carried the baby upstairs to sleep. She came back down and said, "That dog's up there watching cartoons."

Within ten minutes, D'Lisa started crying.

"Here I come. Here I come."

Riding MARTA home, standing in the middle of a crowded car, Walt Robinson was spoken to by a woman sitting in front of him. She had stared at him and finally said, "You're, you're, that doctor at Grady."

"Hi," he answered.

"You're my daughter's doctor, aren't you?"

Robinson nodded. "How is she?"

"She's at my house recuperating. She had that operation. Dr. Lowry is trying to get her to go to her clinic. She wants her in there—Whatever." She looked at Robinson apologetically, as if she perceived he felt badly about losing a patient.

Robinson leaned close to her and said, smiling, as if to reassure her he was not offended, "I'll be there a lot longer than Dr. Lowry."

Every Wednesday morning, the OB/GYN department gathered in the old Grady auditorium for Grand Rounds, a lecture or presentation of medical cases. Midwives, physician assistants, nurses, and clinic assistants were urged to attend. They sat in old wooden curved-back chairs, with small retractable desks that folded down between chairs. This Wednesday, it was finally a sunny, cool day. The hot summer was fading and fall arriving. For those walking to Grand Rounds, the sun felt refreshing, not oppressive. In the auditorium, Dr. Wayne Denson introduced Dr. Charles Holcomb, who would speak on medical ethics. A resident sitting in the auditorium who had been on call the night before fought to keep her head up. She put her head in her right hand, elbow on the armrest; her head slipped off her hand, and she jerked it back up.

Dr. Holcomb presented general information about the study of ethics: do you concern yourself primarily with the consequences of actions and choices, he asked, or the rightness of the action itself, separate from the consequences? He defined a series of terms: honesty, non-maleficence, beneficence, justice, autonomy. Then he summarized the issues related to maternal/fetal rights, new reproductive technology, and health care for the indigent.

The resident who had been up all night switched from leaning on her hand to leaning back in her chair, her mouth sagging open. Three more residents nodded to sleep, two leaning back, one forward.

Holcomb gave reasons that might justify legal intervention in a case, say, where a Mennonite mother refuses medical treatment for her newborn. He also presented criteria for ethical analysis and pitfalls to avoid (don't rely too much on the law; avoid using religion to explain your opinion). Finally, he told a story about a woman who planned a home delivery, but the baby was in a breech position. She was brought to Grady. One foot was about to come down the birth canal, a risky position for a baby that should be coming head first. What if one leg snagged, and the other kept coming? The woman insisted on a vaginal delivery, despite the warnings given to her by doctors. Holcomb called on someone to present the case for the woman's autonomy and another to present the case for the right of the hospital legally to force a C-section to ensure the baby's health.

Then the floor was open for questions. Someone wanted to know if there was a hierarchy within the list of terms Holcomb had defined. Someone wanted to know if there was time to get a court order when a C-section was needed.

"You can get them quickly," a voice from the auditorium said. "The question is whether it's a good thing to do."

As the questions came to an end, someone asked what happened with the woman and the baby. Dr. Holcomb said, "Oh, the baby was fine. She delivered vaginally, in bed."

A patter of applause carried faintly through the auditorium. On the right side, about halfway back, two midwives were clapping.

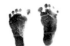

Managing Labor

A resident's agenda, working sixty to a hundred hours a week, is to start at point A and get to point B and be trained in this specialty so they can go out and practice OB/GYN. But it can't be just residents who run like elephants through Grady Hospital for four years and the rest of us just stand frozen to the side of the wall until they get through. Residents are not just a bunch of elephants running through Grady to just suck up all this knowledge. There are other people here. You'll learn a lot if you listen.

—*Dr. Wayne Denson*

Sitting in the cafeteria, third-year Emory University Medical School resident Timothy Crews explained resident roles in Labor and Delivery. "First year, you do triage, evaluate whether to admit. You do uncomplicated C-sections and vaginal deliveries, forceps deliveries. You're at the bottom of the heap, the front-line man in the trenches. You get shit on. You do paperwork, and you don't do much. You're at the beck and call of everyone, constantly presenting to people above you. You make no decisions about patient care. The good of that is you can always call someone above you and shift the responsibility. You don't sweat over the plan and decisions. Brawn but no brains."

"Second year," Crews continued, "you treat pre-eclampsia, do complicated C-sections, manage a pregnancy induced for a dead baby after twenty weeks. You are in charge of those not yet admitted. You do more, and your responsibility increases. You take call by yourself. You do less scut work, but you're still between first-year and upper-level doctors. You're chomping at the bit. All your second year you want to do surgery, and that's in short supply. Usually the third- and fourth-year have dibs. For the first time, you think, 'I'm the boss.' The nurses treat you a lot different between the first and second year. You don't admit patients, and you're dead if you think someone should be and you don't call an upper level. The second-year schedule is horrendous compared to a nine-to-five job. I came in on Sunday to work nine-to-seven, and I thought, 'This is only ten hours, not bad.' But I worked seventy hours that week.

"The third-year runs the delivery board, oversees all laboring patients. Preterm labor. They work the hardest. The fourth-year helps make the decision to admit but after she's admitted, the third-year is responsible for management. It's a big step. You're running Labor and Delivery. You decide if a C-section is needed, if forceps are needed. It's a big responsibility. Forceps—everybody could do a few more. To learn, you want to do it when it's easy, on a multip and the baby just about falls out. You want it to be easy, but you want it to be necessary. That's the problem. If it's a big baby and a tight perineum, you don't experiment on that. Your responsibility quadruples. It takes a lot to get used to worrying about a bad baby. You see those decels and you're tempted to cut and get a good baby. But a bad strip does not necessarily equal a bad baby. And you don't know which. You think of that strip being blown up on a courtroom wall. Some bad strips are OK. There's a big division between second and third year. The faculty treat you differently. You can talk more intelligently about problems. Your third year, you begin to think, 'I'm a doctor.' You've had all this experience, and the different cases come together. Sometimes you have to defend a decision, and if you have a rational basis, you're OK.

"The fourth-year is a consultant. He assists the first- and second-years with C-sections, or other operative deliveries: vacuum, forceps. They manage OB-ICU patients. For most services you're the one ultimately responsible. It's nice to have three years of residency beneath you, and you don't get bothered with scut work. You can say, 'Get him to do it.' But your final year is the most stressful. You're worrying if you're getting enough surgery. Everybody worries about not doing enough. No one gets too many."

Crews explained this after he had just met with his "team," a first-year, second-year, and two medical students who were all on the same rotation under his supervision. To the medical students he said, "Someone's going to get an assignment. Pick a number between one and ten." "Nine," one said. "One," the other. Crews held up two fingers. The "one" was told, "Go find us something on TOAs. Make us copies today." The winner nodded obediently.

"There's no such thing as 'low outlet forceps.' It's either low or outlet." Timothy Crews instructed the first-year at the beginning of a day in Labor and Delivery. At 6:30 a.m. he had reviewed the charts from the night shift, then made his way to the residents' room on the fourth floor. "It's important to call it the right thing in the charts. Very important."

The exiting third-year summarized the current cases on the labor board for Crews, who had been reading a book on an aggressive style of managing labor common in Ireland. He was ready to try it himself. He went to 19, pushing the mobile ultrasound machine in front of him. He needed to check the position of the baby. The patient clutched the bed rails with both hands until a contraction passed. Her mother began instructing Crews.

"Mom," the patient said, "they know what to do."

Mom sat in a chair by her daughter. "I know they're well-trained," she sighed. But she watched Crews's every move as he spread the gel and moved the transducer around on her daughter's belly. Mother and doctor watched the screen. The patient moaned when he checked her cervix.

"I'm sorry," Crews said in his soft North Carolina drawl.

Squirming, she grasped the rail again.

"If you move, he can't check you," the nurse said.

After he examined her, Crews said to the nurse, "Don't push her yet."

The patient begged for a C-section, but they ignored her, both writing on forms for her chart. She turned on her side and closed her eyes. Just above her head a sign from the pathology department reminded them, "Remember, collect an extra tube of cord blood." If anything went wrong, pathology wanted to analyze everything they could. Her mother sat quietly on the sofa while the monitor thumped and two pens scratched on paper. As Crews left, the patient moaned and grasped the rails. Together, her mother and sister said, "Don't push."

Crews walked to 20 and asked her which baby this was.

"Fourth."

He put on gloves, smeared his right hand with gel, and checked her cervix. He told her not to push yet. "Are you having contractions one after the other?"

The nurse answered, "Every two to three minutes."

Speaking of terbutaline sulfate, a uterine relaxant that they called "terb," he said, "We're going to give you some medicine to stop the contractions, OK? Your baby's heartbeat went down some. If we can't stop it, we may have to have a cesarean delivery, OK?"

She looked at him but did not answer.

"Dr. Crews, please come to the doctors' room for doctors' rounds."

As Crews entered the room, attending physician Dr. Mildred Hankins, using a model of a woman's pelvis and a small brown fetus doll, demonstrated a delivery technique for the residents and students. She sat in the middle of the room; they were around her, watching closely.

To Julianne Bass, the first-year, Hankins said, "You need to read the Woods article about the Woods maneuver. You're here to learn. We all make mistakes. What's important is to learn and not make the same mistake again." To Crews, she said, "Let's go down the board." For each patient, she asked questions or made suggestions. About one patient that might require a C-section, she said the most experienced person should do it. "If you have to go through the placenta," she warned, "it needs to be quick."

"I tried my managed labor today," Crews told her, "like in the book you gave me, but it looks like she'll need the C-section." He said about one patient, "She had a deceleration when she came in. We gave her some terb, and she's doing a little bit better. Variability has been good. The variables are getting a little deeper and getting a little slow to recover. Her problem is she has an uncontrollable urge to push, and she was pushing at six and five."

Hankins warned about possible laceration of the cervix and added, "That's the reason you don't push people until it is complete."

"This lady," Crews continued, "every time she had a contraction, she held her breath. She said, 'I'm not . . . holding . . . my . . . breath.'" He chuckled lightly. "I said, 'Yes you are; you just can't help it.' I turned her on her side and gave her Fentonil, which didn't help a whole lot. Her husband was in there, or her significant other, trying to help her blow, with mixed results. I really feel she'll deliver this baby vaginally because she—"

"If she doesn't get too much distress, yeah," Hankins said.

"A while ago she had several contractions that were—let me put this up on the screen—boom boom boom right together, and I gave her some terb back here, to space them out a little bit. They're not as close together now."

Still holding the fetus doll, which she had curled into a ball, Hankins asked questions about all the patients on the board. Crews and Paul Namath, the fourth-year, responded, while the first- and second-year residents and the students listened. Moreso than with the other attendings, everyone listened carefully to Hankins, whose knowledge and teaching skills were worshipfully respected.

"Let's make sure you know the things you do for a decel," she said.

Crews answered, "OK, first you do a pelvic exam," and listed several more steps. The first-year asked a question about prolonged decels.

Hankins said, "Prolonged decels will most often lead to fetal death, so check for appropriate variability."

First-year Bass asked what to do if she's ready to deliver and feels the cord prolapse, which is when the cord falls into the birth canal.

Crews and Namath said, "It depends on the position of the head."

"There are no hard rules for that," Hankins said. "You have to make a decision." She explained several possibilities.

About the last patient, Crews said, "I feel like I'll be calling you about her, because, unfortunately, I feel she's going to have a cesarean."

Hankins urged him to review the charts the next time he manages a patient that winds up having a C-section. "Go back to the notes and see exactly what happened. Put together what you learned." He nodded. Clutching the fetus doll, folding and unfolding its body, forehead to ankle, Hankins looked at the board and noted, "We have no normal deliveries up there." She drew a diagram of the vagus nerve in the brain and explained the impact of atropine, which is sometimes given for general anesthesia. She asked who knew what the parasympathetic nerves released. Only the third- and fourth-years did. Hankins continued asking questions, which only the third- and fourth-years answered, sometimes hesitantly, sometimes confidently.

After Hankins left, they attacked the food spread on the desks: quiche, cheese ball, lemon cream pie, Doritos, Lays potato chips, crackers, and cheese dip that Randall Lee, the second-year, heated in the microwave oven perched on the refrigerator. Stone ate some dip and said, "This needs to be heated more."

Lee, defending himself, said, "It was bubbling on the sides."

Waiting on the reheating dip, third-year Karen Olsen looked behind the refrigerator. "Have you seen all this shit back here?"

"Ignorance is bliss," Namath said.

Olsen asked Lee, "Did you hear about the tumor conference? It was the best one yet. Five residents showed up, and six pizzas."

Bass came in and said she was trying to decide what to wear on a date. "He said it was semiformal, and I asked him what to wear. He said, 'Just dress sexy.' I thought it was degrading. I'm going, but it's the last time."

Crews checked on 20, then 21. He returned to the doctors' room and told the other residents about the book he was reading. "In Ireland, they monitor frequently. They know when they come in they're going to deliver in twelve hours. Regardless. They don't admit them unless they're in labor. And they manage labor. Eighty percent of the pregnant women take extensive labor classes. Here, with high numbers and with little support, they don't know what to expect. Family support is not as good. In Ireland, there are fewer requests for epidurals. If they're less than a centimeter per hour, they start oxytocin or Pitocin. If delivery is not imminent in twelve hours, they do a C-section, but the C-section rate is only five percent."

He went to room 8 to see if Pitocin was helping. He told her, "We're trying to fool your body into thinking it's in labor. That's hard."

"Dr. Crews, please come to the doctor's lounge."

Walking back, he said, "We also tried Prepodyl to ripen her cervix, but it's hardly changed at all. She's here because there's no fluid around the baby, and we decided to induce her. She could be leading to a C-section if the induction doesn't work."

"Thank you, ma'am," Dr. Crews said in his soft drawl to the house-keeper who was vacuuming the carpet of the residents' room floor. "We appreciate it." He moved chairs around for her. The floor was littered with paper and food crumbs, rather like the OB clinic waiting room at the end of a busy day. "We're in and out and eat in a rush," he explained, "and food and stuff gets dropped. Some of us are better at cleaning up than others."

A student returned from McDonald's with breakfast. Crews said, "That smells good, but my wife has me on a diet. I'm clocking in high these days."

The midwife came in and showed Crews a strip. He unfolded it and said it was OK to send her home. He asked a medical student to accompany him to 20, where he checked the patient's cervix. He reminded the student about not pushing a patient too early. The room was dark, the shade pulled down; only a slice of sun shone in. Walking back to the residents' room, Crews illustrated with his fingers how he estimated the cervix's dilation. He put two fingers side-by-side for one measurement, then spread his fingers apart, like calipers, for a wider measurement. He told the student, "One finger is about one and a half. Two is three. It's like reaching inside a box and feeling of the shapes in there to determine what they are without seeing them."

A nurse announced over the intercom, "Prepare the OR for a C-section."

Crews told the student about assisting a doctor at a private hospital who had diagnosed placenta previa—the placenta lodges between the fetus and the birth canal—but when he cut for the C-section, the placenta was where it belonged. "He had the ultrasound picture upside down. I always double-check to see where I am. I couldn't resist. When the doc said, 'The baby must have turned,' I said, 'And took the placenta with him.'" Crews relished the little victory over a more experienced doctor, at a private hospital where residents usually stand to the side, unlike at Grady, where they run the show.

An EMT rolled a woman by and said, "She's about to have this one."

Crews went to the nurse's station and wrote on yellow progress sheets. Loud moans came from 19 as a grandmother opened the door and left the room. She shook her head and muttered, "Lordy, lordy." Crews took the notes back to 20, where he told her, "Don't bear down when you push. That's not good. Are you sure you don't want an epidural?" She shook her head. He quickly checked on 19 and wrote in the chart. Back at the nurse's station, he said, "Nineteen may require a C-section. If nothing happens in a couple hours, she doesn't need to continue."

From 19 he heard Lee, the second-year, instructing the woman, "Push push push push push push push," in a soothing tone, which was interrupted periodically by her loud desperate scroans. "Yeah, like you're squatting," Lee said gently, just before she scroaned again.

Walking to 20, Crews said, "I want to see that strip again." The husband was saying, "Blow, blow. Don't hold it. Blow, blow." Crews encouraged the woman to get an epidural, saying, "I normally don't push it, but I think it will help. Think about it."

He returned to the residents' room, where he told the other attending about the patient in 20. The attending was convinced she needed an epidural. "Tell her it's not for her comfort," he instructed Crews, "but out of concern for the baby. Tell her she's this close"—he put two fingers together—"to a C-section, so she'll need one anyway for that, plus it might help the baby." He said this confidently, apparently sure it would convince her.

Crews punched some keys at the computer and 20's strip appeared on the large screen. Something he saw sent him scurrying outside. A tall young man with long strides, he moved down the hall easily and quickly. "I'll check her first," he said. "I'm real uncomfortable pushing an epidural like this." The soothing "push push" and the patient's wailing scroans still echoed from 19, as Crews returned to 20. He explained to her what an epidural was and what he expected it to accomplish. He left 20, and the first-year showed him the strip of a woman thirty weeks pregnant with twins who had fallen in the tub and came to Grady. He unfolded the strip and glanced along its length. "She looks good. You can send her home. Just make sure she's not having contractions."

"Ah-oh-oh-oooh-aaaagh!" A long scroan filled the hall, coming from 19. Crews checked in there, then came out. "No progress. We'll have to cut her if there's no change in an hour."

He returned to the residents' room and spoke with Dr. Hankins about the patient in 20. "I told her significant other that I feel she'll deliver vaginally." They pulled her strip up on the screen and talked about the pattern they saw. "She still does not want an epidural," he added.

"Well, you can't give one to somebody who doesn't want it," Hankins said, and reviewed with Crews how to determine if she would need a cesarean.

"Dr. Crews to 20."

He checked on 20, then walked to the residents' room, where another third-year had come to eat lunch. Crews told her about the book he was reading and said he was trying it out but was disappointed. "It looks like there'll be a C-section in 19. She's been complete for two hours and hasn't done anything. We'll have to cut. She wants her tubes tied, and the grandmother wants her tubes tied, but she won't sign the papers, so we can't do it."

He returned to 19 and told the grandmother they could not tie her tubes without the patient's written consent. He told her about the Depro-Provera shot. "It'll cover three months," he said, "and give her time to talk it over and decide." He explained how a C-section worked.

"Dr. Crews to 20."

He went there and examined her again. Next door, an anesthesiologist entered 19, to prepare the patient for a C-section. The grandmother walked out of the room and paced the halls. Crews returned to the residents' room, where Hankins was questioning residents and students. "Who's going to do the C-section on 19? What's happening with 20?" Crews brought 20's strip to the screen. Hankins asked if she was on Pitocin. Crews said she was not. A nurse entered and told Crews that 20 had agreed to an epidural.

Another nurse came in, closed the door, and said, "I have a lady who was here in February and April with negative pregnancy tests and is trying to convince herself she's pregnant. She's complaining of abdominal pain times two weeks. She thinks the baby is moving around. Somebody other than me is going to need to talk to her." She looked put out.

Hankins said, "I think the ultrasound machine might talk to her."

Crews walked with the nurse to see the patient; along the way another nurse asked him to come to 12 to see if the patient should be sent home.

"I've been trying to eat for some time," Crews said, to no one. He saw those patients, then checked on 8. He told her he would check again later and send her back to antepartum if nothing had changed. He went to 21 to see a new patient, then to 20. At the nurse's desk, he called the WUCC to let them know the patient who thought she was pregnant was on her way down. "We checked her and didn't find anything," he said. He walked from exam room to exam room, looking for an Intrauterine Pressure Monitor. He said it monitored the strength of contractions, whereas the external monitor only told when they happened and how long they were. "We can also use it to add fluid inside," he added. He found one in 16 and went to 20 to attach it. He came out and said she had quieted down since she got the epidural. "Her cervix has swollen from the involuntary pushing." He saw Hankins down the hall and said he was going to fill her in on 20. Dashing down the hall, he said, "I'm going to take advantage of her being here." After talking with her, he went to 12 to see the woman with twins who had fallen in the tub. He held up the strip and said, "These babies look beautiful. What concerns me is that you're having contractions this often when you're only thirty weeks. These babies are beautiful. We're going to clear your bladder, give you a shot—it's our smallest needle—and possibly send you home."

Second-year Lee, in the residents' room, completed paperwork for a C-section to be performed on the patient in room 3. She had had previous surgery on her uterus, which put her uterine muscles at risk, so Lee, not the first-year, would perform the surgery. It would be delicate. "Your first C-section," Lee said, "takes a long time, but you get faster as you go along." Lee finished writing and handed the chart to Bass. "Get her medical history," he said. He walked to 3 to explain the C-section. He went to anesthesia to make sure they were ready. He also asked, "Anything interesting in GYN?"

"Nah."

Lee returned to the residents' room and asked the student what field he was interested in.

"I thought that I'd love pediatrics. I've done peds, and I did love it, but I'm not sure. I liked OB and didn't think I would."

"I'm not the most money-conscious guy," Lee said, "but peds, they do the same training but get two-thirds the pay."

"Yeah, someone told me she did all that training, then got in practice and it's, like, all common colds."

At 2:15, Lee emerged from the C-section in the OR and walked to the residents' room, where he picked up a piece of pizza.

"Microwave that first, bub," Namath suggested.

But he put it right in his mouth. Olsen came in and asked him, third-year to second-year, "I know you got the Smith C-section next, but can you help with triage? But eat first."

He quickly took two big bites of cold pizza and darted out. He worked with the medical student in 12, then 14, then 15. After triage became manageable, Lee returned to the residents' room and finished his cold pizza. A sign next to the pizza box said, "Pizza today compliments of Dr. Olsen and the Antocin study. Thanks for your help."

Julianne Bass, the first-year, said into the phone at the nurse's station, "This is Dr. Bass. . . . Uh huh. . . . What kind of reaction? . . . I can't evaluate that over the phone. If you feel you need to come in, we'll be happy to see you. . . . All right, bye." She continued writing. "It really bugs me that nurses don't screen calls. I wouldn't be picking up the phone like that if I was in an office. It slows down my work." She was not even the boss of nurses. On the way to the residents' room, she was stopped by third-year Olsen.

"You were supposed to admit the patient in 2."

"Oh, sorry."

She hurriedly returned to 2, her ponytail swishing. "This always happens. We try to triage them as quickly as we can. It stresses the third-year out if the board isn't clean. And if you want to piss off your upper levels, admit someone who hasn't yet ruptured. Being a first-year is very political. You have to please everybody. You have to please the nurses, keep triage clean, make sure the deliveries go well. We have to—" She stopped talking as she passed the fourth-year, who was walking the other way. "We hold up the basement. . . . No, that was me as a med student. Now I'm holding up the first floor. But it's good. Everybody goes through it."

She returned to the residents' room and was promptly paged back to 2 for the delivery. Deep, full scroans emerged from in there. Nurse Ella Davies's face emerged through the door. She said, "Big meconium, page peds." They always called pediatric residents when meconium, bodily waste from the baby, was present.

"Got it," the nurse at the station said. She punched the code on the telephone buttons. Fourth-year Namath walked down the hall and went into 2. Two pediatrics residents scurried in. A baby cried. Two women walked to the room; one knocked gently.

"I'm her mother," she told Davies. "What did she have?"

"A boy. The baby had a nasty bowel movement and is having trouble breathing. You can see your daughter when we sew her up."

"She didn't tell me she was pregnant."

"She didn't know. I'll call you when you can see your daughter."

"That was a thrash," Bass said, leaving 2. "I've never seen meconium that thick. The placenta was disgusting. It looked like pea soup." She added, "There's no way somebody can think a baby kicking is indigestion." She passed the registration desk, where a woman on a stretcher, escorted by an EMT, told the clerk her doctor was Dr. Walt Robinson. Bass stopped abruptly and turned that way. "He's not a doctor," she corrected. "He's a mister, one of our PA's." She resumed walking. "I get called a nurse a lot," she commented.

In the residents' room, a doctor at Emory on a fellowship ended a phone conversation with, "OK, I'll be there." Sensing something interesting, Bass asked, "What's going on?"

He waved dismissively. "Oh, some ovarian cancer in the OR."

Olsen came in and asked Bass, "Are you sure Duarte is ruptured? I'm not going to be surprised again, am I?"

"No, I checked," Bass assured her, then said, while leaving, "I better go see this preterm patient. I thought this was going to be a slow day. We just got three new ones. As soon as we let one go, a new one comes in."

Crews returned to the residents' room and spoke with Hankins about

20. They agreed to do a C-section if there was insufficient progress by 5:30.

Crews said, "If this was in Ireland—"

Hankins finished for him. "They would have done it already." She told several stories about deliveries that did not progress, how deliveries used to be done years ago, close calls she had had. In awe, residents always listened to every word she said.

Crews returned to 20 and explained to them why the C-section might be necessary. He assured them the baby was doing fine, that he did not want to try Pitocin because the baby might not be able to tolerate making the contractions harder. He asked if they had any questions; they did not.

"It's important to have a plan," Crews said in the hall, "and to let the patient know what it is. Tell them what you have done, what you might have to do. That's one thing the book on labor in Ireland stressed."

At 4:30, he took out his lunch, pasta his wife made for him, a low-fat recipe in Oprah Winfrey's cook's book. Before he could eat, a first-year asked him about sending someone home who had been given terbutaline. He answered him, then a medical student mentioned that he had not seen any forceps deliveries that week. Crews said, "My first week, I had three, and I've had none since. I had to hunt around for them."

"Yeah, you have to hunt around for those," the student echoed.

The first-year had said Crews's pasta smelled good, and so had the student. Now a nurse walked in and said, "That smells good."

"I wish it had some sauce on it," Crews said. While he ate, he reviewed two cases with the second-year.

A resident about to leave looked in the room and said, "Smells good." Hankins came in and asked about 8. Crews stopped eating, and they went down there. On the wall in room 8 a sign said, "In Search of Placentas Live and Healthy," followed by a beeper number. He returned to the residents' room and updated the board information for 8. "I'm going to check on 20," he said. "I'll see if she needs a C-section. I've expected it all day. Now I'll go, and she won't be cut." He examined her and went to report to the fourth-year. On the way, he said, "The baby is still high. If she's changed, it's only a hair. We're gonna cut her."

Before he could get a word out, the fourth-year said, "She's the same."
"Yeah."

"OK, get her ready."

She called Dr. Hankins—primarily as a courtesy, as Hankins had already approved the C-section. Crews wrote in 20's chart, "Failure to Progress" and "Arrested Dilation." He told the patient they had decided a C-section would be best. "Ma'am, I've talked it over with my boss. It's not an emergency. It just needs to be done. I'll send another doctor to explain it more." He returned to the residents' room to review C-section procedures for the first-year, who had not done a C-section yet, as all the sections that had been done on his shift were either emergencies or on patients with previous C-sections—both situations requiring a more experienced doctor. Crews told him what to write on the progress sheets and said, "Make sure the forms are dated today." He reminded him of everything he needed to tell the patient. He added before the first-year left, "And check to make sure the head is not right there, ready to pop out. It happens." Crews phoned anesthesia to see if they were ready.

"Prepare the OR for a C-section," he announced over the intercom.

Crews wrote a few more notes on progress sheets, and said, "My work is done. The next shift will do the C-section. Hopefully, I can go in five minutes, if my replacement gets here." He had arranged to leave early; normally, his shift was seven-to-seven. His replacement, the third-year he had replaced early that morning, entered while he was out changing clothes. One of the two medical students in the room said to the other, "Which one of us does the C-section? I've done two. You?"

"Two."

"Flip a coin."

Crews returned and went down the board with the incoming third-year. She pointed and recalled from that morning, "She's had two reasonable-sized kids."

The phone rang, and Crews answered it. He listened and said, "He's right here." He handed the phone to the second-year. Grinning, he said, "I love being the third-year. I get to pass along calls if I want."

The incoming fourth-year, Mary Lowry, looked through a drawer for a carryout menu from a nearby restaurant, so she could order food. She pulled out a KY Jelly tube. "What's this doing here? With the ketchup and sauce?"

The first-year came in and said about 19, "She wants her tubes tied, but her papers are with the rest of her stuff in the security office."

Together, Crews and the incoming third-year said, "Go get them ASAP, or we can't do it."

Before Crews left, he looked over the board and said, "No normal deliveries today." He added, chuckling, "But I do so few now, if I had to do one, I might not know what to do."

In her apartment, Robin James said about the previous pregnancy of her oldest daughter, Pauline, "She lost that baby, but we don't know if it's because of the car wreck she been in. It's hard to talk to her about that. The doctor at Grady said if she got pregnant again, they'd have to sew her up down there. She'd have to spend most of her pregnancy laying down. So we been trying to figure out how to help her have a baby; the only way is if she marry a rich man who can afford to sit her down while she pregnant. Pauline know a lot of rich folks. That's what worry us. She kinda act like 'em. She swear she don't like how they is, but them the kinda folks she hang around. She knew a lot of Falcons players. Deion Sanders. That Dominique man. She go to their houses, know where they live and stuff. Scott Marvin, he with a team in California now. The Falcons traded him, especially after he took pizza from the pizza boy that time. We all were happy she got pregnant; we were hoping she would have somebody she could boss around instead of us. She try to run all of our life and hers too."

Robin was not clear about Pauline's relationship with her current boyfriend. "I don't think it's somebody she would like to have a baby by. That's what we think, just between me and Cheryl, we talk. We love him if she love him, but we don't know. One minute she's cussing him out and the next minute she can't be without him."

Robin said of Pauline's first pregnancy, the one that ended in miscarriage, "That devastated her. It wasn't her fault. Her husband beat her real bad and used to would leave her all the time. We don't contribute that miscarriage to health."

Robin said she was skeptical of a Chicago lawyer who told Pauline he wanted her to have his baby. "She met him through Andrew Young's brother. She doesn't want to have his baby because he's too old. He's married, he's old, and he isn't telling Pauline everything, so she doesn't trust him. He wants to pay Pauline twenty-five thousand dollars to have his baby. But Pauline said she probably couldn't tote the baby. So he told Pauline that if she asked my other daughter, Cheryl, could they artificially inseminate his seed and Pauline's egg and for Cheryl to tote the baby. Pauline called and asked me about it, and I said well what about the baby? He said he would set up a million-dollar trust fund, if the baby made it and everything. She said, 'Mama what you think,' and I said, 'Pauline, I don't want to talk about this foolishness. I don't like foolishness.' I'm gon' say it. This man getting old. He fixing to die, and he don't want to leave all his money to his wife. He wants a child real, real bad, and he likes Pauline. Pauline don't know he done checked her out, but I know that a man with his age on him, you know he done checked, he seen that Pauline just somebody that's trying to make it and stuff like that. If he just asked Pauline to get pregnant, he know she ain't going to want to get pregnant by an older married man? But if he offer all this money—"

Maybe so, but Pauline was eager to have a baby, especially after losing the one born prematurely earlier in the year, in addition to the others. "When you get a certain age you start wondering," she said in her apartment. "I'm thirty-two now, and I wonder am I ever going to have kids. I was glad I was pregnant last time, but if something was going to be wrong, I was ready to say to God, whatever. Then when it didn't live, we all held it. I didn't want to let him go. I was so sad, and he was so big. If you had seen the baby, you would have said he could have survived. He was long. They said he was longer than most newborns, too. But anyway, I survived." She said she and her sister Cheryl were considering a plan in which Cheryl's daughter would provide a surrogate womb for a baby that would be Pauline's. "She's thirteen years old, and they really want me to have a baby. They don't want when I died, they don't have anything to remember me by. Any of 'em. They really want me to have a baby, and not be upset anymore that it might be a stillborn or miscarriage. A doctor told me one possibility was to find someone else to carry the child for me. They said they want her to carry the baby. She wants to do it. She wants to do it. Carry my baby. I was worried. I think a lot, would it look like me or her?

"I don't have to worry about the expense because—it's not that I just go out with guys that have money, but I only date rich men. For things like that. I know what I need to be doing. It's not that I just go out and look for men that have money. But I can't afford to mess around with a poor man because I'm not that healthy, and if I have a child or get pregnant by them, I want the father to be able to afford the doctor bills. I couldn't make plans like that with a poor man. I want him to be able, if the child has health problems, he can afford to put them in the right hospital."

On the Chicago lawyer, she said, "He is like, 'I don't care what it costs or what I have to do. I really want to have a child by you.' He knows how bad I want a baby, and he can afford it. He's nice, too, but I don't love him. But he can give me what I want. He can help me have a healthy child. That's one of the goals in life that I haven't succeeded. I'd have to have somebody cover my bills that whole time, or I can have someone else to carry it. My sister was thinking she would do it, but her tubes are tied. But if I found a person who never had a pregnancy, it's more of a guarantee. So my niece was thinking, why don't I do it? She really wants to make me happy. They see every holiday they all get together with their families, and I'm the only one that don't have anyone, a living child, and they want to help me out. They want me to have something that I left here on earth, that was mine.

"He asked me to move up with him in Chicago. His family has wealth from years and years ago, hundreds of years ago. But I would have to do what he say. He'd take the child away because he wants a baby really bad, too. His children are older. He's older than I am. My mom doesn't know how old he is, but she knows that he comes down to see me. He says you need to come up here with me and let me take care of you. The rules I would have to follow are not me. I won't do that, just for the money. He's the kind that whenever I need money, I call him and get it from him. But he really respects my feelings. He takes me out on trips, and I don't have to worry about anything. But I don't want to be married anymore. I was really hurt last time. And I don't want to do it again.

"I thought about adoption. I could get a baby just like that." She snapped her fingers. "I know so many people, the area where my sister lives, lots of women they don't want the baby, and they are looking for someone to give it to. They'll sign it over to you right away. A lot of those moms use drugs and have alcohol problems, and you know right away there's going to be problems with the baby. Physical or mental, or both. I'm not that desperate yet. I really want my own. That's why you wonder why don't I get married first and pray about it, and maybe it would happen, but something else is more important—the business I want to start. I can't worry about a husband or anything else. I won't have that time to put into the business if I'm married. Most men, you know, I don't want to say this, but most black men don't want a wife that works as hard as I do. They want somebody that works maybe not that much and do what they say, basically. That won't work for me."

Jan Dorman sat in an empty office in the OB clinic and looked at the floor while she talked. Like nearly all of Dr. Holcomb's patients, most of whom only recently became infected, she looked healthy. Twenty-one years old, her smile made her plump pasty face pretty like a child's. She did not smile often.

"I kept telling the guy I'm pregnant," she said. "He said no you're not. I said yes I am. I can feel my body. Whenever I'm pregnant—I had a bunch of miscarriages—I always lose ten to fifteen pounds the first month, then I gain it back. He thought I lost weight because I was on drugs. He asked around, 'Does that really happen when women are pregnant?' I told him women are different. When I went to the clinic, we had broken up, and when I showed him the paper, he grabbed it and hugged me and said, 'You got to come back.' We had fist fights. He had even went to jail. I expected him not to want to see me no more." She chuckled a bit and said, "But he showed the ultrasound picture to people he works with. 'Look at my baby.' And it was only a spot there. It's funny. I didn't know his real last name until I was four months pregnant. He told me one name, and his uncle called and asked for him and said a different name. Then I met his sister and found out his real name. He was marrying women under various names and taking their money. He thought there were warrants out on him, so he changed his name. He had a sheriff friend run it through, and there were only traffic warrants. But if it wasn't for him, I wouldn't be here today. He got the money for me to take the bus. He borrowed it from his boss. The hardest part about this pregnancy is the HIV, and he stood by me through that, too. I remember, I was five months pregnant. I had been tested for HIV before, every six or seven months since I was fourteen."

Jan related all this with a flat monotone, a voice as soft as her pale white skin. She sat motionless in an office chair. The story flowed steadily, a story that was just there.

"I had been raped at fifteen. I got gonorrhea, and it messed up my eyesight. I had started the HIV tests as a precaution. They had always come back negative. I thought I was clean. The baby's father used to be a pimp and used drugs. He was real wild. We don't know who got it from who. He still won't go to a doctor. He said he would probably hit a doctor.

"I started crying. My body went weak, and the doctor said, 'Do you need a hug?' I said, 'No.' 'Is there anyth—' 'No.' I wouldn't let her finish. She was telling me the percentage of the chances and all about the baby, but it didn't comfort me at all. I had walked over to the window. I just looked out and was bawling. I started saying the baby hadn't even had a chance. She said the baby has a better chance than you got. It still didn't ease me. When I went in I saw a little pamphlet in her hand, and I was thinking it was gonorrhea or chlamydia, which I was famililar with. I said, 'Do I have gonorrhea or chlamydia?' She said 'No, did you expect to?' I didn't have no symptoms, so I didn't figure nothing. She said it's far worse than that. She tried to work her way around it so it would be easier to say it, but point blank still, when you look at it, bam! there it was. She handed me the pamphlet first. I was like, 'No.' She goes, 'Yes.' " Jan said the "Yes" very softly.

"He knew something was wrong because I had told him to come back with me, and she said no I need to talk to you by yourself right now, and you can get him if you want later. And he knew then something was wrong, but he couldn't figure out what it was. When I came out he had a big thing of my juice that I brought to take up there so they could do the ultrasound. I said, 'You got a cigarette?' He said, 'What?' I said, 'Did you bring your cigarettes?' He could tell I had been crying because I had makeup on when I went in and I came out and I didn't have none on because I had to wash my face because I had been crying so much. He said, 'Yeah.' I said, 'Let's go.' I took my juice from him and walked out the door. I walked outside, and I was going to wait until we got back to tell him. But I couldn't. I told him right there in front of the doctor's office. He said, 'You gonna stay with me or what?' In a way, I believe he had AIDS and didn't tell me. He swears he had a test done right before we got together, and he had been negative, so we're not putting the blame on either one of us. But he had his own little way of asking questions. I told him as long as we're together it would be all right. Walking home, he kept me away from the street. I guess he could see on my face what I was planning on doing. It was on my mind to jump in front of a car. With it raining, they wouldn't be able to stop. They would have slid. If it wasn't for him, I would have been dead right now, most likely, because I would have jumped out in front of a car. Pregnant or not.

"I'm down a lot about it. It takes everything I've got not to let it show. I'm not scared for myself but the baby. I've done everything I want to do—except travel the world." She laughed at the notion. "We decided we're gonna do home schooling. We don't want no public harassment. He brought that up. I hadn't thought about it. I wanted a baby for a long time. Now that I got one, I had to find that out. My mom called it my miracle baby. A doctor had said I probably wouldn't get pregnant because my tubes were too scarred from the gonorrhea and the miscarriages, but he just figured that."

"Jan Dorman to exam room 1, please."

She went to see Holcomb and returned to the office. She said it was a routine visit. He measured her fundus, listened to the fetal heartbeat, checked glands in her neck. "He reminded me to take the AZT, but I don't remember. It's been hard to take pills since I was fourteen, when I tried to commit suicide. Since then, I haven't been too fond of pills. It didn't kill me, but I had to walk with a cane for two months. Now, if I walk too much, my left side feels like I'm going to give out."

She had been seeing a doctor near the hotel where she lived, until the positive HIV test. Then the doctor said, "You should go to Grady." "She seemed to have the heebie-jeebies," Jan said, again sitting motionless in the office chair. "I didn't want to come to Grady at all. I know it's one of the best hospitals in Georgia, with the best doctors, but it takes too long to get in and out. Plus I don't know my way around Atlanta too well. But I'm comfortable with Dr. Holcomb. And I don't like too many male doctors."

She returned to the subject of the father of her child, Carl, a young African American man whose deep walnut skin sharply contrasted Jan's pale tone. "A lot of times I'm down, and he asks what's wrong. I say nothing, but he knows. I can tell he doesn't want to talk about it. Sometimes he'll ask me, 'Do we have long to live?' I look at him and smile and say, 'You're going to outlive your mama.' He'll sit there a minute, then smile, and say, 'Yeah, you're right. We can't let this stop us.' "

She said she sometimes stays all day in her hotel room, where she lives. "I go out and do laundry and people come over here to see me, but otherwise I don't go out too much, except if my mom comes and gets me. Or my stepmom. . . . I go see her once in a blue moon. Me and the baby's daddy will go to the pool hall. I'll get me a glass of lemonade, and I'll watch them shoot pool or whatever. It's right down the street."

She said her stepmother copes with a stepdaughter being HIV-positive by thinking of it as cancer. Her father, she said, does not talk much about it. Her mother has asked her to see a counselor, but she will not go. "It broke my heart when I told my mother. She said that if I die first, I should be cremated, then when she dies, she would be cremated, and have the ashes mixed. She said, 'You lived your life alone, but you shouldn't spend eternity alone.' She said, 'Your life has been so hard, and now this.' She calls the AIDS hotline a lot, to ask questions. She's just now able to talk about it without crying. For a while, she would change the subject after a few minutes because she was about to cry. We were together last Saturday, talking and all, and she reminded me how I treated my family before I found out. She said, 'I knew you loved us, but you never showed it.' Now, I tell them I love them. Mom says I grew up real quick." She smiled a bit and said, "I used to be an instigator, instigating fights. Now I try to stop people from fighting. They don't realize how precious life is. I know I didn't. Not until then.

"I used to be a really serious bitch. If I knew my friend's boyfriend was messing around, or their husband, I would tell 'em. I started doing it to piss them off. Hah hah. I used to use people for what I could get out of 'em. Like money, a place to stay, clothes. I used to didn't care about life. Like, I'm here, I don't know why, and I don't care. But now, I still don't know why I'm here, but I know God put me here for a reason, and if this was it I'll find out. It used to be I didn't want to be around my family too much, and now I want to spend a lot of time with 'em. My mom used to give me, give me, give me, and I used to take, take, take, never give back. And ever since I found out, I give, give, give now, too. She was at the point where I didn't really love her. That's how much I had used my mom. When the doctor told me that, I sat back and thought about my past and I realized how I had treated my mom and my family. I literally cried about it, and I regretted it. It was time to make it up before it's too late. Used to, like if it was raining, I was like, oh God, another rainy day, and now I'm not like that. Now, it's like the rain is pretty to me now. Thunderstorms, everything, is just pretty to me now. I just thank God I'm here another day. It's real hard. But when you got a mother that loves you as much mine does, see her hurt knowing about it, it's painful. Really painful."

Later that night, Jan dreamed she had a little boy. In the dream, she thought, They were wrong about me having a girl, and we bought all that girl stuff. The baby was not deformed, as in the first two dreams she had had about it. In the first, it was born with hair as thick as a dog's fur. In the second, the baby had some deformity, the specifics of which, in the haze of the next morning's groggy awakening, she had not been able to recall—only the notion that something was terribly wrong.

Who Have Money
Is Very Strange People

In the apartment she shared with Kenneth, Azi Torres said, "Kenneth can't find out right now. It would be too complicated. He can't stand Jeff." She was speaking about the fact that she and Jeff had gone to Chattanooga, Tennessee, a month before and gotten married. "Jeff says to try and live here a while and we'll see. Kenneth is jealous about Jeff because Jeff is rich, and Kenneth work. Can you imagine being jealous about?" Incredulous, she said, "I am be jealous about Michael Jackson? Because he is rich and he has nose like aah." She pinched her nose. "That's some attitude that I no like."

Before they married, Jeff had felt compelled to introduce Azi to his grandmother. For months, Jeff had told Azi she should meet the widow of the man who built the business whose profits the family now enjoyed. Several times he had said, "Let's go meet my grandmother," but had backed out. Each time, Azi had recalled her sister's eerie prediction about Jeff's grandmother.

"I never believe Jeff," she said, "and when I come back from Florida, he said I want to take you. I think he wants his grandmother meet me, the approval for she like me or not, what impression she has of me. Show the baby. I always hear from him, 'Oh, I take you and meet my grandmother,' but he never did, so I didn't believe. I thought at the last minute he would say no, let's do another day, but I was prepared with one nice dress, more serious. My hair was made, was not messy, won't be like you see today. I was well dressed and put lipstick. I didn't put makeup because I can't stand. I just put a little bit."

Azi dressed Robert cutely, worried that this wealthy matriarch would recoil at the thought of her great-grandson being a Grady baby. The grandmother lived in a mansion in Buckhead, Atlanta's richest neighborhood. "Her house is really beautiful," Azi said. "Inside something else, and have an elevator. Is not funny? My mother's house have steps. I ride in the elevator when I get there with the baby. Is very nice. Telephone inside. One of the women, housekeeper, the secretary, answer the door, and he went upstairs and talked to his grandmother first and then they went there and called me. Then he said this is my son, and he put in her arms. 'Oh, ohohoh.' She was very surprised and very emotional. She looked him, and he was laughing and laughing. He did just exactly right, look like he knew. He said, I will make these people melt their hearts. She said, 'Jeff, how come you hide something so adorable?' " Azi imitated Jeff's grandmother with a high-pitched voice. "She's treating me very well, understand? We talk little bit. Jeff said, well, Grandma, this is something that I should tell you a long time ago, and now we gonna get married. She said I am so happy for you. It's good you have to take care of this child. She was in love with Robert completely. You feel that she mean it."

Then the grandmother asked the question: "Where was he born?"

Azi thought about Grady's reputation, about this woman's stature in Atlanta, and she thought about her sister's message from a spiritist medium. She said, "Grady Hospital."

The grandmother replied, "Grady saved my life."

She said that twenty-four years ago she was in an automobile accident. The woman next to her was killed, and no one expected her to live, either. Her body badly damaged, she was whisked by ambulance to Grady, where she was treated and healed.

Azi also found out that, like her, the grandmother had eloped. "She wasn't pregnant," Azi said. "She just did. Then I know that she likes me. Uh-oh, he make poo-poo. She is one of the wealthy people in this city, but she is not a snob. She is just very wealthy because her husband left her heck of money. He's dead long time, and then she is a woman that is on a board of a lot of things. The woman worth eighty million dollar. She mention about Jeff's mother, like she no behave well, her daughter. This is Jeff's mother's mother. She want to say that's the way Jeff's mother is, like she was behaving bad. I thought, ooh. She called her after we left, I think shake her little bit.

"My friends said, They have a heck of money and they should be paying you private doctor. But nobody in his family gave any support. Nobody thought it could be a serious relationship. His brother was asking how could he communicate with me. Like I could just make love with him, not even talk to him. Is like a prostitute. I just go in bed with you and make love and not even talk to you. I was not able to speak fluent to them, but I was communicating well with Jeff because he all the time with me, twenty-four hours. But they meet me and expend no more than thirty minutes with me. Or twenty. And they judge me. I am foreign, and they are very prejudiced about. They probably really want Jeff marry somebody from here. Can you imagine when this woman die, they probably each one will get ten million? This without what they have already." She laughed. "My friends kid with me, 'You crazy?' I was telling my friend that Jeff wants marry me, and she said what are you doing that you didn't married yet? And Jeff drove one month with his tuxedo, in his car, and try convince me to get married. Was whole August, September, that he ask me to marry him. The first time he ask me, I tell you exactly, because I wrote it down." She looked at her calendar. "I put here in the paper, was in July, I think. Let me see. Yes, July."

Azi remained in Kenneth's apartment because the day after their wedding, Jeff traveled west to go hiking with friends. After his mountain adventures, he decided to find a job in Seattle, and suggested Azi move there with him—in fifteen days, they agreed. So Azi was arranging to put her belongings in storage. She had too many things to do and said she would tell the rest later.

It was a beautiful, sunny, cool day in the fall, a day that made one glad to live in Atlanta. The sun felt warm, the breeze cool, the hot, buggy summer forgotten. Jan Dorman's shabby hotel was just off Cleveland Avenue, a street notorious for drugs, prostitution, and strip clubs. It was next to a satellite airport parking lot and across the street from a bland industrial park, which gaped with ports for unloading eighteen-wheelers. The roar of I-85 thundered through the trees behind the hotel. A bumper sticker on an old Ford in the hotel parking lot said, "If Guns are Outlawed Only Outlaws Will Have Guns." A hotel worker walked by the Ford, a still-folded garbage bag hanging out of his back pocket, in his hand two boxes of rat and mouse poison. The hotel called itself a conference center but looked like no place for a conference.

The peephole in Jan's door was missing; the hole was stuffed with paper. She opened the door to a room crammed with a small apartment's worth of things. The area around the sink was the "kitchen." The TV was tuned to a soap opera. She sat on the double bed by the window, the sunny day kept out of sight by thick floor-to-ceiling curtains.

"A lot goes on in this hotel," she said. "Tee hee. But I'm scared to get government housing because they try to put you in the projects." She had come to live in the hotel the previous December and had met Carl. She said, "We've been together off and on according to how we get along family-wise and physically." She said he rarely goes with her to the hospital. "If I ask him he says he's too tired. I can't blame him. He's tired from working. I cuss him out sometimes and throw things at him. 'I didn't have this baby by myself!' But I understand where he's coming from. He works here. After the second visit, when we found out, he's been too scared to go back, I believe. Hee hee."

It was he who had convinced her to get a job at a strip club. When conventions are in Atlanta, glitzy strip clubs are packed with corporate men with expense accounts. One national directory of nude dance clubs ranked Atlanta among America's elite cities for its upscale clubs and top-quality dancers. Some local companies pay for private VIP lounges. These clubs help attract conventions, which bring hundreds of millions of dollars. Conventioneers come for the hospitality, the airport, the large convention center, and the naked women gyrating for money. These clubs feature marble foyers, sophisticated sound systems, large ornate dance floors, and fancy dressing rooms with body-waxing services. No wonder they can choose the most alluring dancers; the dancers remove money from their garters and count thirty thousand to seventy thousand a year that ogling men have slipped in.

Jan did not dance in any of those clubs. Hers was a small joint on Cleveland Avenue where no moneyed men came to impress corporate customers. "The baby's daddy," she said, "knew people at the clubs, and it took him a good month to talk me into it. I figured he was trying to pimp me. He let me know right then that whatever money I made was mine. He didn't want none of it. He said, 'I want you to have your own money.' I had had friends trying to get me into it, and I was too ashamed of my body. When I was dancing I still felt ashamed, so I had to get sloppy drunk where I couldn't even stand up." She laughed, saying that. "Just the thought of stripping your clothes off in front of people you don't know.

"You just get up there and do your thing, basically. If you want help, you ask another dancer to show you moves. But I love to dance. It was just the problem of getting to where you could undress." She tittered her little laugh again. "It takes a lot of guts to do it if you're ashamed of your body. You couldn't make too much money. The club had gone downhill. You don't get no hourly wage. You just make your money off tips, and you have to pay the club a certain amount of money before you can leave, for letting you dance in their club and for your taxes and all. There's good money in it; you just got to know where to go. The best clubs are where all the white men are at. They love women. And they're not too tight with their money. Black men are greedy. They don't like to give you nothing. They like a free peep show and that's it. Drink a couple of beers and leave." She thought a moment, then added, "My second night when I was working, I made about two hundred and fifty dollars in four hours, off one black man. You know the next day I blew it." She laughed at herself. "I got some clothes and outfits to dance in. He was very drunk. He thought I was a prostitute like a lot of the other girls. Thought he could pay me a lot of money and I would go home with him. He snatched me off the stage because I wouldn't talk to him. They had to throw him out. I was drunk, had five inch heels on. Tee hee. I fell on my face, just about.

"You don't mind if I smoke, do you?"

"You know that's bad for your baby."

"I couldn't give up both alcohol and smoking.

"Ever since I was eight I wanted a child. In fact, this is the eleventh pregnancy. The others were miscarriages. Because the guys all beat on me." She repeated that she did not know if her current baby's father was HIV-positive. "They said if the father's positive too, then there's a better chance of the baby having it. They say the immune system of the baby, when it's first born, has the mother's immune system and on down the road the baby's flushing out the mother's immune system and creating its own so that's basically how most of them get rid of it. And a lot of times the baby don't make it past the age of two. So that's what's mostly scary about it. I had this talk with my mom before you came in. She said, 'With your brother and his baby, I was excited, but with you, I'm scared.'

"I'm trying to be real strong, but hearing her cry makes me cry. Me and my mom for a while weren't close and this came up, and we got a lot closer. I have to thank God for that much. It's still hard, though. The baby's daddy don't like to face up to it, so I got to be strong for both of us. It seems like I have to remain strong for everybody. If I let myself get down and cry all the time then everyone else is going to get upset. Today in fact I walked to the store down the street—got some bread and stuff—I don't know why, but when I was coming back across the bridge, I just slowed down and started looking down below, thinking about it, and that thought crossed my mind again, and it took everything I had to drag myself across the bridge. I just wanted to jump off. That's scary. But after I got across the bridge I was all right."

She said she told her mother about the positive test soon after she learned the results. "Either that night or the next day. I waited about three or four days before I told my brothers. My one brother, he started crying. He couldn't even talk on the phone. He said call me back. He was upset with Mama because she didn't tell them. He asked her why, and she told him, something that important, if it was you, you would want to be the one to tell. Then he understood it. But he won't talk about it at all. If he does, he cries.

"There's a lady downstairs who is full-blown who's sick a lot. I would go and visit her, but I haven't told her. She didn't tell me, but I know. I found out from the grapevine. She'll talk you to death. Otherwise, she's a sweet lady. She has to have a shot every day."

Here is how Azi Torres said her marriage came about: James, the policeman, invited her to go on vacation in Florida. She told Jeff, who feared she was going to marry James there. Frantically, he called her repeatedly, saying they should get married. When James and Azi returned home to James's house late at night, Jeff called her there. She told James, "Tell him I'll see him at home." She arrived at her apartment and found a dozen red roses and a romantic note from Jeff. She spent the next four days with Jeff in a hotel. He had moved out of his apartment and was planning to leave Atlanta for the West any day. Finally, he said, "We need to get married tomorrow in Chattanooga." She did not think he would go through with it, but she bought a new dress and made plans to drive to Chattanooga. They went to Kenneth's apartment to prepare for the drive.

Kenneth did not know what was going on, but he was not happy. He confronted Azi outside the apartment, with Jeff inside getting Robert. "He said to me, we gotta talk, you no have time to me. He start yelling with me. I could not talk to him. I knew that we were about to leave to Chattanooga, and I said tomorrow night we talk."

She was surprised to see that Jeff knew exactly where to go in Chattanooga and that he knew the routine. She thought, "He plan this all out." At the courthouse, she thought he would back out at the last minute. They were filling out the form, and still, she wondered. "I was thinking he would fill up the paper and do this"—she made tearing motions—"and that's it. And even after he did everything I thought he could say never mind. Understand? They say in America it's five minutes to marry, two to divorce. So I didn't know."

They got married, and the next morning he drove west, without Azi, to go hiking in Montana. "We didn't have one day together," she said. "No honeymoon. No first night. Nothing. He left because friends was waiting. He should be left three days before, and he was here, and then he desired to get married. He is a mess. Was more quickly than the weddings in Hollywood."

Azi told this story sitting at the dining table in Kenneth's apartment, Robert in her lap. He reached up and played with her necklace, which tickled Azi. "He's so funny now. Silly stuff. He's discover hands. It's so interesting, children at this time." Partly packed cardboard boxes were in the living room. Spread in front of her were pictures Jeff had sent, of him and his friends hiking and camping in the beautiful northwest mountains. He had been there over a month and was currently staying at a cabin in a park near Seattle, Washington. His plan was for her to fly to Los Angeles, where he would meet her, and they would drive back to Washington.

"Jeff said he went to see what is good, what is not, what cities, what they look like, what have to do. He probably spend one or two days in each city, and he been in Canada already. Now he's in Seattle."

Meanwhile, there was James.

"I couldn't hide it from James. He knew something was going on, and he wanted to talk about it. By this time, he's more like a brother to me, a good friend. He rent a hotel room, so we can talk privately. I told him I married Jeff, and he cried a lot, but eventually he accept it. He said if you love him, there must be a lot of good in him. James is a wonderful guy. He accepts me as I am. He accept my decision, not like Kenneth."

Soon after she told James, Jeff's mother called Azi and said they needed to talk right away. She would be there in two hours and would call back in an hour. She did not call back in an hour. Azi thought that meant she was nervous. She appeared at Azi's door, and Azi displayed Robert. "Robert is funny," Azi said. "He laugh, just what you want, almost like he know he was supposed to be do well for the mother-in-law." Jeff's mother wanted to know if they had signed a prenuptial agreement. Azi said they had not, which did not please her mother-in-law. She also asked how Azi could marry Jeff when he did not have a job. Azi said when she met him he did not have a job, and he was important to her back then. Jeff's mother also asked, If your son got married would you want to be there? Azi said yes.

"Then how could you marry my son without me there?" she asked.

"I said well it's unfortunate. I didn't believe that would happen. I did not think we was about to do that. Really. I told her, don't think I make Jeff marry me. He was driving with his tuxedo in the car for almost thirty days waiting for me get in the car and take me to Chattanooga and marry him. I told him if you better off, I will leave and you find somebody else. That will please your mother and will be nice to this society to you. Will have more to do with you, not foreign, or anything. I told her, and she just listen. They are funny. I learn something. In this country, who have money is very strange people. Very funny. Understand?

"I get help from my sister, and Jeff's mother give me a suggestion, to hide from him. Don't say to him that I have help from my sister, but in reality I didn't tell her the truth. I have some help from Jeff, too. I didn't want to tell her. I wanted her feel bad, because the help that I get from him was nothing, understand? Was nothing. When I was working, I was paying his bills. She wants to find way to make Jeff working, understand? They want he work even for free, for any money, even volunteer. Because in reality if he no want to work in life, he doesn't need to. What he did in school was something in recreation management." Mockingly, incredulous, she waved her hand in the air. "What is recreation management? What is that? Did you know somebody that make money doing that? I don't know. This is kinda funny. He did make money once when he was working for a shop that sells equipment, to cars, things like. He can sell well. He's good. But he want something that he will be happy with. I am sure if he goes to work in Kroger, he no will be happy with. But his mother—it doesn't matter. She want to know that he is working. That's disgusting for a mother. She is pretty bad mother to my belief. Only thing she can do is leave him alone. No pick on him. Each time they get together she is finding his mistakes and tell what he did. That's her whole history repeat each time. How you think he is supposed to be? Frustrated. That's why he get to me, he no get happy. He get very frustrated and complain and just take everything to me like my fault. That's why he screw up everything."

Azi feared that if she told Kenneth about the marriage, she would have no place to stay. "He will no find out from my mouth. He will find out couple months down the road. I need his help. I am sure if I say that, I have to be out the door completely. He will be so angry. And Jeff knows that."

On a dreary October day, Jan Dorman looked out her hotel window. Rain poured down heavily; the outside was a dull gray mess. She had a prenatal appointment that afternoon but said to herself, thinking of the two times transportation services had not showed up, "I'm not going to stand out at the bus stop in that rain." So she did not go. The next day, she lay in a bed in the Labor and Delivery ICU. Outside the window behind Jan's head, traffic rushed by on I-85/75; MARTA trains rode by on the elevated track in both directions; a freight train rolled slowly past. Jan shared her room with another woman, whose baby had just died, right after a C-section. The woman's mother told Jan that they had had the baby shower the night before. She said, "We had just gotten every-thing for that baby." When the woman awoke from the C-section, she was told her baby had died. Groggily, she had said, "No, it didn't. I heard it cry." But she had heard Jan's baby, who was also delivered by C-sec-tion. At the nurse's station, across from Jan's room, nurses and doctors spoke softly. A clerk wrote in a notebook labeled "Stillborn Records."

Fourth-year Dr. Ernesto Miguez rolled the crib with the dead baby down the hall and asked at the station, "Is there an empty room I can use? I want to draw some blood." A few minutes later, a chaplain entered the room. Jan's family and friends visited her one by one. A pathologist arrived at the desk, and a nurse told him, "She verbally agreed to an autopsy, but she can't sign it. Her hand is still trembling."

Clinic aide Patricia Duncan, who had been paged to deliver the dead baby to the morgue, asked, "Where is it?"

"Down in that next-to-last room," the nurse said. "I see you got a running partner with you today." A hospital volunteer walked behind Duncan. They walked to the room, where the baby was wrapped tightly in white cloth. The volunteer said, "I can't carry it. It breaks my heart." Duncan cradled it as she would a live baby. She wrapped it further, with two "Patient Belongings" bags, to cover it more. As she walked by the station, the nurse told a resident who had just arrived, "She's carrying the baby"—she glanced at the several rooms with new mothers in them—"to the you-know-what." The volunteer followed until Duncan told her to stay, reminding her of the time she had fainted upon seeing a gruesome sight. The volunteer remained behind.

During Jan's labor, the doctor had discovered one foot emerging, which would mean disaster for the baby if it was delivered with its legs split apart. Worried, the residents peered at a fuzzy ultrasound screen, seeking the baby's other leg, until they finally found it in a posture that did not immediately threaten the baby but might later. So they opted for the section. They put Jan's mother, Teresa, in a chair behind Jan's head, out of view of the bloody tugging and struggling that produces a baby from the womb through an incision rather than the birth canal. A curtain blocking her view of her own torso, Jan turned silly. She said, "I want a cheeseburger and French fries. I want a cigarette." A young resident entered the OR, and Jan said, "He's cute." Teresa gently scolded, "Jan, your stomach's wide open, and you're talking like that." Teresa admired the new baby, its face pristinely unmashed by a vaginal delivery. She comforted her daughter, who cried when they brought the baby to her face. Light-headed from medicine, she looked at the baby, which had dark body hair all over—a sign of premature birth—and said, "My God, what did I give birth to, a human or a monkey?" Later, she would remark sheepishly, "I was drugged up, wasn't thinking." Teresa was told to sit back down. They did not want her to watch them pull the uterus out, plop it on Jan's belly and sew it back together, so Teresa caressed Jan's head. Jan, though numb below her chest, felt a vague tugging and jerking among her insides. Teresa was shocked at how the doctors and nurses seemed oblivious to the deadly virus in Jan's body fluids. She remarked later, "I've always heard you'll get the virus from blood and stuff, but nobody seemed to be too concerned. I think it was more like if you have a needle stick or something. The doctor that found the foot, all that fluid and stuff went up in her glove and she wasn't the least bit concerned about it."

Patricia Duncan returned and said the morgue was more organized than what she remembered of old Grady. "When I first took one down, I had to step over this and that. I'd open a refrigerator and they're lying around on a shelf. Now it's remodeled, and they have someone in there to assist you. The babies are on this shelf, and adults are on stretchers. I see different kinds of limbs in containers. Sometimes I'll ask, 'What's that?' I'll see 'em cutting on things, going to get plastic bags or fluid." She said she had come to accept carrying a dead baby as merely a part of her job. "You just do it. Once it got to me, though. It was a term baby, a full seven-pound baby. That got next to me. Just today, this volunteer has a small baby herself. At first she was geared up to do it, but when she saw how small it was-. . . ."

Duncan pulled out of a drawer a "Request and Authorization for Disposition of Infant Body" sheet. She said, "Pull the yellow copy out. That goes to a black notebook. The top copy goes in the patient records. This copy goes to Pathology." Duncan wrote her own name in as an example. She wrote "infant remains of Patricia Duncan" in the blank after, "This will be your authority to deliver the body of." She signed her name below the statement that said she "holds the hospital harmless against any claim that might be made on this request." She showed how to fill out a "Georgia Fetal Death Certificate (Spontaneous Abortion or Stillbirth)" form. It requested the sex of fetus, pregnancy history, cause of fetal death. It asked the immediate cause of death on line A, then "due to (or as a consequence of)" on line B, then "due to" on C. It asked for "fetal or maternal conditions, if any, giving rise to the immediate cause, stating the underlying cause last." Part II of the section on the cause of fetal death asked for other significant conditions of fetus or mother contributing to fetal death, but not resulting in the underlying cause given in Part I. A space was checked to indicate whether fetus died before labor, during labor, during delivery, or unknown. "We fill it out to here," Duncan said, pointing. "All this, the doctor fills out. Next, I'll show you four forms we use if the baby comes in dead, DOA. Like if she delivers at home and it dies."

Azi Torres went to the second floor of the clinic building to get a new Grady card, as she had done when she was pregnant. They told her she had to go to the third floor; this office was only for pregnancies. But they wanted to see the baby. James, the policeman, came along to help her, and he lifted the carrier so they could see. "He looks just like the father," they said, remembering Jeff. As Azi left, they said, "When you get pregnant again, come back."

She said OK, but she was thinking, "No way am I going to get pregnant again."

She got her new Grady card, and they walked to the waiting room. When she was called to a room, James kept Robert and talked about helping Azi. "She is not a cautious person," he said. "I caught her once leaving Robert in the car, the car running, and she went into a convenience store. I got all over her for that. I remind myself she's from a rural part of another country, so I have to be careful how I correct her. Since I'm a policeman, I see a lot of bad things. With what I see eight hours a day"—he glanced down at Robert—"I don't know if I'll ever raise him or not, but when you care about someone like I do about him, it makes you scared of what might happen."

James was stuck. He cared for Azi and Robert; he was reliable, employed, but she was married to someone who was in Seattle, Washington, looking for a job. "You never know what Azi'll do next," James said. "I've given up predicting. Right now I'm in a hover mode, just waiting to see what happens." Robert stirred awake and whimpered. James said to him, in a soft voice, "You're going to be crying for a bottle soon, aren't you? It amazes me how fast they change at this age. When I don't see him for three or four days, sometimes I'll see what I think is some significant change."

Carmen Santander, an Ecuadoran woman Azi had met at Grady, entered pushing her baby boy, Andrew, in a stroller. She picked up Andrew and held him near Robert. She spoke in a baby voice on Andrew's behalf: "Hey, Robert. Howya doing, little boy?"

"Do you see how big he is?" said Azi, who had returned.

"Yes, he's big."

Azi looked into Carmen's eyes and saw dark half-moons underneath. "You look like you no sleep too much at night."

James began feeding Robert with a bottle. Azi picked up Andrew and said he weighed about the same as her boy. They compared the thickness of the boys' hair and how often they used a pacifier. They swapped breastfeeding stories. Azi said her right breast was small. She pressed her hands around it, tightening her shirt so Carmen could see. After Robert finished feeding, Azi and James walked to the pharmacy to get her subscription filled.

After Azi and James left, Carmen said, chuckling, "That's great about Azi's three husbands. If number one doesn't work out, go to number two. If number two doesn't work out, go to number three." She gently jostled her son, looked adoringly at his face, then stared away, looked deeply into Azi's three-men situation, about which she had just chuckled, and saw darkness. "She's gonna have problems," she said. "She's playing games with people. That's not right."

In a postpartum room, Jan Dorman whimpered as a nurse tried for the ninth time to find a vein in her arm for the IV. Jan's mother, Teresa, fed the baby with a bottle. "Your veins are very fragile," the nurse said.

"I feel like a pin cushion," Jan said.

The nurse picked up the small chuck that had been placed under Jan's arm to catch whatever dripped. She wadded it up and walked toward a small garbage can. Teresa lifted the lid with her foot and the nurse tossed the chuck in. The nurse returned to give Jan an injection.

"Little bee sting," she said as he pushed it in her arm. Pressing the plunger, she said, "Big hurt, big hurt, BIG HURT." Jan grimaced all the way through.

"I wonder if they could put the IV in her neck," Teresa said. "They did that with your brother once when he kept pulling it out."

"Not in my neck. I'll walk out of this hospital first."

Teresa asked the nurse if Jan could eat yet. She had been on a liquid diet since the C-section. The nurse said she would ask the doctor. Jan asked if she could clean the incision with alcohol pads.

"Don't do that. You can take a shower or wipe it with hydrogen peroxide, but you don't want alcohol down there. It'll burn you up."

The second-year resident came in. "I understand we've been having problems finding a vein." She snapped on gloves and examined Jan's arms. "I don't see any good places. Your veins are rolling. Look at that. And we need the IV back in. It's been keeping your fever down." She pressed Jan's soft skin with her fingertips.

Jan became whiny. "Every time I think everything's going to be all right, something else happens." She wiped tears from her eyes.

Teresa said, "I'm sorry, hon."

"Let's send for Marcia Fisher," the doctor said, like she was calling in the cavalry. Fisher was a longtime Grady labor and delivery nurse who was legendary among residents. Even fourth-year residents often followed her advice, and first-years frequently said, "Marcia Fisher saved my ass," after a timely suggestion or reminder. A first-year in labor and delivery was usually told, "Whatever Marcia Fisher tells you to do, do it."

After the nurse and doctor left the room, Jan admitted she had eaten a piece of apple pie and a Honey Bun, though she was on the liquid diet. "They were good," she said, sighing. The resident returned, accompanied by Fisher, who peered at Jan's arms through half-glasses perched on her nose.

"Let your arm stay low, baby," Fisher said. "Can you move back in your bed a little? Ease back? I just need to keep your arm still."

Jan moved back slowly, wincing. Fisher said, "I don't like these needles. They're no damn good." She glanced at the baby. "Isn't she cute? These veins just go up and down, don't they?" She left to get a different type of needle, and returned to Jan's side. "Are you ready, little buddy?" She spoke to Jan gently. As she tried for a vein, she said, "I'm sorry. I'm sorry." Then, "Can you give me a tight fist? Oh, so good."

Jan stared at the ceiling and gritted her teeth.

"Hang on, baby. I'm so sorry. Hang on. Be strong. Be still for me. We got one, OK? Maybe it should last a while."

Teresa reminded the second-year resident to see if Jan could eat. The resident listened to Jan's bowels through her stethoscope. "They sound good, but you need to stay on liquid foods until you pass gas from below, OK? Your bowels are just not ready for solid food yet. We have to go slow. Probably late tonight or early tomorrow. Thank you, Miss Fisher," she said as their last hope triumphantly returned to Labor and Delivery.

Teresa helped Jan get comfortable in the bed. "Just sit back and relax."

Her voice tinged with disgust, Jan recalled the day's meals: for breakfast Jello, coffee, and juice; for lunch broth and juice. She added, "They're saying I might go home in three days if I don't have a fever."

Teresa put a pacifier in the baby's mouth. A ribbon tied to the end of the pacifier was clipped to her shirt; if it fell, it would not hit the dirty floor. Teresa said, "I read you're not supposed to use one with a long cord like this. It might wrap around the baby's neck. We'll cut it off. It'll be ugly, but it'll be safer."

Jan reached into her suitcase on a table by the bed and moved clothes around. "Mom, where's my bra? I can't find it in here."

"Are you sure it's not wrapped up in the covers or anything?" Jan felt around the covers; Teresa searched a closet shelf. "I got it, hon," Teresa said and sat back down and stared at the baby. "I know their arms and legs are supposed to turn purple, but it scares me every time I see it. Some people say newborns are boring, that they just lay there. But I don't." She picked her up and looked in her eyes. "Look how she's trying to see you. They say they can see good eight to ten inches. And she tries to listen." Teresa noticed the baby's diaper needed changing. She took her to Jan, but a nurse came in to take Jan's vitals, so Teresa changed it. She pulled the diaper away, saw urine still dribbling out, and put it back. "You're not through yet, are you?"

"I need to examine your incision," the nurse said.

Jan, who was sitting up, said, "Now I got to lay the hell back down and struggle to get back up."

"Well, it's got to be done," her mother said.

After the exam, Jan sat up and tried to hold the baby to feed her. With the IV needle in, she could not hold the baby in the crook of her arm. Whiny again, Jan said, "I don't know why they put that there when they know I have a baby to feed." With Teresa's help, she lay the baby on the bed and held the bottle in her left hand. After the feeding, Teresa slowly lifted the baby to her shoulder and patted her back until she burped. The nurse returned to take the baby's vitals. The baby fussed when her temperature was taken, the thermometer tucked under her tiny arm.

"When I held her, she tried to get through my shirt," Jan said.

"She smelled that milk," Teresa said.

"I wish I could," Jan said, aware that it was not considered safe for HIV-positive mothers to breastfeed their babies.

Jan's stepmother arrived, and Jan told her, "They said if I don't have a bowel movement, they'll have to flush it out with water. I don't care what they say. I'm about to get that hamburger. When they brought that lunch, and it was chicken broth, I started crying. I was so mad." She added, looking at the ceiling, "Lord, please, let me have a bowel movement."

The next day, Jan got more bad news. She might have to stay another week, due to persistent infection. She said she wanted a cigarette. "I'd go outside to smoke, I want one so bad. Of course, her weight would have been up if I hadn't smoked."

Her mother held a pamphlet titled "HIV and Your Child." A row of snacks lined the narrow windowsill: Honeybuns, cans of "Lite Fruit Cup," fruit, and gum. Her mother said, "I want to know what to look for in a child because it takes so long to know." She looked at her daughter and added, "Most pregnant women will test positive for HIV, but since Jan was tested twice she probably has it. But I want her to be tested again."

"As depressed as I've been," Jan said, "I'll sue them if I turn out negative. And they keep talking about my bowels, but I had no bowel movement before I was pregnant, for two or three months."

Jan's mother smiled and shook her head. "If you did that, you'd be sick, real sick. You must have lost track of time." She stroked the baby's fine brown hair. "I'd love for her hair to stay that texture."

"She cried last night," Jan said, whimpering, "but it hurt so bad. I couldn't do nothing but cry. My baby wanted me, and I couldn't be with her."

"Keep taking your pain medicine on time," her mother told her.

A nurse arrived to take the baby to the nursery for AZT medication. Teresa left to get a cup of coffee.

After they left, Jan said, "If you give AZT while the baby's still creating its own immune system, it decreases the chance of developing it. I'm comfortable with her getting it, but I was drugged up when I signed the authorization form. They had me sign so many things, I would have signed one of my checks."

Soon the nurse returned with the baby. The baby's father, Carl, came in, carrying a small television. A male friend walked in behind him. Jan had continued talking about AZT until she saw the friend, then stopped abruptly.

"Did you bring my soap and shampoo?" Jan asked.

"Dang, I forgot," Carl said. He slapped his thigh. He walked down the hall with his friend, who was leaving.

Jan shook her head and said, "His friend better not have heard us talking about HIV. He doesn't know. None of Carl's friends know. His family don't know. If they found out, he'd be so mad."

Teresa returned. "Those rude nurses are back. They won't even look at you if you speak to them." She said she liked the day shift nurse best, the one who had felt badly the day before about not finding a vein in Jan's arms. "She's sweet. She has a southern accent, but she's black. And that nurse who put in the IV yesterday, she said the needles down here are crap. I like a nurse who tells it like it is. You feel like you can trust her."

Carl returned alone. "They won't tell me nothing here."

"It's because you're not married," Teresa said.

"They said, 'If she won't tell you, we can't.'"

Jan said, "You can't be mad at them for respecting my privacy."

He asked if she was eating; she sneered, "If they'd bring real food."

Carl picked up the baby and sat on the bed, by Jan. He said, "They make a funny face when they go to the bathroom."

"Not all the time," Teresa said. "Sometimes they just scrunch up their face. Sometimes they look like they're going to cry, then they smile and laugh." Carl handed the baby to Teresa, who cuddled her until she smiled. "Some people say it's just passing gas, but I don't believe it. I can see she's trying to listen. I think there's more to it. You know how later they'll say, 'We were wrong,' and that's what I think this is."

Carl pulled a pillow over his face and Jan's, and leaned closer to her. They whispered to each other.

Damn Stupid Guy

"Hello, I'm Renee Lindley, your nurse. Are you having contractions?" Lindley asked this in Labor and Delivery room 8. The patient said she was, and Lindley explained to her about getting pain medication through an epidural or a narcotic in the IV. She explained the problems meconium—bodily waste from the baby—can cause if the baby inhales it. "When the baby is born, it might breathe"—she gasped quickly, imitating the baby's instinctive first breath—"so we need to prevent that. When we say don't push, that's so we can suction the meconium. Otherwise, it can get sick or cost his life. You'll be uncomfortable, but do that if you don't do anything else. For the well-being of your child, understand? Consider the epidural. Don't worry about people saying you'll be paralyzed. Those who said it, they're not paralyzed. All my patients, they're not paralyzed." An LPN brought in the suction tube.

The patient's sister said, "That's what's gon' get out that stuff?"

"Yes, when we deliver the baby."

"You're going to deliver the baby?" the patient said, eyeing Lindley.

"No, a doctor will come."

Lindley walked to the nurse's station and told Cleo, the other nurse, "Tell 'em don't call me unless my patient is delivering. Honey, let me heat my coffee." She walked to the break room, where she heated her McDonald's coffee in the microwave and recalled epidural stories.

"One chick said it would leave her paralyzed. Two friends had it and told her that. I said, 'Your friends are paralyzed?' 'No, but that's what they say.' 'Can they walk?' 'Yes.' 'Then they are not paralyzed.' I said, 'Anybody that wants you to lay up and hurt, I wouldn't call them friends. You need some new friends.' I tell my son, 'Be quiet. You're passing on ignorance.' "

She munched on a Danish and said, "One lady said she didn't want it because she had it before and she slept until the nurse woke her up and said it was time to push it out. I asked what was wrong with that. She said it put her to sleep, so maybe you'll put something in there. I said she fell asleep because she felt good. This lady at my other job went Exorcist on me. She had this doctor who, for religious reasons, doesn't like to give epidurals. He gives pain medicine only. She asked for an epidural, and I told her her doctor didn't allow it. A few hours later, I'm rubbing her back, and she starts waving her arms." Lindley lowered her voice to a deep guttural. " 'I want an epidural. You tell that religious maniac I don't give a fuck what he thinks. I'm paying for this.' I got that doctor, and she said to him, 'I am hurting. I want an epidural, and I want it now!' " He said, 'OK.' " She imitated the doctor with a meek little peep.

Lindley continued, "I try to get a big suction to get big pieces of meconium. Sometimes the pieces can be this big." She broke off little chunks of her pastry, pointed at them, then ate them. "And with that epidural, she won't be feeling that pain and want to push so much."

Lindley said she had gone from Grady nursing student to Grady employee. "I had always said I would go back to school and be a newborn nurse practitioner, so I decided to work a little of it and see. At first I went to the ICU nursery, but I got tired of sick and dying babies. I went to term nursery, postpartum, and back to term nursery, then labor and delivery. It was never my intention to stay at Grady. But I like what I do, so I stayed and stayed."

She grew up in Bogalusa, Louisiana, and attended a Catholic high school in nearby Chatawa, Mississippi, "a small town large enough to have a Confederate graveyard." She added, "Nuns are good con artists. The graveyard was off campus, so it was considered a 'privilege' to go clean it. If you got too many demerits, you lost the privilege of cleaning the Confederate graveyard. All the bad things I didn't have any business doing—smoking, cussing—I learned in Catholic school. When I went from Louisiana to Mississippi, they used to make fun of us for being Catholic. But I learned a comeback: 'If it wasn't for the Catholic church, you wouldn't have one.' I learned to be mean." She looked at her watch. "I got four minutes left on my break. I'm gonna run outside and smoke."

She returned from her smoke break and entered 8. The patient's sister and a man were pacing the hall. The sister said, "I'm scared." She peeked in the door. "They said the baby's having a hard time breathing, that when the baby comes out, they gonna have to suction. It might get pneumonia." Lindley waved them back in the room, then asked the patient, "Do you want an epidural? Remember, I told you it was a little catheter they put in your back. You're breathing too fast. It's important for oxygen to get to the baby. There's no use in going through all this and have a baby that can't breathe."

Lindley walked to the nurse's station and called home. After she hung up, she said, "Whew, I'm gon' whup some stuff tonight." Dr. Nancy Brownlee, the third-year resident, came to the station and said, "Miss Lindley, I've decided to rupture Miss Howell, to get this induction on the road."

"You'll have to wait just a minute while I finish this report."

"OK, no problem," Brownlee said, smiling. "That's why I waited until you finished your phone call."

After Brownlee left, Lindley said, "They're just practicing. They don't need to rupture her yet. That's why I'm in no hurry to help her. If my baby was in trouble, I'd go. But they're just getting in their practice." Still writing, she added, "I'm so pissed. I've never had my wages garnished before. I've been in contact with these people forever. If they say I owe them, let us work out something. If I say I'll pay two hundred dollars every month, I'll pay it. And payroll. I can't believe they did that to me. I don't conduct my business that way. Why should they treat me like that? I'm gonna write a letter to the CEO." She made a call to see if the accidental deletion of eight hours she had recently worked had been straightened out. "I need that for my son's tuition," she said on the phone. "OK, bye." She called the head nurse and said, "They told me you and me got to work out something."

She heard from a room down the hall, "Hold onto those handles. They're your best friend. Almost there. One more push like that, and it'll be out."

"I'm pushing, goddammit! It ain't coming out!"

"It's right there. Do you want to wait on the next contraction?"

"I want it out!"

"One more big push, and it's out."

Grunting and screaming, the patient pushed again, and demanded, "Pull it out! Pull it out, dammit!"

"That's it, let's do it, push."

Four murderous screams later, the baby was out, and the room was suddenly serene.

"Yeah, it's common," midwife Lauren Foley said of pregnant women who snarl during the delivery phase called transition, or hard labor, when strong painful contractions may come with no pause between them; some women also experience vomiting, leg and buttock cramps, hot and cold flashes, and heavy perspiration. Plus, there's this baby pushing through the vagina. Don't worry, some pregnancy manuals say, transition rarely lasts longer than an hour and a half. Foley sat in the midwife office. A sign on the bulletin board announced a midwife-friendly practice opening in Chattanooga, requesting recommendations of fourth-year residents. "Churchgoing choir ladies scream words they would never say. Some women that are real coy get uninhibited. They yank sheets off. Sometimes they have bizarre personality changes. I told my husband I didn't want an epidural, then before I went in labor, I warned him that I would ask for an epidural when labor got painful. I told him he'd say, 'No, you don't.' Then I'd say, 'Forget what I said.' I told him not to let me, though I'd say forget what I had said.

"So, I said it. He said, 'You told me you'd say that.' I said, 'Forget that shit! I want it!' It's amazing that marriages survive fathers in childbirth. I ran him off. 'Send my daddy in here.' I was a typical southern girl. 'My daddy'll get it for me.' Then afterwards, I was pissed off at my husband for letting me have that epidural. My second child I was an asshole, a real bitch. I went to a midwife, which I didn't the first time. But I got sent to a doctor for an induction because of high blood pressure. I curled up into a ball and said, 'Get away. Don't touch me. I'll tell you when I'm ready to push.' I wasn't even a nurse yet, so I only knew a little about childbirth. I was the kind of patient that annoys me now. They read one thing. But the delivery was fine and wonderful. And no epidural."

Lindley finished writing and helped Dr. Brownlee with the rupture. She returned to the nurse's station to write and watch the monitor where her patients' strips crawled across. "I went to Parisian," she said to the other nurses, "with two gift certificates. In that fancy Phipps Plaza. I bought some socks and things, then this cashier said"—she imitated a snooty voice—" 'You have to get a gift certificate for your change.' It was about ten dollars. I bought some more things with a different gift certificate and went to another cashier, and he said he didn't have time to do another gift certificate and gave me change. So I said, 'She gave me this for change; can you cash it?' I walked out of there with thirty-seven dollars. Heh heh heh." She slapped her hand on the outstretched hand of another nurse, also laughing. "That first lady treated me like I didn't have no money, like I was there only because I had a gift certificate."

"Yeah, like you had food stamps."

Lindley returned to 8 and told the patient she would be giving her an antibiotic through the IV. The fourth- and third-year residents came in and looked at the strip. Lindley left to get a bag of saline solution, to flush out more meconium. "I know where I'm going," she muttered. "Already. We're headed toward the OR. I knew it when I saw the strip." The room buzzed: four OB doctors, the anesthesiologist, medical student, Lindley, the LPN, the clerk giving scrubs to the patient's boyfriend, who would accompany her to the OR. The door swung open, and the patient was wheeled down the hall, surrounded by all those people.

Lisa Dean said Dwayne was around somewhere, getting his affidavit ready. He had been arrested for driving without a license or insurance, and he was trying to get a public defender. But she was trying not to think about him. "Do we have to talk about this?" she asked.

"Not if you don't want to."

"I don't. Other than that, everything is OK. D'Lisa is six weeks old. She's lifting up, turning over, almost sitting up. She's real alert to everything." Using baby talk, she spoke on D'Lisa's behalf. " 'Yes, everything I hear I have to turn around and see.' She knows who I am. When someone else has her and I walk by, and she smells me, she wants me."

Cuddling D'Lisa in her large arms, she recounted her daily routine. "First, when I get up, on weekdays, I get my son ready for school. I get him up at seven, seven-thirty, and she'll wake up with us, and I dress her, give her a bath. Rob goes to Head Start. Cheryl takes him with her baby boy." D'Lisa gurgled, and Lisa again spoke for her in a high bouncy voice. " 'I like to try to talk to people. They can't understand, but I try.' Say, 'My eyes changed colors.' " D'Lisa cooed a soft ya-a-a-h, ya-a-a-h. "Then I fix the bottles. I have to make sure all her bottles are cleaned in boiling water. She greedy. She don't always want breast milk. At night she'll settle for it but not during the day. Say, 'Yeah, yeah.' Say, 'I'm so alert.' She'll get frustrated when I breastfeed her. I guess it don't come out fast enough for her. She'll go 'Oooh oooh.' She get upset." Lisa sang, " 'I get so upset.' "

Dwayne came in, picked up D'Lisa and kissed her. "What's up, Boo?" He said the diaper smelled like it needed to be changed, handed D'Lisa to Lisa, and left. Lisa continued, "Then I have to cook, get myself dressed when she'll go to sleep. When she sleeps, I clean up or lay down and go to sleep. Say, 'I sleep better when I have a fresh bath and I'm in my jammies.' " D'Lisa reached toward the kitchen table. "Are you trying to steal my potato? Rob gets home about two. He rides with Ms. Cheryl. He says, 'Give me my baby sister.' " She imitated him by lowering her voice: " 'Can I go outside?' Heh heh. I let him in about seven-thirty for dinner. When it's time for bath, 'Let me take a bath in the morning. I just want to stay stink.' Heh heh. After his bath, I just make him get in the bed, so he'll sit up there and watch TV and in about thirty minutes he'll be asleep."

Her friend Leslie dropped by to talk about the next weekend. They were planning to spend Lisa's birthday at a hotel. "We need a break," Leslie said. "We're going to get in the hot tub, sit by the pool. Cool out."

Lisa added, "Mom will take care of the kids. We need a mental health break from boyfriends, kids, all that kind of stuff. Mental health break. Without me having to make bottles, change Pampers. Sometimes we need that. That's when people have breakdowns."

"Stress," Leslie said.

In the postpartum unit, Jan Dorman's mother, Teresa, explained that Jan had been taken back to the OR a few days after her C-section. Jan lay next to her. Her infection had persisted, her stomach was red and hot, and they went in to repair the fascia, the membrane around the intestinal cavity, which had ruptured. The incision was left open, rather than sutured shut, to allow air to help it heal. "I'm taking the baby home," Teresa said. She spoke in her gentle, high, steady voice. "She'll be in a place where she won't just be fed, but will actually live." She added, "They said there's no infection in the womb, but her vagina was swollen. Some kind of fluid buildup. It looked like a cow udder with no teat. The labia quadrupled. The nurse said some swell up so bad they can't walk. I would have never thought. . . ."

Jan said, "What's so funny is, Carl, the baby's daddy had a feeling something was going to go wrong. He would say so. The Lord helped me through it. Overnight the fever went down. I got to where I could get up and go to the bathroom. It's a miracle. For a while I thought I was going to die."

The next day, still in postpartum, Jan whimpered, "My baby got to go home, and I got to stay here. Last night I started crying. I didn't even want to hold her. And I got this thrush in my throat, which is supposed to be one sign of HIV. It's like a rash. The baby's got a better chance than I got. And I was scared—this bug I got—I was going to give that to her. Every time something starts going right, something goes wrong." She said Carl had not been able to sleep much. "He's been more worried about me than the baby. I knew he loved me, but I didn't know he loved me that much. I'm all he's got." She sobbed lightly. "He loves me, and he's got nothing at home. He's had a hard life. His family doesn't have nothing to do with him, unless they want something. They abandoned him when he was a few months old. They found him in an empty house. He was raised by a foster family. He watched his foster mom die, the only mom he really knew. He saw his daddy the first time a few years ago in a nursing home, and his dad didn't know who he was. That hurt so bad he couldn't go back. He has aunts and uncles here, but he used to smoke lots of cocaine, and any time something comes up, his family throws that in his face. They shouldn't do that. That was his past. He did real good. A lot of people have to get professional help, and he did it on his own. He's been clean for four years, on his own. He tells 'em, once you hit rock bottom, you're as low as you're gonna hit, and when you do, you'll know it. They just throw it in his face. They don't think about the fact that he quit on his own. He put his life in God's hands. He said he prayed to God to help him, and God saw him through. And with this right here"—she pointed at her incision—"he prayed to God again and promised God that if he let me live, he would start going to church again. And he would have me and the baby go, too. He'd been walking around moping, crying and everything. Nobody's ever seen him like that. Nobody knows him that much. He's shy. We're gonna start going to church every Sunday now."

Azi Torres bemoaned life with a baby. "I woke up yesterday, today, so dizzy. No sleep before three in the morning. One week straight I woke up the whole night because the baby woke up. If I have to change him, is hard to sleep again and then I expend a lot of time to him in the morning. So I no have get much sleep at all. Yesterday I took two Tylenol PM, then went to sleep about two-thirty. I just woke up nine-thirty. That's when he was crying, and even if he cry before I didn't heard because I was really deep sleeping. And then I woke up and give him a bottle and he slept again. I was laying in the bed, and I sleep again little bit but then when I woke up I was so dizzy. I am up almost two hours but I still feel dizzy, like you want to be in the bed and sleep whole day."

She was still preparing for her trip to the West to join Jeff but was getting frustrated. "I have been packed a lot but slow, slow. I am tired to pack. I got to change Jeff's storage, five-by-ten to ten-by-ten, to have more room to fit my stuff, and he said, 'Oh no, Azi, go to my storage and throw some stuff out.' I cannot throw his stuff out. I don't know what throw out. Everything cost money. He have old sofa that. . . . My friend, Ester, who does nice job with sofa, she cover sofa. You can't afford throw things out anymore. I grow up not throw anything out. I repair things. In America people just throw out. Is like throw money out. I no like the idea to move there without anything here."

She said Jeff wanted her in Washington so they could choose an apartment together. "He no work well alone, understand? Right now, he is waiting for some money because his money is out. And me, too, because when get some money in his account, I will go over there and get some. He have to wait for his mother, put money in his account. He ask her some extra money because he rent a cabin, and he said it no have anything in the cabin. Just a bed. He don't know where he gonna go. He not start work yet because he want drive to San Francisco to get me. He said have some kind of job, kinda two different jobs that he can get, but I am sure he no will work until I get there. I will sacrifice me and the baby right now for him, but I will make sure if he no find something to do there very quickly, you will see me very soon back Atlanta. I am too old, understand? Too tired."

"I'm ready to go up there and raise some hell. This is ridiculous." Jan Dorman pointed toward the front desk at the Women's Urgent Care Center. "I've been here since twelve-thirty." It was 4:00. She was waiting to have a doctor check her incision.

Mother Teresa said, in her flat, gentle tone, "She doesn't wait very well."

"This doesn't make any sense, having me wait like this."

"I know. I know. But it's not life-threatening, so we have to wait. One area I'm concerned about is that they said to check for smoothness, color, and smell. One part of the incision isn't smooth. It's puffed out on the edge." Watching the baby sleep, Jan fuming next to her, Teresa said, "I'm sure she dreams. I see her eyes move, smile, and frown. I have a month-old grandbaby, and I'll massage her while she's sleeping. I can tell. She'll go from a frown to looking content."

"Miss Jan Dorman, please come to exam room 10."

Jan shuffled out, followed by her mother, who carried the baby. Teresa said, "Sometimes she doesn't understand all they're saying, and I want to know everything they say. And she tends toward exaggeration." They were not happy to discover they had to wait again, in chairs in the hall outside the exam rooms. Two other women sat waiting, and two stood, leaning against the wall. But Jan and Teresa laughed together, watching the baby's face change as she slept. Teresa rearranged the baby's white lace headband, decorated with small green and red flowers. "These things are useless," she said. "All they do is push down on her ears." Teresa said the baby had gained weight. "They said to look for—signs of HIV—ear infection, pneumonia, diarrhea, and no weight gain."

Teresa pulled a photograph of the incision from her purse, and they looked at it, a swollen pink line across Jan's broad white belly. A towel covered her crotch. Jan was called to a room, walked down the hall, and was told they made a mistake. They were to change her gauze, which required that she be in room 1 or 2. Both were occupied. She returned to her chair.

"This is ridiculous," Jan fumed, "having to wait all that time, then coming back here and waiting."

Teresa picked up the baby and cuddled her. "When Jan was immature, she used to say, 'If I get pregnant, I'm going to give it to you.' And I almost wish she would. Do you want to hold her, or should I?"

"You hold her." Jan handed her mother the bottle, and Teresa fed her. "OK, Miss Dorman."

Jan walked down to room 2, passing the nurse's station, on which a statuette of Uncle Sam pointed, the caption below warning, "Have you taken your pill today?"

At 7:00 they emerged from the room. "Everything looks good," Teresa said.

Jan said, "I'm going home this weekend and take care of it myself. I'll be Dr. Dorman." For the first time that evening, she smiled.

Walking to Central Stores to get more gauze, they recalled being in the recovery room after the C-section. "We tried not to talk too happy," Teresa said.

Jan recalled, "I heard them tell her they tried everything to get the heart going. She was all drugged up from the C-section. She cried, 'Oh, my baby.' Her sister and mother were crying, too. That one nurse tried to tell them not to bring her in there with us, but they did. I almost cried. I felt so sorry for her. I heard the nurse say her baby was well-formed, no signs of anything wrong."

They arrived and waited at the counter. "It was hard to be happy,"

Teresa said, "knowing she had lost her child. I can hear her all over again."

Jan held a large box of Disposable Underpads that had been handed to her.

"That's too heavy for you," her mother said. She carried the box, and Jan carried the baby. They walked to the parking lot under a steel blue sky, the scattered clouds lit pink by the sinking sun. Lights from McDonald's, the parking deck, Grady, and the health department added a soft white glow. Teresa said, "At least the traffic will be light, now that we've been here so long."

Lisa Dean arrived for her six-week checkup at 11:30, her voice hoarse, her face in a scowl. "She's been fussing," said her friend Marian Thurston, who accompanied her. A few weeks before, Marian had returned from a long visit with her boyfriend in Alabama, and told Lisa—whispering while walking across the parking lot at Floral Acres—"I'm pregnant."

Lisa checked in and was sent to the lab. "I hate it when they stick my finger," she growled.

Marian said, "I hate it when they say, 'It won't hurt.' You're a damn liar. Everything hurts me."

Lisa let them draw blood, returned to the waiting room, checked D'Lisa 's diaper, fed her apple juice. D'Lisa cried when the bottle was removed. "She don't mess around when it comes to eating," Lisa said and restored the bottle. "You're greedy." D'Lisa finished eating; Lisa burped her; D'Lisa spit up on her bib. Lisa removed that bib and put on the spare. D'Lisa cried; Lisa gave her a pacifier. Lisa picked her up, cuddled her, and rocked her slowly. She cradled D'Lisa's hand. "She's got hands like mine and feet like Dwayne's."

Marian said, "I saw this girl checking in who looked twelve years old."

"She probably was," Lisa replied. She was called to have her blood pressure taken. Passing by the scales, she said, "I'm so glad I'm not pregnant no more." To the enormous woman ahead of her at the blood pressure station, Lisa said, "Are you having twins?"

Laughing, she answered no. "I'll be glad when it's over. I'm due soon."

Recalling her eighth month, Lisa said, "Whew, honey, I remember.

Boy, my nose got so big. I was miserable." Back in the waiting room, Lisa told Marian how much she weighed.

"You're breastfeeding. That's your problem."

"Yeah, they're fat."

"That's all titties is. Fat."

Lisa said she was glad she no longer wore support hose on swollen legs.

Marian said, "You looked like some old white man going to play golf."

D'Lisa opened her mouth wider. Marian interpreted: "She's saying, 'I want some titty.' " She turned to Lisa and asked, "Did you have an epiderman?"

"No, that slows the heart rate down." Suspecting something, Lisa squinted and asked, "Did you have an epidural when you made the baby?"

"Hell, no."

"Then don't have it when you deliver. You got to take the pain." Remembering her own delivery, Lisa laughed. "I'm talking some shit, the way I was." She also recalled Dwayne at her delivery, and her laugh turned to a frown. "He looked so stupid in there."

Watching a woman walk by, Marian said, "Your butt was like that when you were pregnant."

"It was not. Her butt is humped up. Mine was just big."

D'Lisa raised her head and looked around. Another woman walking by said, "Look at her hold her head up. You're going to have another one next year. She's getting out of the way for the next one."

A tape on AIDS and pregnancy came on the TV. Lisa said, "You know, God works in mysterious ways. He works in mysterious ways. If a baby dies from AIDS, there's some reason for it. He works in mysterious ways."

Recalling her own AIDS test, Marian said, "That doctor scared the crap out of me, looking all serious and stuff. I thought I must have AIDS. She saw me and said, 'Don't worry; it's negative. I'm just having a bad day.' Those were the scariest days of my life. I was thinking, 'What if?' They asked if I had sex with someone who was bisexual. You don't know that. I thought if I got AIDS, I'd go to Africa or somewhere and live out my life. I was happy with the results. Now I'm gonna be celibate."

Lisa looked at her and crossed her eyes.

"I'm going to try as hard as I can."

On the TV, a man rolled a condom onto a banana.

"Lisa Dean, to exam room 7, please."

Marian looked after D'Lisa. A sign on the bulletin board across from her announced that Emory University Hospital was seeking sexually active women for a study being conducted.

Overhearing a teenager talk behind her, Marian said, "I hate that phrase, 'baby daddy.' That's ghetto. I wouldn't want to be called baby mama. If you say 'baby daddy,' that's saying that's all you think he's worth."

At Grand Rounds, boxes of Krispy Kreme doughnuts were passed among the residents, who sat bunched in the front middle. Luscious coos emerged from everyone reaching for the fried sugar wonders. A scowling medical student said to his neighbor, "I'm cold. I worked all night. I'm grumpy. I went to the vending machine for coffee. All I got was hot water. It was terrible." Chief resident Paul Namath carried a box of doughnuts over to attending doctors Bishop and Cawthon. "Like a doughnut? They're still warm." Bishop took one. The two medical students, whom the doughnuts never reached, watched Namath serve his superiors. One chuckled and said, "No doughnuts for students."

The Grand Rounds speaker, a medical malpractice lawyer, began, "I'm sure a lawyer is one of the last people you wanted to speak, but I defend doctors, not sue them. We're the good guys, not the bad guys." She put a definition of a doctor on the screen: someone who makes sick people well enough to sue for malpractice. "Malpractice," she said, "is part of your practice like managed care. You have to live with it." Her topic was writing in charts.

The more detailed and precise, she said, the better it will serve you later. When the patient goes to a lawyer, the first thing they do is pore over the chart and find something glaring. When you give your deposition, all you have to go on is the chart. You'll be asked about every detail in it. The jurors have your chart blown up on a big screen in front of them. It's not enough to say, "I gave appropriate care." You need proof.

Ask yourself when you are writing in a chart: (1) How will this chart withstand the scrutiny of a lawyer? (2) How will the jury react?

She put on the screen a sexist drawing of a female patient, with ample curves, breasts, and nipples. Don't, she said, draw something like that. Keep it professional.

The rule in litigation is, she said, if it's not written, it wasn't done. Now, you *know* plenty is not written down, but try to write it all. Write what instructions were given to a patient, so they can't say, "I was never told that." Make a carbon copy of the instruction sheet with a referral on it. That will go a long way to help you win a case. If you tell someone to get a second opinion, and they don't, but you didn't write down that you told them to, they'll say you didn't say it. Write legibly and date entries, and put the time.

She put two examples on the screen. One word could have been either "pregnant" or "frequent"; another, either "routine" or "positive."

Most of you, one of these days, she said, will have to defend yourself in court. All they need is a hundred dollars and a willing attorney. Don't write in the margins later on, and don't leave long spaces in between. It will come back to haunt you. They look for doctored charts. Chart in ink only, not pencil. Avoid changing pens in one entry. Never erase, white out, or alter what you've written. That's good patient care, and it's good in case there's a lawsuit. If you make a correction, make sure it's clear it's a changed error, that you're not hiding something. Show it's in good faith.

For you nurses, don't write, "Sleeping. Sleeping. Found dead in bed." Instead, write, "Rigor mortis noticed. Doctor called." Avoid editorial comments. Don't say the patient was a complainer. Even hypochondriacs do have something wrong sometimes. If you have to write on something other than a chart—say, a bedsheet when you're in a hurry—make sure it's transcribed. Don't make any comments that are irrelevant to patient care. Don't write, "The doctor looked tired that night."

Avoid pointing fingers. Attorneys love that, watching you shoot each other, and the jury blames you both. Don't circle the wagons. For example, anesthesia may blame OB in a bad baby case. If there's an equipment problem, don't write, "Defective equipment." Put some statement other

than that. Don't put confessions in a medical chart. If you realize something later on that could have been done differently, it's OK to have that
thought, but don't put it in the chart. The jury will judge you on what
would have been done *then* according to reasonable standards, so don't
add what could have been done. You may have done what's defensible,
but there's still a bad outcome. You used good judgment. You can win
that. But if they see a doctored chart, they'll hold that against you, award
a higher amount, and set you up for punitive damages. You don't want
that.

She concluded with an adage on the screen: "A chart is a witness who
never lies and never dies." Then she opened it up for questions.

Dr. Ernesto Miguez asked what to write when something was not
done as ordered—blood analysis, for example. She said to write something like, "Lab work pending." If you point a finger, it'll point back.
Someone asked about being paged but not hearing it until it is repeated
later; and the chart will say the doctor was paged. She said if you are
concerned about that period of time, write that you were advised to see
the patient at such and such a time. That doesn't point fingers.

Dr. Wayne Denson said that physicians are under tremendous stress
when they face a lawsuit. He said he knew of one who died of a heart
attack while testifying, and another who suicided. He said an attorney
can be your best friend for a while. Do you know of any strategies for
dealing with stress? She said she didn't know of any support groups and
that we tell you you can't talk about it with your colleagues or business
partners. You'll have to tell who you talked to and they'll go ask them
questions about what you said. Talk with your family, but attorneys don't
want to spend time listening. No conversation is protected, except between you and your attorney, priest, or psychiatrist. Talk to them and
your family. Only those are legally protected. You can talk with colleagues about the fact that you've been sued, but I'm not aware of any
strategies to help you that won't come back to hurt you.

Azi Torres said she was slowly preparing to meet Jeff in California. "I no
go there without Jeff working first. His mother said she would send him
money for an apartment, but she never send. He took applications in

Seattle, but now he is stuck two hours away in the camping ground. He told his mother he is supposed to get work in Seattle, but he never get back there because he could not leave the campground without pay, so he lost opportunity to work. She try to prove point. If he no work will come back. But he no want come back right away. This is very hard time for him. He applying for work, but not much work in recreation management. He tried store, like REI, Home Depot. They didn't have anything available. And they want experience. I think that's Jeff's problem, no experience. His last job, who gave him job was relatives. Another job, he was related to the owner."

Azi said she moved Jeff's belongings and most of hers from a small storage unit to a large one. Both James and Kenneth helped. "I have two great guys. I'm lucky. I have no family, so have friends that are important." Kenneth still did not know the full story of Azi and Jeff. "I told Kenneth I'm traveling with Jeff for a while in the West. I don't know if I come back or exactly what I'll do there. I no go and risk living in the car with a baby. Very cold there and no playing with this. If he no do anything, I visit and find a lawyer and get on with my life. I got to leave this apartment anyway in two weeks. Kenneth is moving."

Azi also revealed that the visit she had made to Piedmont Hospital the year before—when she felt she had been treated poorly because she was a foreigner on Medicaid—was for a miscarriage. Earlier, she had simply said she had abdominal problems. "I knew I was pregnant, and I get sick sick. I could not walk. I lost twelve pounds. One day I start to bleed and my friend said it might be a miscarriage. Some peoples took food to me, almost a month. Jeff feel guilty because he work and couldn't help me very much. I did forgive him to that. He should be with me more after work, buy food, and bring to me more. I could not make food to eat. I felt like old people that somebody left, and they are about to die and no have anybody to take care. I never told my family. If my family know really what happen, they gonna hate Jeff. He's a damn stupid guy sometimes. And his family try accuse me, they ask me why you get pregnant? Was accident, both times."

This second accident, however, produced a child, upon whom people—in grocery stores, in parks—would remark that he looked exactly like the father and hardly a bit like Azi. After a while, Azi became weary of it. "All the time they throw this in my face. The man who come fix things in the apartment. 'He look just like his father.' "

"I wasn't real happy because I didn't know if it was going to be a black or Mexican baby." In the living room of her home, Jan Dorman's mother, Teresa, talked about when she first learned of Jan's pregnancy. "I didn't particularly want her to be black, you know, but it doesn't matter now at all." She chuckled lightly. "I just love her. When Jan found out it would be the black baby, she didn't call for a while. I guess she thought I would be unhappy. And now it doesn't matter."

Teresa also recalled the change in Jan's attitude when she tested positive for HIV. "I've been expecting it for a long time, but when I heard it, it was still a shock. You hope you never have to hear it, even when you think you probably will." She laughed again. "I'm sure she's told you the kind of lifestyle she was leading. You just pretty much expect it. She had a street kid attitude, real tough, and now she's a lot more sensitive. You feel like you could get closer to her, you know what I mean? But it was self-protection, a lot of it. She's had a hard time.

"I think she's kinda in denial. She doesn't want to face it 'til she has to. A couple of months ago she said she wanted to have one more baby, and I told her, 'Jan, you don't have that right. It's playing Russian roulette with another person's life.' She knows deep down she's gonna face it. She doesn't talk about HIV very often. And I don't want to bring it up too much. I don't know if she's ready. Some of Jan's relatives won't see her. They're so afraid of HIV. They won't educate themselves. I don't see how they can watch TV and not learn something."

She gently ran her fingers through the baby's hair. "I've kept her here a few times, like I brought her home from the hospital. I've kept her four times since then just so Jan can get some rest. Her body's been through so much. I don't want to keep her too often because she needs to have bonding time. Really deep bonding happens in the first few months."

She said the baby, so far, was healthy and, she hoped, free of HIV. "They have to ask the parents' permission to give AZT. Jan was kinda scared to, and I told her, 'What if she does have HIV? You may live long enough for a cure and the baby may not. How would you feel if you refused her medicine?'

"I feel bad now about some of the feelings I had earlier about the father being black, because now I love her like she was my own. There's no difference at all. It seems like a petty thing I was taught growing up. My husband was not warm to the baby at first, but by now, he's eager to hold her and be with her." She stroked the baby's light-brown skin. "She'll probably darken up some, and then when she starts playing in the sun, she'll tan, I'm sure. But she's a beautiful baby. And she's serious. She doesn't grin—like my other grandchild who when you talk to her, she grins—but she listens. She'll lay there folding her hands and just look around. People don't tend to think of babies as humans, and they are human. My other grandchild, when she wants attention, she sits there a while, then cries, but Deanna"—she called Jan's baby by her name—"she cuts loose. Right from the start, she cries hard."

Teresa said she was not happy when she learned Jan would be going to Grady Memorial Hospital. "This may seem small-minded, but I knew it was mostly black. That's the reason. But my mother-in-law read they were one of the top ten in the nation, but I think that was only for the ER. I wasn't real happy about it. But Jan found out Dr. Holcomb is supposed to be real good with HIV; I was happy about that. The first and third shift I was happy with, but not that second shift. I kept telling the nurses that Jan's stomach didn't look right. We're just regular people. We have enough sense to know that if the red is rising and it's hot, something is wrong. That nurse kept saying, 'It just looks like a reaction to the Benadryl or tape.' We kept on, and she finally said, 'I'll call a doctor.' She obviously made him think it was a rash or the Benadryl without seeing her, so he must have taken her word for it. The infection got worse. If the doctor had come and seen what we saw, her care would have been different. They would have given an antibiotic or something. That second shift, I guess, well I don't guess. She experienced some prejudice about her being with a black guy. It was real obvious. The looks and unfriendliness. Jan would say she needed pain medicine, and they wouldn't bring it. I told 'em and TD told 'em she needed pain medicine. Then her boyfriend would come and raise Cain about it and then they'd jump; they'd do their job, but they'd be looking at him like they hated his guts. I watch eyes. I can tell a lot from eyes, and they did not like it. And she needed ice for her vagina, and they wouldn't bring ice. The first and third shift were great about it."

Thirty years ago, Grady Hospital would have been in a quandary trying to determine on which side of the hospital to place this baby. Jan would have been taken, certainly, to the front side, and had only white nurses. Carl, if he had been a patient, would have been taken to the back side, and had only black nurses. The hospital had two completely separate sides then. On which side would they have put a baby with a white mother and black father?

Black Appendicitis
White Appendicitis

Dr. Roy Bell answered the phone at his dentistry office and was told a colored woman died at Grady because she was not treated. Bell had no proof it was true, but he believed it. In 1961 Atlanta, the truth of a particular story was not as important as the oppressive grind of segregation, which Dr. Bell faced, and despised, every day. "That was the starting point," he says now. "It was very personal. Grady Hospital, to Atlanta, was a very image of the power structure of Georgia. It was just unthinkable. How can something like this be turned around?" Bell had also been stirred by a chance meeting with a Negro public health trainee from New York. Bell innocently asked, "How do you like Atlanta?" He answered, "I hate it." He recounted how he had been barred from eating with the other, white trainees at Grady Hospital.

Bell was not the first black Atlantan to question Grady's segregation. In 1919 the Atlanta NAACP wrote an open letter to the city protesting the exclusion of black doctors from Grady. Over the years, black doctors had in countless informal ways mentioned to Atlanta whites that a segregated hospital was unwise. But when the "new Grady," which is now called "old Grady," was built, in the mid-1950s, it would have been illegal to build it without separate facilities. Built in the shape of a giant three-dimensional H lying on its back, two identical towers rising sixteen floors into the sky, Grady Hospital had two ERs, two waiting rooms, two Labor and Delivery wards, two surgery departments, two registration areas, two everything—identical, except for color of skin. In fact, before the "new Grady" was built, the hospital had in effect been two Gradys, two wooden buildings facing each other across Butler Street, with a tunnel under the street in case someone needed to cross from the white world to the black world, or perhaps the reverse—which is why even now an Atlantan might be heard saying, "I'm going to the Gradys."

In 1958, when "new Grady" was finished, Ernest Vandiver was elected governor of Georgia. His campaign slogan, referring to the number of black children he would allow in Georgia's white public schools, was "No Not One." By 1961, when Bell received the phone call about Grady, the tremors of opposition to white-imposed segregation were rumbling more and more ominously. The Student Nonviolent Coordinating Committee (SNCC) and other black student groups formed, proposing tactics more radical than those of the powerful older black generation of Atlantans, who had forged a nonconfrontational working relationship with Atlanta's powerful whites. The elder black leaders knew how to get certain things for the black community, in exchange for certain things. They knew when to push, when to ask, when to compromise. They had forged an uneasy relationship with Atlanta's white civic and business leaders that had brought some benefits to the black community without the violence that troubled other southern cities. And they often were put off by militant students who made radical demands. Between these two generations in age, Bell favored the students and their more aggressive methods, a choice which could endanger one's standing in polite society—white or black.

Bell was an intellectual, reflective man with a precise command of words, but when his anger pinpointed a target, he moved—fast, rash, alone, even if ridiculed by his peers. His longtime friend, Xernona Clayton, Southern Christian Leadership Conference associate of Coretta Scott and Martin Luther King, introduces Roy Bell of the early 1960s by telling about one blot on the record of an otherwise admirable Atlanta mayor, Ivan Allen Jr.: the Peyton Road "Berlin" Wall.

Atlanta's growing black population was restricted by segregation to an inadequate supply of real estate. The board of aldermen, for example, would often zone a "buffer" area "commercial" simply to stop the growth of black neighborhoods. (Even now, in areas where black and white neighborhoods once nearly met, few north-south connector roads exist.) A 1929 law prevented a person from moving to a street where the majority of residences were occupied by members of a race with whom the potential buyer was forbidden by law to marry. In the 1940s the Atlanta Planning Commission proposed (but never enacted) a plan for a highway through a park to be bordered by fences to keep the park segregated. When blacks began looking beyond their restricted areas for homes, residents of white neighborhoods near black neighborhoods became nervous, then panicked, as they feared the presence of one black resident would ruin their residential havens. An opportunistic real estate agent could spread rumors that a home had "gone colored," buy houses cheaply from fleeing whites and resell them at a profit. Blockbusting, it was called. It took only one purchase, or hint of a purchase, to start a stampede.

Peyton Road connected white and black neighborhoods, in a region of Atlanta where some blockbusting had occurred. A white neighborhood association, trying to protect their racial homogeneity, proposed to Mayor Allen and the Atlanta board of aldermen that Peyton and nearby Harlan Road be barricaded. With those two roads blocked, driving from one area to the other would be inconvenient. They'd stay on their side; we'd stay on our side. No more white flight panic. The barricades were eventually approved by mayor and board, the official reason being to maintain stability.

The tactic was futile, arrogant. Stop a burgeoning black population with a barricade that blocked two roads? A year and a half before, the Berlin Wall had been erected in Germany, and Atlanta's version came to be known, as incredulous reporters from newspapers all over the country continued to call, as "Atlanta's Berlin Wall." The East Germans at least knew how to build a *barricade*. It kept people out, and in. These two Atlanta barricades were nothing more than a slap in the face of every black person in the city. Picketing began immediately at City Hall, as well as at the barricades. A lawsuit was filed, calling the barricades illegal and arbitrary. Many blacks began a "selective buying campaign" designed to boycott West End businesses that supported the barricades. Picketers held signs announcing, "We Want no Warsaw Ghetto—Open Peyton Road." During the Christmas season, white residents decorated the Peyton Road barricade with Christmas paper and ribbons. Someone wrote "Thank the Lord" under the "Street Closed" sign. In February white residents discovered a hole in the wooden barricade. Angered, they chopped down trees and underbrush and used them to cover the hole. Police heard reports the KKK were on their way to the barricade, but the Klansmen never appeared, and the city rebuilt the torn portion of the wall. Mayor Allen said he deplored the fact that "anyone or any group has seen fit to take the law into their own hands."

Who would do such a thing?

For Mayor Allen, the barricades became an embarrassment. Even some whites in the Peyton Road area were annoyed by the extra five miles they had to drive to work or to the grocery store. Because of the barricades, *Atlantic Monthly* nearly canceled its glowing feature article, "Retreat of the Rednecks: Progress Goes Marching Through Georgia." The barriers stayed up for only three months. Eventually, a judge ruled them unconstitutional. (Lawyers for the city had argued that it was not unconstitutional for the city to barricade public roads like Peyton and Harlan because once the city voted to barricade them, the places where the barricades went up were no longer public.) The day of the ruling, Mayor Allen had a crew at the barricades, radio in hand. Twenty minutes after the ruling was handed down, the barricades were gone.

But during those three months, black Atlantans, whose support was crucial to Allen's election, seethed. An Atlanta minister says now, "We were shocked, even more because it was Mayor Allen. Nothing had happened here like that before." One prominent black minister said at that time, "These are the darkest days I've seen in Atlanta as far as race relations are concerned. Atlanta is the first town in the South to build barricades across public streets." Crowds had gathered by them, to talk about the latest court ruling on the barricades, or about the second vote by the city council on the barricades—which had kept them standing.

No one fumed more than Roy Bell, a respected, well-paid medical professional whose town was largely off-limits to him. Before the barricades came down, Bell had had enough. He drove his yellow Cadillac through one of them. "It was silly," he says now, but many black Atlantans approved. Bell did not make the papers; word spread person to person. Constance Currie, who worked at the Atlanta Anti-Defamation

League, heard the word passed down the halls, "Roy Bell drove through one of the barricades," and a cheer went up in the office.

Some black leaders heard about the incident and were skeptical, wondering if the tale was apocryphal. They thought, "It's a major barricade. You can't drive through it. He might have driven around it. . . ."

Bell's response? Chuckling, he says now, "It dented up my Cadillac a little bit, but I made it through."

After the disturbing phone call, Roy Bell's target was Grady Memorial Hospital. Bell and other young black professionals in their early forties, eager for the end of segregation, were chronologically and tactically between the two vastly different generations. Bell's generation was more forceful than their seniors but less explosive than the students. Activist college students fiercely and publicly demanded immediate change; their elders arranged deals in private meetings. Atlanta's public transportation was integrated, for example, by a lawsuit engendered not by a boycott by Atlanta's blacks, but the arrest of black leaders who had boarded a bus and sat defiantly in the "whites only" section, an arrest that was fully coordinated by Atlanta's white chief of police. The arrest and lawsuit had been planned at a meeting of Atlanta's white and black power structures. The students, on the other hand, picketed, sat in, boycotted, and demanded the end of segregation with no regard for the cooperation of such white leaders. The gulf between the generations was so wide that a Student-Adult Liaison Committee was formed to facilitate communication between the students and the dignified older black leaders. Roy Bell, drawn to his elders by his intellect and savvy, was eventually drawn to the students by his intemperance and impatience.

Bell simply demanded that he be heard; he marched into places, alone, and expressed his rage. Journalist Hal Gulliver recalls Bell speaking at a legislative committee hearing that had been announced as "open to the public." "It was possible," Gulliver says, "for a candidate to run a big ad in the paper saying, 'Come meet the candidate,' and everybody understood it meant black people were not invited, and the people that ran the ad wouldn't even give it a thought. They just made the assumption that everybody understood it would be just white people who came. Bell went down to the state capitol to the hearing and testified. It was startling to all the legislators, who were all white. There was a lot of courtesy in that time that is hard to explain. Even though people were very segregated, there was also a lot of civility at some levels. These legislators, while totally stunned, treated Bell with great courtesy. He said I understand there's going to be testimony, and I want to testify and the chairman probably swallowed but said, Dr. Bell, would you please be seated, explain who you are and why you want to testify. That became a major news story, 'Black Dentist Testifies Before Committee.' " Reporters asked Bell how he had the courage to speak before them, and Bell turned on his charm. "He was really bright, witty. He said, 'Well, I was sitting down this morning having breakfast with my wife and I heard on the radio that this committee was going to take testimony, and I told my wife I'd go down to the state capitol and testify.' "

Bell's independence could be frustrating, even to his own compatriots. A plan might be carefully set by a group of civil rights workers, only to have Bell spontaneously create his own plan, sometimes compromising their efforts by his wildcat tactics. He says of himself now, "I was out of control."

Student activist Charles Black recalls, "He was one of the few black professionals who was supportive of the students. He knew what he was talking about, but he was very impatient, radical, to say the least. Bell was not of our generation, though he was at least as radical as we were, so he appeared even more radical. He gave advice, loaned his car for travel, donated money. His being a dentist, identifying with the students was important to us. But he was sometimes not satisfied with the pace of things. We had very democratic committees; we'd meet sometimes two or three times a day. There wasn't a place for a maverick like Bell; he wanted to act quickly and on his own. He would have what he had to say, and we would have what we had to say. We made it clear we spoke for ourselves, though we were supporting him. Bell would say, 'We gonna do such and such' without us necessarily saying we were going to do that. We had to clarify that sometimes."

A white doctor who supported the student movement says of Bell, "He was always saying inflammatory things. One big debate was whether to infiltrate or confront. Bell wanted to confront. He was very aggressive, like he had a chip on his shoulder. He treated me like dirt because he was so hostile to anybody white, no matter what they were. He was civil but very hostile." Black saw the hostile Bell also: "He did react bitterly to whites. He was crude, I thought. He was not concerned about anybody else's feelings."

Jondelle Johnson, a civil rights activist who later became director of the Atlanta NAACP, says about Bell, "He had no finesse, at a time when it was dangerous not to. We had problems with the police, the Klan, but he didn't care. He said what he wanted to say and did what he wanted to do. He jeopardized his family and his practice. Most of us feared for our lives, but he went beyond the limits the rest embraced. He would go anywhere. Everybody said he was crazy. There was a way of doing things so not to alienate the whites, but Roy did it his way. Quite a few blacks didn't want to associate with him, for fear it would jeopardize what they had." But Johnson also says about him, respectfully, "He was well-read. He was brilliant. He was one of my heroes. I guess he was ahead of his time."

Bell even turned on the SCLC when he felt it was necessary. Once he publicly accused the civil rights organization of changing its tactics due to their acceptance of money from New York governor Nelson Rockefeller, and once he said they were exploiting Martin Luther King Jr.'s image. Again and again, Bell's friends would hear of yet another outrageous deed of his and shake their heads. What would he do next? There he goes again. White Atlanta leaders considered him an irresponsible rabble-rouser. But he was smart.

"It was always humorous for me," he says, "to hear something like that because it helped the movement when men were goaded. 'The audacity of this colored boy.' Heh heh heh. 'I have never heard of such a thing! Preposterous!' Some of the people I confronted were arrogant, and they played right into my hands. They formed a perfect platform for outrageous dialogue. It made for good press coverage. As an adversary, strategically, sometimes you had to say outrageous things, but it's a different thing saying outrageous things and believing them."

Once Bell determined Grady Hospital would be desegregated, he was relentless. He might appear anywhere and say anything to bring attention to Grady. He went before the Atlanta City Council and called them killers and murderers for endorsing a policy that discriminated against sick black citizens. He addressed the Georgia legislature, and hounded mayoral candidates for their position on Grady. He telegrammed the Georgia Attorney General, suggesting that, as Emory Hospital was segregated, the Attorney General should give an opinion as to whether Emory University's tax-exempt status should be revoked. He sent a similar telegram to the Assistant Attorney for Civil Rights in the U.S. Department of Justice in Washington, D.C. Bell wrote many letters: to President Kennedy, President Johnson, the Presidential Civil Rights Commission, and city, county, and state politicians.

Obstetrician Dr. George Lawrence recalls once rescuing Bell from one of his protests: "Roy Bell lay down on the floor of the white Grady waiting room. A white man walked over and spit on him and Bell beat the S-H-I-T out of him. Bell was around two hundred pounds and over six feet tall. He went to jail and I got called to get him out. I called other doctors, and they didn't like him so much, so I went by myself and got him out. I said, 'You can't do this by yourself. We got to do this together.' "

But Bell could be respectful. In August 1961, before the Fulton County commissioners, he gave a logical, statistically well-researched plea. He said Grady's separate facilities lowered the quality of services for all, but particularly for Negroes. By having two hospitals in one, he argued, Grady is costing taxpayers too much money. He pointed out that there were no Negroes among the five hundred visiting medical staff. Atlanta, he said, has four thousand hospital beds, but only six hundred eighty of them for Negroes. The three private hospitals for Negroes were not fully accredited. "Please explain why public funds are used to operate two Grady technical schools," he pleaded, "neither of which admit Negroes?" He appealed to the county commissioners, the Fulton-DeKalb Hospital Authority (FDHA), which oversaw Grady, and "all responsible humane citizens, Negro and White, to immediately do something about these deplorable conditions." He said it should not be necessary to use court action and hoped they could settle the matter among themselves.

The Atlanta-based regional director of the U.S. Health, Education, and Welfare administration, Pete Page, who discreetly helped black doc-

210 Black Appendicitis White Appendicitis

tors desegregate Atlanta's hospitals, recognized that Bell's infuriating tactics could be good strategy: "He had a pattern of making some outrageous suggestion about what to do, sometimes making people very angry, which would elicit useful responses from people who would do something a little less explosive and more practical. He was different, but on balance he earned his way. He really did."

Bell decided to picket Grady every day possible, and for picketers he turned to the restless, energetic black student activists at Atlanta black colleges. They, however, had heard of the loose cannon Roy Bell and were leery. They were involved in desegregating lunch counters, hotels, restaurants, the state capitol; why include a public hospital in an already hectic schedule—especially if it meant trying to tame Roy Bell?

Morehouse College student Charles Black, director of the Committee on the Appeal for Human Rights (COAHR) and, later, editor and columnist for the *Atlanta Inquirer*, once, with James Foreman of SNCC, led a march to the state capitol in downtown Atlanta. En route, Georgia Governor Vandiver issued an executive order prohibiting picketing on state property while the legislature was in session—which it was. Confronted by Atlanta police empowered by the order, Foreman and a portion of the students turned around, as if to go back; Black led another portion on a circuitous route that ended at the capitol, where they found state troopers surrounding the capitol building, shoulder to shoulder, billy clubs in hand. Black walked forward and was shoved in the stomach with a billy club. He asked for an audience with the governor, the message was relayed inside, and the governor said he would see only Black and Foreman, who had worked his way around to Black's side. Black said to Vandiver, "We want you to rescind the executive order that outlaws picketing on state property, and we want you to issue a new one that outlaws segregation in the state of Georgia." Vandiver declined. "That's the most ridiculous thing I've ever heard," the governor snapped.

With such dramatic activities filling their lives, Black and other students didn't see joining Bell as very urgent. The hesitant students changed their minds when a small boy was hit by a car a half a block from their office, a ten-minute drive from Grady. They called the Grady ER and were asked the boy's race. They said Negro and were told there were no Negro ambulances available at the moment. Forty minutes later, an ambulance arrived. The students fumed, and many said, "This is a matter of life and death. Let's work with Dr. Bell." They joined the volatile Bell on the Butler Street sidewalks, sometimes picketing eight to ten hours a day, carefully avoiding any interruption of hospital services. Sometimes Bell had six students, a dozen; often it was him alone. More drastic actions were planned but not enacted, such as faking an emergency in the picket line and carrying the black person into the white ER. COAHR sent students to twenty-five churches to ask for donations and picketers. Black asked Negro citizens to report mistreatment at Grady so they could compile a list for future use, possibly for a lawsuit.

With demonstrations occuring all over Atlanta at restaurants and public accommodations, picketing at Grady recieved little press attention, most of it from the *Atlanta Inquirer*, which had been founded by civil rights activists. A typical headline in the *Inquirer*, which reported on a range of racial issues, was "Bank Maid Upgraded to Clerk." One ad in the *Inquirer* for United Dairies said, "Buy milk from the dairy that hires Negroes." During the Grady picketing the *Inquirer* ran a cartoon that featured a boxer with "NAACP" on his chest, knocking out a boxer whose chest was imprinted with "Segregated Hospitals." The caption said, "Forever the Champion." Bell repeatedly called the *Inquirer*, requesting that a reporter be sent down to Grady. In one story when the picketing first began, Bell said he hoped this was the first of a series of demonstrations all over the country. He held aloft a sign that said, "Disease and Death Know No Race—Give the Other One-third an Equal Chance to Live." Other signs said, "Forward Atlanta, Grady's Policy is Backward," "Grady Has 75% Negro Patients, 0% Negro Staff Physicians, 0% Negro Interns, 0% Negro Board Members, Why?" When Grady announced they might get their first Negro intern, the *Inquirer* reported that Bell, "Atlanta's crusading dentist," responded that having one intern would be tokenism, a ploy to avoid full integration.

Atlanta Constitution columnist Pat Watters interviewed Bell and wrote that Bell wanted someone with power to listen. He said Bell had been before the county commission, who listened but said they could not tell the FDHA what to do. The FDHA would not grant him a hearing.

Uninvited, Bell went to an FDHA meeting to speak. The FDHA said they would appoint a committee to look into the matter, but gave no date for the committee's report. Thereafter, they would respond to questions about desegregating Grady, with "We're working on it." Bell threatened to sue. He tried to meet with all five mayoral candidates; one responded, another sent a representative. Bell told Watters he had been falsely branded a radical troublemaker, had received vicious phone calls, and there appeared to have been some tampering with his car. Watters commented that he thought Bell's lack of bitterness remarkable. "Being heard is one of the most important of the things he wants," Watters wrote.

Bell also turned to a medium that decades later would become a powerful force: talk radio. For a time he conducted two weekly programs on two black-owned AM stations, and occasionally appeared on a talk show called "Open Line" on another. Black and white listeners called and responded to Bell's provocative rhetoric. On one show, he blasted Negro critics of the student movement, the Atlanta school board (including one Negro member), the Fulton County Commission, the Atlanta administration, and the black-owned *Atlanta Daily World* newspaper. One white caller asked why Negroes wanted to "punch in" where whites lived, and he explained how Negroes were cramped into a small area. One suggested Negroes deserved less because they paid less taxes, and Bell said racial discrimination kept them from owing more property taxes.

Often Bell's broadcast partner was surgeon Clinton Warner, who was as smooth and respectable as Bell was fiery and uncontrollable. Former State Senator Leroy Johnson, the first black elected to state office in Georgia after Reconstruction, says, "Warner was a stable, influential force, respected for the soundness of his approach. Bell was as opposite as night and day. He was a bull in a china closet. He was rash, boisterous, everything you can think of—that was Roy Bell. His goal was the same as Warner, but his methods were different. Warner's adversaries would accept his presentation on desegregation, and they would resist a presentation from Bell. Bell was irrational, unpredictable, good at verbal abuse." Despite his respectability, Warner was one of the few wealthy black professionals who supported the activist students, much as Bell did, providing money, transportation, and physical exams for movement workers. He was chosen Man of the Year in 1961 by the influential Butler Street YMCA, due in part to his support of the student movement. During breaks on their shows, Warner would often shake his head and say to Bell, "Why do you call them honkies? They know they are, and we know they are."

On one show Warner and Bell said there was a conspiracy to keep Negro doctors out of hospitals. Hospitals required membership in the local American Medical Association, but the local chapter would not accept Negroes. Bell said of Emory University residency programs at Grady, "White doctors practice on Negroes to get their training and later do not want to touch them or have them come through the back door or after their white patients leave." One white caller asked why Grady should be desegregated, and Warner answered, "There's no such thing as a black appendicitis and white appendicitis. There's just an appendicitis."

But inside Grady, the daily, hourly insults of segregation persisted.

Former Grady nurse Ernestine Kelsey remembers the resentment she felt when black employees got a letter from administration that read, "I am happy to announce that your salary has been increased by five dollars a month." "Not a week," she stresses, "a month. It wasn't worth the paper it was written on. He made a big deal in those letters about five dollars a month."

The author of those insulting letters, the hospital superintendent, Frank Wilson, was a gregarious man, a University of Georgia graduate, teller of hilarious stories, classic southern back-slapper, wily maneuverer among Atlanta's powerful whites. Former city councilman, former vice president of a lumber company, member of Druid Hills Baptist Church, he was credited with Grady's growth and impressive national reputation. He served a term as president of the Georgia Hospital Association. Known to favor white suits, a thin black tie, and white Panama hat, he was overheard by Ernestine Kelsey saying, "I'll die and go to hell before Grady Hospital is integrated." But he was politically astute. A white doctor who served his residency at Grady tells of Wilson once acceding to the black community: "One night Grady was jammed with people, and a black woman with a stroke was brought in. The policy then was that if someone like that could swallow, you could send them home. They told her family to take her home, feed her, clean her, have her move some to keep up her strength. They were shocked. 'You're not going to let her stay in the hospital?' But there were no beds. We got a call from Frank Wilson at midnight. He said to admit her. I told him there were no beds. 'Find a bed. We don't turn away school principals,' and he hung up on me. She was a black school principal with friends in powerful places. He responded to political pressure from somebody."

In September 1963, a Negro worker at Grady went to the colored laborers' cafeteria without her meal ticket. She sent for it, but the white supervisor called for a security guard, who roughed up the worker for forgetting her ticket. Almost three hundred workers—maids, aides, porters, housekeepers, kitchen helpers—signed a petition saying they would walk out if nothing was done. They included a list of grievances, among them that most made fifty cents an hour, less than half the federal minimum wage of $1.15. They were allowed to use only the basement bathroom, and only at specified times. Dr. C. Miles Smith, president of the Atlanta NAACP, presented the petition to Wilson, who agreed to open all restrooms to all workers and to hire a Negro supervisor for the laborers' cafeteria. Smith reported that Wilson was gracious to him. The security guard was fired. Wilson also said he would submit a pay increase suggestion to the hospital board.

That colored laborers' cafeteria, which Smith called a "segregated segregated cafeteria," was a cruel insult. There was a white cafeteria and a colored cafeteria, with their own degrees of higher and lower status; below them both was the colored laborers' cafeteria. A small, dingy place, it was the only dining area for the lowest-ranked workers in the hospital. Kelsey, who resented the smaller slices of meat on the colored side, says the laborers' meals were worse: "When they served roast beef, the whites had chunks. We had it thin like sliced bologna. If we got thin roast beef, the laborers' cafeteria got, maybe, grits and collard greens."

Under Wilson's administration, black nurses were addressed by title, "Nurse Kelsey." White nurses were addressed as "Miss," a small but nagging reminder that one counted more than the other. According to Kelsey, during a week-long site evaluation by a hospital accreditation agency, switchboard operators were instructed, for that week only, to refer to all nurses as "Miss," regardless of color. The hesitant operators were assured the previous policy would be restored after the evaluation. All that week, when a black nurse was paged as "Miss," Kelsey shook her head and thought, "This is stupid."

A white instructor in the Grady nursing school decided one day that it was foolish for her to teach the exact same class twice, once for white students and again for black students. She combined the two classes, saving time, until two city officials walked by the classroom, saw the mix of students, and demanded that they return to segregated classes. They did.

The *Inquirer* listed these reports from Grady personnel: Blacks had to make arm boards out of plywood, while the white side had custom-made boards. Blacks sometimes had to make chucks out of paper padding. They did not have enough blankets. Doctors still called black patients by their first names; whites they called Mr., Mrs., Miss. Blacks had a shortage of diapers while the whites had extras. Black patients without ready money, who had to wait on someone to bring money before they went home, were put on stretchers in the halls instead of being placed in empty rooms on the white side. Negro student nurses put their laundry in the chute on one day, whites on another. The Grady blood bank even had separate shelves for "black" and "white" blood.

Joseph Wilber has a gentle voice, a low chuckle rather like Lisa Dean's. Retired, he lives in a large home in the north Georgia mountains, overlooking a small lake. A graduate of Harvard Medical School, he began his residency training at Grady in 1954. He recalls seeing Negro patients served their food with only a spoon—no fork or knife. He saw Negro women asked to undress in a room full of people and asked to sit, unclothed, on an exam bed and wait. Local physicians made rounds at Grady each week—a contribution of time that carried some prestige— with the residents presenting cases to them. "Mr. Jones here was brought in last night," Wilber began one such round, "with a headache and nausea—"

"What did you say?" the local doctor asked.

He repeated himself. Three times the doctor asked him the same question, and three times he answered the same way.

"What's your name?" the doctor asked the Negro patient.

"Bill Jones."

"Dr. Wilber, you are no longer in Boston. To you, this man is Bill."

Wilber continued, refusing to disrespect Mr. Jones, "The patient came in last night with headache and nausea. . . ." The doctor glared at him.

Sometimes the insult was the exclusion of blacks from decisions that affected their lives. In September 1961, it was announced that a just-completed Negro nursing student dorm would be named "Mississippi Hall." At a time of intense civil rights activity, the new Negro dorm would be named after the most defiantly segregated state in the country, a state whose murderous backlash against desegregation was called in Howard Zinn's book on SNCC "special savagery," a state which Martin Luther King's friends would later beg him not to visit for fear of his life. A 1955 NAACP report on Mississippi was titled "M is for Mississippi and Murder." It was also announced that the existing Negro nursing student dorm would be renamed "Alabama Hall." Local black doctors protested. Grady officials denied that the dorms had been named yet, but the NAACP president called the Grady switchboard and asked for Mississippi Hall, and his call was transferred to the new dorm. Grady backed down, and the dorms were eventually called Piedmont Hall and Armstrong Hall, for the streets next to them.

While the marchers walked up and down Butler Street, one person watching them from inside the building was Rev. Charles Gherkin, head of the Grady chaplaincy. He came to Grady in 1957, just before the new building was completed. Gherkin, who had been born and raised in Kansas, asked the search committee if he would be chaplain to the whole hospital, not just the white side. The committee, which included Frank Wilson, assured him he would minister to all of Grady. Later, Gherkin wished he had gotten that assurance in writing. Soon after he arrived at Grady, Wilson summoned him to his office and said, "Them niggers over there don't want you. Stay on the white side of the hospital. Let the Negro preachers take care of them." At that time Grady was still two Gradys, on opposite sides of Butler Street. Gherkin, ignoring Wilson's instructions and Grady tradition, walked freely to the colored side, ministering to patients as they needed him. "Conditions on the black side were absolutely atrocious," he says. "They were so close together that when they did a procedure they had to pull that bed out into the aisle like a file drawer, then push it back."

Gherkin did agree to segregated worship. "I knew I couldn't have integrated services. Part of the agreement I made with the committee was that I would conduct services for blacks in the auditorium and whites in the chapel. But Wilson vetoed it and said I had to get black ministers to conduct services for blacks. So I contracted with a young black minister."

Gherkin once met with black nursing students to answer questions about chaplaincy. After several questions, a young student in the back raised her hand. "This was a real honest question," Gherkin recalls. "She was not a militant girl." He nodded to her, and she asked, "Do you think we're inferior?" He replied, "No, you are one of God's creatures, like everybody else."

Eventually, Wilson heard that Gherkin was not obeying him. He spoke with some pastors of white churches, to see if they could have Gherkin sent back to Kansas. "Fortunately, he approached the wrong ones," Gherkin says. They said they would not vote to fire him. "Over the years, we learned to have a certain respect for each other," Gherkin says of Wilson. "We of course disagreed. One day at lunch he said, 'Chuck, you mean you would like to have these Negroes up here eating in the same dining room as us?' I said, 'Sure,' and he just shook his head. He could not comprehend that."

Gherkin often looked out the window of his office and watched Bell, and others marching on Butler Street. His office was opulently furnished with antiques donated by a prominent white Atlanta woman. When Gherkin held meetings with students in that office, an administrator told him he had desecrated the donor's gifts by allowing students to sit on them. Amidst his fancy furniture, watching the protesters, Gherkin wondered, "Should I be out there?" "My conclusion," he says now, "was that I won't be able to do the job I was brought here to do. And, two, I think I can do more good for integration where I am. I've never been absolutely sure about that. I didn't go to Selma. . . ."

In February 1962, Roy Bell arranged a big event. A group of students was at a municipal courtroom, where a hearing was being held for eleven activists who had been arrested for demonstrating at the state capitol. After the hearing, Bell convinced many of them to walk over to Grady and conduct a sit-in. Twenty-three people, including Bell and Black, were arrested for disorderly conduct, for refusing to leave Grady when asked. The *Inquirer* reported that, singing, they were taken away in a paddy wagon. Students not arrested telegrammed President Kennedy and Atlanta Mayor Allen, protesting the arrests.

Bell says that while in jail they cleaned the place. "It was very dirty, smelly, so we decided we'd clean it up. We secured mops and brooms, hoses, and that jail has never been so clean. We sang; some had beautiful voices echoing throughout the whole cellblock, reverberating against the steel bars and walls in different tones and sounds in perfect harmony. It was like an opera, in quadrophonic sound. Beautiful."

Charles Black and another student eventually arranged a meeting with William Pinkston, assistant director of Grady. They prepared a presentation of their demands and their reasons for making them. Pinkston greeted them warmly and welcomed them into his office, where he had a surprise for them: Daddy King, Martin Luther King, Sr.—father of the famous preacher activist. Daddy King was one of the prominent older black leaders whom the student activists deemed too compromising. It was not uncommon for white leaders who were irritated with students to turn to leaders such as Daddy King for help. Black began explaining why they were protesting and what their demands were. They were interrupted by Daddy King, who told them not to kick a man when he's down. You're being too hard on Mr. Pinkston, he said. He has shown good faith, and he will do what is right. You need to give him time. Pinkston then called on King to say a word of prayer, which he did. The prayer ended the meeting.

"We got nothing accomplished," Black says. "I blame Daddy King for that."

A few years later, Black, as editor of the *Inquirer*, opined that a dinner meeting of civil rights activists to report on a boycott of downtown was hypocritical because it was held at the downtown Apparel Mart. Why spend that money downtown? Daddy King called him and chewed him out for forty-five minutes, demanding a retraction. Black replied that he would not retract the truth. King then demanded that Black pay them back for his meal ticket.

After the meeting with Pinkston and King, many students were demoralized. To push Grady further would require that they regroup and find ways to increase the pressure—in a battle that got little support from the black community and little visibility in the press. Black says, "It was a lonely vigil." And it was a vigil that was publicly associated with Roy Bell, the fierce man who might embarrass you if you stood next to him. The students returned to other demonstrations, and from then on, when Bell picketed in front of Grady, he marched alone. The *Inquirer* called Bell a "one-man gang" and "the militant dentist."

Grady was not Bell's only target. The local chapter of the American Dental Association (ADA) was closed to him due to segregation, and membership in the local chapter was a prerequisite to membership in the national body. He and another dentist presented a resolution at the National Dental Association, the association for black dentists, criticizing the granting of federal funds to segregated medical research institutions. They urged nonviolent action at the next ADA national meeting. Bell said that while the ADA called itself democratic, Negro dentists were educated and evaluated by ADA standards while being barred from membership in twelve states. Bell for three straight years picketed the Hinman Clinic, an annual dentists' scientific conference held in Atlanta that did not allow black dentists. He and a group of medical students picketed the meeting of the Georgia Dental Association. He sent a telegram to HEW protesting the president-elect of the ADA, who was from Atlanta, for being a member of a racist society, the GDA. He traveled to Miami, and picketed the national ADA meeting.

Two months after the arrests in the white waiting room, Bell, working with the NAACP Legal Defense and Education Fund, filed suit against Grady, to force the hospital to desegregate. Bell filed as a dentist who might potentially practice at Grady. He also put together the team of plaintiffs. One was Warner, who asserted he should have the same privileges as other Atlanta MDs. Ruby Doris Smith, a Spelman College student and SNCC activist, who had picketed Grady, sued as a potential patient and potential nursing school applicant who would want to attend on a nonsegregated basis. Five other persons were coplaintiffs, also as potential patients. They sued not only Frank Wilson and the FDHA, but the local and state chapters of the AMA and of the ADA for barring black members.

Ruby Doris Smith, a Grady baby whose mother had seven babies at Grady, was an activist from her first days at Spelman. Determined, an ardent believer in nonviolence, she was one of several protesters arrested and dragged from the state capitol, after being denied food in the cafeteria and sitting in in the governor's office. She also sat in at downtown restaurants. She was jailed for sit-ins in Rock Hill, South Carolina, and Jackson, Mississippi. In Jackson, she and the other protestors were taken after two weeks to Parchman State Penitentiary, where, when the women sang, guards took their mattresses away. They sang more, and their sheets were taken away; more singing, and their toothbrushes and towels were taken. The men were greeted at Parchman by sneering, spitting, swearing white guards who used cattle prods. In jail, Smith filled her day reading novels and the Bible, writing letters, singing freedom songs, and practicing ballet. In August 1960, she participated in "kneel-ins" in Atlanta churches. At First Baptist Church, she was denied admittance, then sat in a chair in the lobby and sang hymns with the congregation.

Before the suit was filed, there was a bit of intrigue within the NAACP between their Legal Defense and Education Fund and the legal counsel of the NAACP national office—two separate legal entities—over which would file the suit. Bell had been working with Jack Greenberg of the Legal Defense team when he received a phone call that sent him into quick action. Someone mistakenly told him about a meeting with the NAACP legal counsel to plan the suit, a meeting about which he was not supposed to know. He immediately called Greenberg and said, in a mock innocent tone, "You told me you were preparing a brief. Why would you send your people down here without contacting me?" Bell knew Greenberg was unaware of the other meeting, but this ploy let him know. It worked. Greenberg flew from New York to Atlanta the next day and the suit was filed. Bell had not lost his moment.

The defendants responded with a flurry of motions to dismiss the case. The dental association cited the freedom of association, claiming, "This is not a Constitution for the minority only." They added, "Private practices, however discriminatory, however repugnant, do not fall within the Constitutional ban on racial discrimination." Grady claimed the lack of black doctors was Emory's choice, not theirs, for Emory supervised the residency program. The medical associations reported that they had already rescinded a category of membership that had been particularly odious to black doctors: scientific membership. This category was created in 1952 to appease black doctors who wanted less to be a member of the local and state associations than to gain its benefits: membership in the national AMA, group malpractice insurance rates, privileges in Atlanta hospitals. Scientific membership involved no dues or voting privileges; it allowed admittance to scientific continuing education sessions but not to regular meetings or social gatherings. You may hear a lecture with us, the category communicated, but you may not sit down to a meal with us, or make decisions with us. Invitations were mailed to local black doctors; all declined. They said we'll accept full membership or nothing. The national AMA once advised the chapter to eliminate the scientific category, and an Atlanta member once made a motion that they follow that advice. The motion won in a secret ballot, but it was later voted down when more members were present. Influential black businessman Jessie Hill wrote the local white doctors' society and requested that at least emergency room services be nonracial. They responded: We defer to local hospital boards.

Conflict over scientific membership had led to one of Dr. Warner's arrests. (He would also be arrested in 1964 at a hotel sit-in.) In 1961 Warner and seven other black doctors were arrested at the Biltmore Hotel, at an educational meeting for physicians. The black doctors went to eat in the hotel cafeteria with the other doctors, and hotel management—to whom the white doctors had deferred on this decision—denied them entrance. We'd be breaking Georgia law if we had integrated dining, they said. Eight black doctors refused to leave the cafeteria. The police were called; the doctors were arrested for violating Georgia's anti-trespassing law. The black doctors who were not arrested were served lunch in the hotel's hospitality lounge by the Women's Auxiliary of the white doctors' society.

The scientific membership was a branch in a thicket of obstacles that prevented Atlanta's black doctors from practicing medicine fully. Lack of membership meant no hospital privileges. Black doctors seeking to join as full members were thwarted by the application for membership's requirement of two endorsement signatures from current members. Finding two white doctors willing to sign was a chore. The medical societies could truthfully claim no one had submitted a completed form. Similarly, some hospitals required two letters of recommendation with an application for privileges. Emory Hospital required doctors to be currently in a practice that already included Emory Hospital doctors. Well, all the doctors were white; their practices were all white. Some hospitals required donations to a building program. Some required doctors to practice in a certain area, while black doctors were segregated into limited parts of Atlanta.

In one deposition, Bell was asked if he had spoken with Frank Wilson about hospital privileges. He replied that he had, that Wilson was cordial but said, "Well, let's be frank with one another. I know what you want. You want to have Negro doctors controlling Grady Hospital and before I'll see Negro doctors down here, I'll die and go to hell." Bell said they both laughed; Bell said, "Well, we'll see," and left.

While the suit was being argued, other related actions were taken around the country. The NAACP picketed the national AMA meeting in Atlantic City and the AMA national office in Chicago. President Kennedy sent a telegram to the American Hospital Association urging them to address discrimination in hospitals. He also directed the Justice Department to associate itself with the NAACP in suits against federally-funded hospitals that discriminated. Some AMA chapters began asking the national AMA to revoke the membership of AMA chapters that were segregated. HEW held an all-day conference on the elimination of hospital segregation.

In late 1963, upset with the slow pace of change in Atlanta, a large group of blacks marched to Hurt Park, where Martin Luther King Jr., James Foreman of SNCC, and others, made speeches, proclaiming that they had only heard promises, editorials, and resolutions, but had seen no action. They called for better job opportunities, improved schools, a public accommodations law, and the desegregation of Grady. The march was coordinated by the Summit Leadership Conference, a coalition of civil rights groups. In spring 1964, the Summit Leadership Conference organized a "Sacrificial Easter," in which Negroes were urged to buy nothing more than food and medicine during Lent, so that white businesses would get the message that change must come soon. In a move that stunned student activists, on a Saturday afternoon one hundred black college faculty picketed Grady, and a group of doctors and dentists led a march through downtown Atlanta.

In early 1963, the local and state AMA chapters were dropped from the lawsuit. They had amended their bylaws to allow membership on a nonracial basis and presented to the judge a list of eleven black doctors, including Warner, who had been accepted as full members.

In May, Frank Wilson claimed in a deposition that though Grady hospital was segregated, no one was discriminated against. About the emergency room, for example, he said the "operation of nondiscriminatory but separate emergency treatment facilities for white patients and Negro patients is in the best interest of the patient care program at Grady Memorial Hospital and designed to preserve said patient care progam for the benefit of and in the best interest of the physical and mental health and well being of all patients at Grady Memorial Hospital irrespective of race." The phrase nondiscriminatory but separate appeared throughout depositions given on behalf of Grady. Explaining why the emergency room operator would ask for the race of someone needing an ambulance, he said they often called on private ambulance services when theirs were all in use, and those services were segregated, so the Grady operator would need to know the person's race, in case a private service was called upon.

Wilson did, after all, have the backing of the national publication of the American Hospital Association. In an issue of *Hospitals*, an administrator from Gary, Indiana, warned about the risks of desegregating hospitals. The professional staffs, he said, would, of course, cause no problems, because they can be depended on to recognize skilled people when they see them. What about Negro trustees? he asked. Since it's uncommon for Negroes to have the status required to be a trustee, there will probably be only one, and it's probable that any discriminatory decisions would be made in informal meetings when the Negro is not present. Prolonged use of this tactic would undermine the board of trustees, and that Negro might be called an Uncle Tom by the Negro community. So desegregating boards would be quite a problem. And in a hospital room, he warned, an elderly white woman with heart problems lying in an oxygen tent could be roomed with a Negro, and the white woman's husband might complain, "She doesn't like Negroes. She does not live with Negroes, and she does not want to start now. Her emotional condition will be aggravated by the presence of Negroes."

What do you do?

"To legislate that physicians and hospital staffs," he wrote, "ignore emotions in patients arising from any cause is to amend the historical right of medicine to make the patient's well-being its most important concern."

Or, he warned, since hospitals often room people together with similar interests—schoolteachers, carpenters—if, in the interest of nonracialism, they simply room people first-come-first-serve, ignoring the custom of rooming like careers together, there might be a scene at the door! Do we really want society's racial disturbances to come into the hospital? It is unfortunate, he bemoaned, that sick people will be asked to face these difficult problems.

The judge ruled against the dental association's request to dismiss, which was based on the right of a private association. He cited the role given the two associations by the state of Georgia to nominate members of three agencies that regulated dentists. They were, in his judgment, under color of law. The result was that only white dentists did the appointing and only white dentists were appointed. The action of excluding Negro dentists from its membership was state action and was a violation of the equal protection clause of the U.S. Constitution. The court added, however, that if not for this nomination procedure, the assocations "would have the undoubted right to admit only such persons as they desired, and could, without violating any law, exclude Negroes."

Soon, Warner and Bell began to notice a difference in their black colleagues, who, now that the judge was ruling continually for the plaintiffs, said they were in favor of what Warner and Bell were doing. Previously, they had been hesitant to associate publicly with sit-ins, arrests, picketing, and lawsuits. Some even said, "I was really for them all along." Reflecting on this change, Horace Ward, one of the plaintiffs' lawyers, now a federal district judge in Atlanta, says, "Mostly Bell was the furthest out of the dentists or the doctors, and they kind of let him go his own way for a while. But his cause began to come together, heh heh, so they joined with him in this lawsuit. He was a catalyst. He's the one that put this together and stuck with it."

The white power structure, as the city's most prominent business and political decision makers were called, also saw where the case was going. According to one black politician, they let Grady's administrators know theirs was a lost battle. Atlanta had made significant changes peacefully; they would not let a charity hospital ruin their image. So Grady began to desegregate piecemeal. First, the emergency rooms were made nonracial; a black intern was accepted; black chaplains were accepted; black doctors were accepted to the visiting staff to make rounds with residents; technician training facilities were made nonracial; the chapel became open to all persons at all times; the Grady card application office was integrated; then the individual clinics: pediatrics, cardiac, dental, surgery, and so on. White and Colored signs were removed from all doors. Black and white nurses wore the same color uniform and same style cap.

After the ER was desegregated, Bell said to an *Inquirer* reporter, "If they are sincere, they could have completely desegregated. The public shouldn't be lulled into thinking progress is made. I'm to appear before the Authority to renew my demands, and if they do not fully comply in thirty days, I will organize a full-scale protest demonstration at Grady. It's strictly an instance of too little too late."

Finally, in February 1965, the judge ruled that Grady must desegregate every aspect of its operation. Only two components remained segregated: patient rooms and nursing school dormitories. They had held out until the last those places where white and black would lie in bed near one another. Grady proposed that the dorms desegregate the next fall semester, in September, and that all rooms and wards in the hospital be filled on a nonracial basis by December 31. The plaintiffs accepted the dorms proposal and objected to the wards and rooms proposal. It was finally agreed by all to desegregate the wards and rooms by June 1.

All through the early 1960s Dr. Joseph Wilber, after finishing his Grady residency and practicing in Atlanta, had tried to change the minds of other white doctors. He once gave a speech to the St. Joseph's Hospital staff, arguing on moral grounds that they make an effort to integrate. At the time, Atlanta was experiencing a hospital bed shortage, which made for a handy excuse: "It's hard enough now, if someone has a bleeding ulcer in the middle of the night, to find a bed. You have to call three or four places. If we add more doctors to the staff. . . ." When all Atlanta hospitals, public and private, were eventually forced to integrate, Wilber suggested the hospitals set up orientation sessions for new black doctors to make them feel welcome. He was usually met with silence or, "Why should they get special treatment?"

Wilber joined the black doctors' association but could barely stay awake in meetings. White doctors had day schedules, but black doctors saw patients from eleven in the morning until around one in the afternoon, took most of the afternoon off, and saw patients in the evening. Their professional meetings started at eleven at night. "They saw patients at the *patient's* convenience," Wilber learned, "during lunch hour or after they got off work." Why? There were no guaranteed job benefits for most blacks. Those who worked for whites were often fired if they missed work to see a doctor.

"I kept at it for five or six years," Wilber says of his civil rights work. "It became clear there were a few pioneering black doctors who would go through the hassles and do it on their own with no help from anybody. It became clear to me that they wanted to do it themselves without any white people involved. I felt pushed out. 'Joe, you're a nice guy, but. . . .' I got tired. So then I joined a dialogue club. Blacks and whites met once a month in couples' homes. We'd eat dinner and discuss issues. I did that for five months. They were real fun, real good. Then toward the end of the seventies, integration was no longer a goal. It's still my goal, but by then everything was opened up—restaurants, movies. Blacks were not as interested in integration but in doing it on their own."

In the white medical society, Wilber said, about five or ten percent were "down deep virulent racists. Most didn't care much about it. They didn't ostracize me. They just pretty much ignored me. Maybe behind my back they called me a nigger lover. The attitude about keeping the black doctors out was sub rosa. No one talked about it. If I asked them why there were no blacks in the society, they'd say no one ever applied. Or they might mention Roy Bell. He was the epitome of what they didn't want on the staff. 'What about that guy Bell? We don't want him on the staff.' " Wilber said they also were leery of Otis Smith, a black pediatrician and a cohort of Bell. "Smith was another firebrand. He spoke pretty rough. Otis Smith was a pain. At times, Bell was a bastard."

But Bell ran for public office. While Grady was desegregating piecemeal, before the judge's declaration that the hospital must fully desegregate, Bell ran for state Senator, against the popular Leroy Johnson. Bell had been a leader of the Fulton County Young Democrats, but for this race he became Republican, which brought instant endorsement from the Republican-leaning black newspaper the *Atlanta Daily World*, along with financial support from the *Daily World's* publisher. In its endorsement, the paper said Bell would show more interest in the masses of the voters and take stronger stands against unjust laws, and that, as a Republican, he would not be subject to pressure from the party leadership. They praised his courage "to take unpopular stands against what he considered wrong." They pushed for two-party involvement in the Negro community. An ad mentioned that Bell received a 1964 award from the black doctors' National Medical Association for "brave and outstanding service to those he served so well." At a rally Bell deplored how local leaders had distorted the image of the Republican Party. He said, "I'll serve with honesty, integrity, and dignity."

Johnson says that Bell continued his maverick ways in the election. "Bell made wild derogatory statements about me, then when he would greet me face to face, he would be friendly and extend his hand as though he had said nothing. He was very irresponsible in his statements and demeanor. You expect a level beyond which no one would descend, but for Roy Bell, there was no level. To him, I represented some kind of authority figure, a power. He was a warrior that wanted to attack any and all that represented authority and power, white or black. I was perceived to have a great deal of power, but I had little real power, just the perception. If he could knock me off, he would be the most powerful black figure in Atlanta. That's what he wanted." Johnson worried none about not getting the *Atlanta Daily World's* endorsement. "They would support an elephant over a Democratic Gandhi," he said. "Bell indicated he was a Republican, and they bought it." Black Republicans were strong in Georgia before the national Democratic Party became firmly associated with civil rights and the Republican Party with opposition to them. In fact, in Kennedy's 1960 victory over Nixon, Nixon received the majority of the black vote in Atlanta.

But, Republican or Democrat, Bell had an image problem. Black says, "Bell had no chance. He had no base of support outside the students. The older generation didn't support him. The younger professionals admired his steam, but thought he was too radical." Bell tried to use his crusade against Grady as a means to get votes. At a Frontiers International Club meeting, Bell told of the events leading to Grady's desegregation as an example of what one man can do. Johnson replied that other people were involved too, not just one man. He showed the names of all the plaintiffs, whom Bell had brought together. He refused to debate Bell, who "wants publicity at my expense." Johnson said he was getting no money from the Democratic Party, but Bell was getting "Goldwater money" from the Republican Party. Johnson said he had ended segregation of summer highway jobs. Bell said he would go to Washington and demand that no federal funds go to segregated institutions. "I will put shoes on black feet and clothing on their back," Bell said.

The *Atlanta Inquirer*, which had lauded Bell's activism, endorsed Johnson. They cited his experience, accomplishments, and sensitivity to the needs of his constituents. They said "the opposition" has easy talk and promises but nothing better to offer. They said Bell was less qualified in knowledge and temperament. Johnson trounced Bell by a 7–1 margin. The next year Bell ran for state representative and was soundly defeated in the Republican primary.

Leroy Johnson says now about his opponent, "Bell was a good soldier for picketing, for harassing the enemy, for causing some frustration for the enemy. He was one you put on the front lines to do the agitating, then when things get agitated, someone like Andrew Young would step in and speak reason to reasonable people for reasonable solutions."

Journalist Watters, who wrote complimentarily about Bell, thinks similarly: "You want him on the front lines, but you don't want him in government after the revolution."

When May turned to June, Grady Hospital performed as instructed. Black and white patients were moved so that rooms and wards were no longer segregated. A seminar had been held on how to handle white patients who resisted, but there was little resistance. A few whites checked out; one nurse recalls an instance in which a female white patient undressed, donned a gown, and, when a black doctor entered the room, screamed and ran down the hall. *Atlanta Inquirer* reporters toured Grady as rooms were desegregated. They observed white and black patients exchanging cordial greetings. They called it "the Tuesday that was" and reported that Pinkston announced, "All phases of Grady are nonracial as of today," but quoted Bell saying, "Since Mr. Pinkston's concept of brotherhood is the same as that of a dollar, I will withold further comment until I can take a personal inspection tour." Later in June, the *Inquirer*, through its sources inside Grady, reported that some white doctors had problems with integration. One white woman raised a fuss when placed with a Negro woman, saying she would not sleep with a nigger. She was moved to another room. Later, another Negro woman was placed in her room; she requested to be moved, was not moved, and she checked out. Chaplain Gherkin had his interns circulate the hospital to defuse any conflict. "I remember going to the ER," he says, "and there were ambulance drivers at a gathering place out there when not out on a call, and I went down to see how they were doing." He remembered that in earlier conversations he had heard them talking about the "rhesus factor," that blacks were the way they were because they came from rhesus monkeys. "But the amazing thing, since integration had become the company line, was they dealt with patients by saying well, this is the way it is. I don't think what they thought privately had changed one iota, but they responded to authority." In July, Bell conducted his inspection and commended Grady for their progress, but said the Negro cafeteria was all Negro, and the white cafeteria had only a sprinkle of Negroes. He also reported that on many wards the nurses were still segregated, whites on one side and Negroes on the other. He said Negro doctors were not utilized to their maximum capacity, and Negro patients still had a "C," for "colored," on their records. He announced that, given the even more segregated condition of Atlanta's private hospitals, perhaps it was time for federal pressure to be applied. As it turned out, that would be his next battle.

In September, the nursing school opened for the fall semester, and the school's administrators had decided that since they had to assign rooms on a nonracial basis, they'd just do it alphabetically. They announced the policy to the students and said that after six months they could change roommates if they wanted to. Bernice Dixon, one of those school administrators, tells this story now and adds, with a tinge of sadness and hurt in her voice and on her face, "A few changed, mostly blacks choosing black roommates. We had a meeting with the white students and told them this was the fairest way to do it. We let them ventilate. There was no anger, some fears. The black students were more disturbed and concerned than the white students. They had a tendency to segregate themselves. We continued the separate graduations and yearbooks for two years, for those already there. The black nurses started the Black Grady Nurse Conclave for alumni, which also granted black scholarships. We worked hard to have one alumni association, but they plain segregated themselves again."

Before all that happened, a year and a half before Grady was fully integrated, several months before they began the piecemeal desegregation, Superintendent Frank Wilson, the man who had said he would die and go to hell before he'd see Grady integrated, had a heart attack and died.

Gherkin called Pinkston, then the interim Grady superintendent and eventually the new superintendent, and said, "We're going to have a memorial service for Frank, and I'm not going to have a segregated service."

"There was a good long pause," Gherkin recalls. "Bill is basically a good guy, raised in south Georgia, a good Presbyterian, and value-wise I think his heart was in the right place. Finally, he said, 'Do what you want to do.'" Gherkin told him he wanted to have two services, one at each shift change. The service would be announced over the hospital-wide intercom, with nothing said about race. "Again there was a long pause, and he said, 'Let's do it.' And that's what happened. The blacks and whites came together, in the chapel on the white side of the hospital. I insisted on that. That was the first integrated worship service we had. You'd think they'd come only if they have a certain respect for the man. If he's dead, there's no penalty in not coming. I never asked them why they came. I thought that was interesting.

"I read Scripture and prayed. The key phrase in the prayer, a prayer of thanksgiving, was, 'We thank thee for all that was good that came from the life of Frank Wilson.' And the ones that knew where I stood and had their own negative feelings about him knew exactly what I meant. It went right over the heads of the others."

Grady Hospital, the local medical society, and the state medical society all desegregated and were released from the lawsuit. Schools, restaurants, and hotels desegregated. Civil rights laws were passed and enforced. The future trend, it appeared, was clear. Facing the possibility of being forced to accept Roy Bell's application, the state and local dental societies, however, fought on. Bell recognized the personal nature of his rejection: "When you're the one carrying the flag," he says now, "you are the target. You come to expect it; you just do it and pay the price."

In court, Bell again found his controversial reputation used against him. Didn't some black dentists say you were not a good person to integrate the white dental societies? the lawyer asked. Isn't it true the black dentists' society disapproved of your picketing? Bell produced a resolution from the black dentists' society endorsing his picketing activities. He said he had never been charged with a felony, only one misdemeanor for his sit-in at Grady Hospital. To illustrate his contention that his exclusion harmed his practice, he said that in January 1965, the Northern Dental Society established a twenty-four-hour emergency dental hotline, but only NDS members could participate, so Negro dentists were not only denied the opportunity to reach new clients, but faced with the real threat of losing current clients. Bell said it was an attempt by white dentists to monopolize dentistry in Atlanta.

Bell was forced to admit that he had not submitted a completed application; he lacked the two endorsement signatures from current members. He replied that the one dentist he had asked declined and he had no intention of going to every white dentist in the city. Bell testified that the one dentist he asked, an oral surgeon, said if he signed the application, he would risk losing referrals from colleagues. The defendants' lawyer objected to Bell referring to his clients' organization as a "white society," so Bell called it "the alleged white society." Bell was challenged on his allegation that the white societies had a "custom and practice" of disallowing black dentists. He was asked "how a group can be said to have a custom or practice with respect to a certain act when they have never received such an application." For example, the lawyer continued, "If no one from Alaska applied and no one from Alaska was in the association, would you say that they don't have the custom of accepting Alaskans?" Bell answered, "That would depend on whether they are black Alaskans or white ones."

The judge ruled for Bell, agreeing with the main charges, and saying "The court finds there was a custom and usage upon the part of the officers and members of the Northern District Dental Society to admit only white dentists, that Negro dentists (except in one isolated instance) were unable to obtain endorsements." He allowed the injunction disallowing the society's discriminatory practices. But it wasn't over. Several months later, Bell returned to the judge and reported that he called the executive secretary and requested an application but was told applications couldn't be mailed because the bylaws required that an applicant be proposed by a member. Bell charged that it was more difficult than before for black dentists to join the society, because they would have to seek out members of the society to propose them as members. He said this caused him irreparable harm and damage in terms of humiliation and embarrassment, deprivation of the opportunity to develop professional skills, and denial of the opportunity to participate in choosing governmental officials for the state of Georgia. "They are doing this to me because I initiated the suit," he concluded.

The judge ordered the dental society to hand Bell an application, allow him time to get the endorsement signatures, and evaluate him in the same manner they would anyone else. Finally, they did, and Bell became a member.

Bell had driven through Atlanta's Berlin Wall. He had sued Grady Hospital, two local medical societies, and two state medical societies. He had run for public office. Next, he would take on the federal government.

Bell and other black dentists and physicians in Atlanta and around the country knew that there was one leverage tool that could quickly elicit cooperation from the most determined segregationist hospital: not moral clarity, not statistics about health disparities, but money. Many, if not all, hospitals received federal grants for construction, research, and indigent care. Civil rights laws had been passed, but Atlanta's private hospitals still found clever ways to deny practicing privileges to black doctors. So a group of black doctors decided to go to Washington, to see the folks at HEW and in the Congress, and to let them know they were spending federal tax dollars on segregated institutions. They put together the Committee on Implementation, which would encourage the implementation of what civil rights laws said should already be happening in private hospitals.

The committee was composed of Bell and physicians Otis Smith, Albert M. Davis, and J. B. Ellison. Their coordinator was Xernona Clayton, a longtime civil rights activist. An efficient organizer, Clayton worked closely with Coretta Scott King. They once protested for two days outside an Atlanta shoe shop that would not hire black salesmen because the shopowners said they feared black men would look up the skirts of white women. Clayton eventually became so close to the Kings that it was often said that if you didn't know Xernona, you couldn't get to Martin. Clayton's most important task may have been harnessing one Dr. Roy Bell. Some doctors were skeptical when they learned Bell was on this committee that was to travel to Washington and talk with politicians.

Privately, to Clayton, they said, "You don't know what he will do. No one can control him."

She could. According to Bell, "Xernona was able to do a marvelous public relations job. 'Say, listen, I got Bell by the nape of his neck. What can he do?' A very light thing, but she was able to bring men together. There had to be a PR job done on my behalf because I had the reputation that no one could control me. And they couldn't. But now was the time to be controlled. You can lead them to the trough, but you can't make 'em drink. Heh heh."

The Committee was, in a sense, the culmination of an effort begun years before by a coalition of civil rights groups and health care professionals. Beginning in the late 1950s, the NAACP, the National Urban League, and the National Medical Association (the black medical society) held an annual Imhotep Conference. Imhotep was an ancient Egyptian demigod of medicine, a priest, scholar, and architect, who designed the famous step-pyramid of Saqqara, the first Egyptian building in stone. The conference was a place to share information and formulate strategy for ending segregation policies of hospitals and medical associations. Bell attended the sixth Imhotep Conference in Washington, D.C., in 1962, representing the SCLC. At the next Imhotep Conference, in Atlanta in 1963, the chairman of the conference noted that no representatives of the major medical organizations (AMA, AHA, etc.) were present. They had occasionally sent representatives or observers, but no major leader. "We've invited them in peace for seven years," he said, "to sit down with us and solve the problem. By their refusal to confer, they force action by crisis. The initiative is no longer theirs to accept." A few years later, when HEW began holding seminars on desegregating hospitals, meetings the AMA and AHA attended and supported, Imhotep Conference leaders said, "We've been doing that for years, but they ignored us."

When Smith and Bell went to the regional office of HEW, they were surprised to find a friend, regional director Pete Page, who was born, reared, and educated in the south. In the Navy he had had close contact with black soldiers. "I listened to their talk," he says, "and learned about their situation, and I had observed what happened in my home area. What really got me aligned in a posture was later when I ran public health clinics in a communicable disease center. Some situations were unthinkable, unspeakable. People were dying, and nothing could be done. In Arkansas there would be cases of early-stage cervical cancer, and the doctors asked the state medical department if they objected to a surgical procedure being done to excise the beginning cancer. These were people brought in on school buses from poor rural areas. The state said no; that goes to private practitioners. But these people couldn't possibly pay a physician. Some had six babies and had never been to a doctor. Experiences like that got to me. It became a part of my way of thinking and working." Once he joined the doctors, he and his family were threatened. He had to install a new phone line because there were times when he couldn't sleep for two or three days because the phone would ring every thirty minutes. Sometimes he would hear people on the other end and sometimes not. He got letters, too—one from a man in Texas who offered to rent a big hall and debate Page about civil rights compliance. A man from Oregon threatened to kill him, his wife, and his five children.

When the doctors picketed outside the regional HEW office—Page's office—he made coffee for them. That night, they met at his home. Page sent telegrams to the HEW when he feared President Johnson might back down from forcing hospitals to desegregate, under pressure from Southern politicians. Page advised the doctors as they maneuvered through the federal bureaucracy. He publicly urged all people to use all facilities and report any discrimination. He said hospitals with records of past discrimination had not only to announce their open policy but take steps to correct discrimination. They must send letters to Negro doctors, doctors' organizations, and civil rights leaders, post their policy in the hospital, and send press releases to the media. Formerly separate facilities must be converted to actual biracial use.

In Atlanta, the Committee helped the regional HEW with spot inspections of hospitals and gathered statistics on black health care and on the obstacles black doctors faced when trying to treat patients who needed hospitalization. Hundreds of doctors had their referral patterns tracked to monitor racial patterns. HEW employees were armed with 441s, minutely detailed Assurance Forms created by HEW to evaluate hospitals.

The 441s requested statistical breakdowns to record racial patterns regarding use of rooms, wards, nursery, labor and delivery rooms, admission offices, cafeterias, toilet and laboratory facilities, waiting rooms, clinics, and emergency rooms. There were questions on staff privileges of black physicians and dentists, membership requirements of city, county, and state medical and dental societies. The major item on the form, from the standpoint of determining compliance with civil rights laws, was the "patient census," a breakdown of occupancy by race (white, Negro, Oriental). Page says, "The in-hospital checks were the only way we could catch the miscreants. Georgia Baptist was one of our toughest and Emory Hospital was no less so, though more civil than the Baptists were. Georgia Baptist kept saying, 'It takes time.' " The inspectors would often discover some practice that perpetuated segregation, and the hospital would be told to comply with the law or face loss of federal funds. For example, they discovered Grady Hospital's practice, continued even after the hospital was officially desegregated, of placing a C on the Grady cards of its black patients and a W on those of its white patients.

A political cartoon in the *Atlanta Inquirer* featured a drawing of Grady Hospital, the front ominously shaded by a tall person standing unseen. His shadow was labeled, "TITLE VI-1964 CIVIL RIGHTS ACT." The caption read, "New Doctor Arriving."

HEW had many compliance inspection teams, most of them working in the South. One team discovered that a hospital administrator had deceived them by having white and black staff members pose as patients and occupy beds in semiprivate rooms. A newspaper ad for one hospital announced, "Effective September 1st, 1965, we are limiting our practice to those white and colored patients and families who prefer the dignity and privacy of segregated waiting rooms. We assure you all that there has never been, and never will be, any discrimination in our treatment of sick patients because of race, color or creed." A Macon, Georgia, hospital was discovered to have converted its formerly all-black building into a facility for welfare patients only, and blacks made up 70 percent of the welfare patient load. Hospital administrators told HEW that welfare patients were assigned to beds without regard to race or color and that

white patients "found the money" to afford semiprivate or private accommodations when blacks were moved into the same room or ward.

The Committee on Implementation also organized a meeting of doctors from around the Southeast. When Bell spoke, he said, "Keep the
Negro doctor out and you keep the Negro patient out." He explained
the most common method hospitals used to minimize the presence of
black doctors: tokenism. After one or two black doctors were accepted,
no more would qualify; applications would be misplaced. The doctors
heatedly attacked Emory University Hospital, which had received nine
applications from black doctors and rejected them all while receiving
almost as much federal money as all other Atlanta hospitals combined.
They said changing Emory would create a ripple emanating out to other
Atlanta hospitals. They noted that Emory had no black interns out of
twenty, no black residents out of sixty, no black physicians out of four
hundred. Bell insisted, "Emory is morally wrong, but the federal government is worse because they disburse the funds that help Emory carry on
its program." Speakers accused HEW of bad faith for certifying hospitals
that had not actually desegrated. They passed a resolution calling on
HEW to fire any staff member who approved a hospital that operated by
the guidelines on paper but not in practice. The resolution also called for
the firing of hospital authorities who set policies that demonstrated negative intentions and hostile attitudes toward Negro doctors being admitted to the staff. An HEW representative who was present promised a
reevaluation of certified hospitals and pointed out that the law required
nondiscrimination but did not require integration.

Once the team of Clayton and the four doctors had gathered sufficient
information and organized it into a compelling presentation of statistics,
stories, and observation, they traveled to Washington, D.C., to confront
the men who made policy and enforced it or didn't. There they would
experience the frustration of political maneuverings and the exhilaration
of apparent victory; and Roy Bell's fiery temperament would once again
be an unlikely tool for promoting social change.

First they met with bureaucrats. One public health official disregarded
their information and said he would have to review his own records,
which, unfortunately, were in Baltimore and would not be available until

the next day, when, the official regretted to say, the team would be gone. Clayton, who normally remained silent at their meetings, said they would remain an extra day. Big smile. (The official was not the only fidgety man in the room. The doctors all had appointments in Atlanta the next day.) Um, er, well, I believe we can get those records this afternoon.

The Great Evader, however, was Georgia Senator Herman Talmadge. Talmadge made jokes, said he had time for only a short meeting, had not had time to look at medical records. When a doctor mentioned that at Grady Hospital a Negro woman who suspected she was having early labor pains might be told that it was not the day for Negroes in the obstetrics clinic, he said, in the drawl that had gotten him through many a small-town stump speech, that he didn't know much about labor pains. Laughing heartily at his quip, he said, "I always left that to my wife." They appealed to his lawyerly concern for doing what is right, but he said a senator had a lot to read, he had another meeting, and he would try to read their materials when he had time. Clayton and the four doctors found him folksy and slippery. But they had a plan, a four-part presentation that was a drama with its own plot devices and climax. Clayton briefly introduced herself and the doctors and, to Talmadge, added, "Certainly, you want to know about injustice in your own home state." Davis spoke next. Intellectual and soothing, he kindly asked the good senator for help with a problem they had discovered. He gave information about Negro health problems, the lack of facilities for Negro doctors. J. B. Ellison, a little irritated that Davis's words were not taken seriously, said, "I don't think you really heard what was said, now," and added more information. After Ellison eased the presentation from a gentle request to a push for something, Otis Smith changed the tale to a conflict.

Smith was a doctor with plenty of reasons to be angry. Years before, sitting in his office, glancing down at an open desk drawer with a gun in it, he had experienced what happens to a self-respecting Negro with no access to power. In 1956, in Fort Valley, Georgia, Smith picked up the phone to call long-distance a patient he intended to hospitalize. The operator mistakenly connected him with a white woman who was making a call. She heard his voice and told him to get off the line. He replied, "You get off this line." She asked who he was; he told her. As he tells it, she said, "'This is nothing but a ol' nigger.' I called her everything in the damn—that I could think of." In a few minutes the white woman's husband called him and said he was coming after him. I said, 'Come on. I'll be waiting.' I ain't never shot a gun in my life, so I called my neighbor and said do you have a gun? He said yeah; he was a hunter. I said I'll be there to get it." He put it in his desk drawer and continued seeing patients. Soon, he looked out the window and saw a police car. A policeman said he wanted to speak with Smith, who said he was seeing patients; they said they would wait. He took his time with his patients. After a while they left, then returned later and, standing on the other side of his desk, said they wanted him to go with them. Smith says, "So I'm sitting there, trying to make up my mind what to do. I got the gun right there in my open drawer. I said if I don't go, they'll think I'm afraid of them. I didn't say anything. After about two minutes, I closed the drawer and said I'd go. By this time the street is full of black folk. They saw the police out there, and I guess the other people in the office told them what was happening, and the street was just filling up with people. Then people followed behind us in cars when we drove off, to see what was happening."

Charged with using obscene language, he sat in the interview room until two black undertakers paid his bond. On his release, Smith remembers, the sheriff said, "I want you to know I cannot promise you anything because I can't go against the people. I told him, 'Don't worry about me. I can take care of myself.' He said OK."

That was Monday. On Wednesday, the local hospital administrator and the chairman of the medical staff called him and said they had heard something about a conversation with a lady. They came to his office, where he explained that the woman had called him a nigger and he had cussed her out. They seemed satisfied and left. By the time he got home that day, a telegram awaited, saying he would not be allowed to practice again at that hospital, the only one in the county, until he apologized to the white woman. On Saturday, the black president of Fort Valley State College, a black college where Smith served as school physician, called and summoned him to his office on Monday. "I didn't realize," Smith says, "the damn governor had been down there and talked to them. I sat down, and he said how you doing and I said doing all right. He said, 'I've been told to ask you to apologize to this lady so we can get everything squared away.' I said, 'Two apologies are due. If she apologizes to me, I will apologize to her.' He said, 'I hate to say it, Dr. Smith, but you are no longer the school physician.' I said OK, and walked out. Within one week's time I was put off the hospital staff and fired as the school physician for Fort Valley State.

"Everybody, community leaders, principals of the schools, got together and said I ought to apologize to the lady. I said no, two apologies are due. If she apologizes to me, I'll apologize to her. So I said I'm going to get me a lawyer." He went to Atlanta and saw a civil rights lawyer and was told he needed to see a lawyer from his town. "Heh heh heh," Smith says, laughing through every word, "But there ain't no black lawyers in Fort heh Valley heh Georgia." He returned home and a white attorney called him and said he would handle the case. The attorney negotiated with the prosecutor and reported to Smith that the charges would be dropped. "It was the first time I'd ever been to a courthouse," Smith says. "There was only one other person in the courthouse, the black guy who cleaned up; he was in the balcony. They said, 'Stand up. I stood up for the judge to come in. The judge came in; he sat down; I sat down. He asked if I had anything to say. I told him what happened. He said is that all? I said yes. I sat down. He jumped on me, talking about 'here you are, a Negro, in Georgia, being disrespectful, cussing out a white woman, and white folk are responsible for you getting an education. Without white folks, you wouldn't be no doctor. You couldn't do nothing. White folks paid for your education, and you were disrespecful.' " The judge had done his homework. Smith was a beneficiary of scholarships for black medical students at Morehouse School of Medicine given in the name of Margaret Mitchell, who, coincidentally, when she was fatally injured by an automobile, was taken to the Grady Hospital emergency room, where doctors could not save her life.

According to Smith, the judge said, incredulously, " 'You're not going to apologize?' I said no. He said I give you eight months on the chain gang. Bam! He slammed that thing down and walked out the damn door. My attorney said, 'Dr. Smith, that's not what they told me. They told me they'd drop the charges.' I had to believe this man because he had pancreatic cancer, and he only had six months to live. I didn't believe he would lie to me, knowing he was going to die. They carried me down to jail and locked me up, and I was supposed to go to the chain gang two weeks from the day I got in."

Visitors continued to urge him to apologize, and he repeated, "Two apologies are due." Finally, he was visited by Dr. Benjamin Mays, the esteemed president of Morehouse College. "He's philosophical," Smith recalls. "He'll find a way to convince you. He said, 'Dr. Smith, I want you to know one thing. The important thing is that you must apologize, but you are not apologizing to her. You are apologizing to womankind. Men do not speak to women like that, irrespective of how disrespectful they are, so you are apologizing to womankind. You are not apologizing to her. Forget about her. Look at womankind.' I said to myself, Here's the man that hooked me up with the Margaret Mitchell scholarship so I could go to medical school. So I said OK. He came out to my house after they let me out. He was sitting up there on the sofa, and he took his shoes off, and he had holes in his socks. I thought, Who would believe, heh heh heh, Dr. Mays got holes in his socks. Heh heh heh."

In Washington, Smith leaned forward in his chair, stared hard at Senator Talmadge and said, "You're not hearing us because you don't want to hear us," and added more information.

Then they turned loose Roy Bell.

Clayton, Davis, Ellison, and Smith were never quite sure what Bell would say. He might slam his fist down and threaten to call in Black Power militants. Bell now describes his role with a basketball metaphor: "Xernona was the orator, the woman. Otis Smith was energetic and forceful. Davis was smooth as dew on a flower, and Ellison was sophisticated. I was called in to commit the hard foul, to foul enough to know you've been fouled but still stay within the rules."

The doctors and Clayton turned to him and waited.

Referring to the late, segregationist Governor Eugene Talmadge, Bell asserted, "Your daddy didn't do right, and you don't want to do right!" Staying within the rules for hard fouls, he sharply demanded that Talmadge use his power to end segregation, performing precisely as his role required. Whew.

Later, at the Washington Hilton, resting after a day of meetings, Clayton blurted to the doctors, "We should see the president. We wrote Johnson a letter, and he never responded." The doctors chuckled, thinking, "That Xernona." She picked up the phone and called the White House. "I want to speak with the president," she said into the phone. Her call was routed to someone, and she explained who they were, why they were there, and why Johnson should talk to them. "He talks about being a decent president and building a Great Society, but he didn't answer our letter." She said they were planning a press conference for the next morning (they were not) and they expected to meet with Johnson before that press conference.

She hung up the phone, and they all burst out laughing. She took off her high heels, changed into lounging clothes, and they all relaxed. Until the phone rang.

"This is the White House."

Somehow, word of the black doctors talking about civil rights was passed around lower-level White House staff, and someone saw it as an opportunity. They met with Wilbur Cohen, undersecretary of HEW, who assured them the president would personally make sure no hospital that received federal money would remain segregated. After a while President Johnson himself spoke to them for a few moments and said he shared their concerns and would do whatever he could. Most of the group were satisfied with the meeting, but not Bell. He would have his press conference. Before they left, he sneaked to the White House press room, announced their presence, and said they would take questions after their meeting with the president. Stunned at Bell's audacity, Clayton and the doctors joined him on the podium. Word spread that a group of Negro Atlanta doctors were holding a press conference in the White House, and reporters amassed in the press room. The impromptu press conference, instigated by Bell, got national coverage. They told the scribbling reporters that the federal government allowed eighteen Atlanta hospitals to receive federal money without full compliance with the Civil Rights Act; they accused the hospitals of token compliance but continued to keep most black doctors out. They named Emory University as a key insitution, as it worked with five hospitals and had powerful Washington connections. They reported how the hospitals continued to keep black doctors out even after they had been found to be in compliance with federal guidelines. The doctors requested that HEW withhold funds from Atlanta hospitals pending full compliance, that Negroes be included on compliance review boards, and that HEW visit Atlanta hospitals on a tour hosted by the Negro doctors. Bell, identified in the *Atlanta Constitution* as chief spokesman for the group, said all they received from politicians was "promises, promises." Bell mentioned Atlanta-area U.S. Representative Charles L. Weltner and said, "Maybe Mr. Weltner's possibly peeping over HEW's shoulder had something to do with this. He should confer with his constituents instead of his friends in Washington." Smith said unless something was done soon, there would be demonstrations and sit-ins throughout Atlanta.

In Atlanta, Eugene Patterson editorialized in the *Constitution* that extremist whites were saying "federal tyrants were out to crucify hospitals with guidelines." Patterson also criticized Negroes for "rushing around Washington telling federal fainthearts they are backing away from enforcement of guidelines." He praised calm meetings of mutual understanding between the medical assocations. "Watch them," he opined, "not noisy exhibitions."

When all hospitals had finally desegregated—and segregation was reduced to the sneaky, unspoken manipulations that would plague many institutions and perpetuate the privileges ingrained by decades of Jim Crow laws and distorted perceptions of white superiority—the victory was the result of both the local acts of detection and enforcement, and of a much larger act, a new federal program that would change hospitals everywhere: Medicare. Before Medicare was enacted, the U.S. Commission on Civil Rights had recommended to Kennedy that they use federal funds to influence hospitals, that they deny funds to those that discriminated, and that acceptance into Medicare be predicated on hospitals operating without racial discrimination. That recommendation became policy, and, in early 1966, with Medicare scheduled to begin that summer, official letters and policy statements were mailed from HEW to all hospitals explaining that compliance with the Civil Rights Act was mandatory for acceptance in the Medicare program. Hospital administrators counted their elderly patients and concluded that big money was at stake. Huge money. Enormous money.

That was when administrators became interested in making sure their 441 forms were filled out and signed. Suddenly, black doctors began receiving polite letters from Atlanta's private hospitals. One letter was mailed to the black doctors' association requesting another copy of the association membership list. "I received this once," the administrator said, "but someway in moving from the old office to the new one I must have misplaced it." It said they expected to comply with HEW regulations and added they had never excluded any physician from the hospital since their opening in 1954. The administrator said, as a matter of fact, he had served as free consultant for one of Atlanta's black colleges. He concluded, "We would love to have any member of your association come by and visit our hospital any time."

Bell and the Committee on Implementation had one last tussle with HEW. After the trip to Washington, the impromptu press conference, all the pressure on Atlanta hospitals, and HEW's promise to crack down on noncompliant hospitals, several Atlanta hospitals in early August were told they were not in compliance, particularly regarding the granting of doctors' privileges and the referral of patients. The hospitals were given an extension. The black doctors felt double-crossed. At a meeting with HEW officials, Bell reminded them that HEW had said they would act on complaints by July 30, and that date had passed with no action. Furious, Bell lashed out, "I wish I could turn you, you, and you into black people. I wish I could turn your children into black children, your wives into black women, and you into black doctors, so you could understand the problems we face. I've spent over a year and a half gathering facts about segregated hospitals." He said he was tired of promises and being disappointed. "You tell us there is a problem, and that you're working on it. I think it's all a bunch of hogwash. I personally am not going to meet with you anymore because I don't have any more faith in you, and I think you ought to resign your offices because you have not shown any fortitude. You have not shown any honesty, nothing but evasiveness."

But by the end of 1966, there were almost no complaints to HEW of discrimination in Atlanta hospitals, and by the middle of 1967 the issue was resolved. Dr. Smith recalls that as he first walked into one private hospital, low-level black workers pulled him aside and said, "We're glad you're here." The activist doctors could focus their attention on treating their patients. Roy Bell, however, remained restless.

"I wouldn't make a good civil rights activist," Bell says now. He speaks calmly, intellectually, jokingly. "My understanding of destiny precludes any type of actions that I would have taken before I became enlightened. I would get a one-way ticket to the nut house if I talked about karma, past life, reincarnation, and the cosmic forces that control us."

In the 1970s Bell became unhappy. Many of his friends said, "You're out of step, Roy, and you just keep on being out of step." He suspected he was exhausting friends' patience and became depressed; his marriage ended. He moved to California, where he hoped his intellect and activism would merge into some sort of political life. He dabbled in local politics, but he experienced a profound transformation when he was introduced to a thinker whose philosophy made sense of all his agony, all the mayhem of the civil rights struggle, indeed all of history and the future. He began to see a reality he had never seen before.

He read the works of Rudolf Steiner (1861–1925), a philosopher, architect, and organic agriculturalist who originated a branch of theosophy called anthroposophy. Steiner, whose life project was to unite science and religion, said anthroposophy was a "spiritual science." It included an esoteric understanding of Christianity, with Jesus Christ being the ideal man. He believed the unseen spiritual world could be seen, just as the physical world is seen. The thought process, to an anthroposophist, is as physically vivid an experience as burning one's finger in a fire. By training one's mind, one can literally see the origin of thoughts, see eternity. Steiner also taught that human history was a succession of epochs that are controlled by cosmic powers and are characterized by new developments in humankind. Bell placed his life in that succession: "When I first met him through his works, I knew I had finally met someone that could guide me to some knowledge and understanding of what this world is all about."

His ideas about civil rights changed, all right. "I look at the scenes that they show on TV about the conditions in the 1960s, and I have a child now, and she says, 'Daddy, what is this?' I have to turn this off because this is something that's dead, something that at one time may have been true, but this is not what all men are like. These programs call themselves praising Martin, but they damn his work by showing something out of context. I guess John Lewis is the most beaten man in the whole world because they keep on showing those pictures. That's not a very pretty sight to look at, but if one has the knowledge that the person who is being beaten is really more at fault than the beater, then how can one say that? Because the person being beaten committed such an inhuman act on another individual in a prior life, to have caused this evolution in his present life."

He's right. If he had told student activists that it was John Lewis's own fault that he was beaten in Selma, Alabama, on the Edmund Pettis Bridge, he would have been considered insane. But that is what he learned from Steiner, who believed karma, an unfailing renderer of justice, causes each human act to echo back to the actor. Bell, who believes in his prior life he was a woman, explains assuredly, "If one says that God is good and God is just, then how can it be that so many people are treated good and so many are treated badly, if God is just? Well now, there's only one way this could be. That's if every person who receives good and every person who receives bad treatment has willed that treatment for himself, and of course, if a person said that to me a number of years ago I would have said he was crazy. He would be insulting my intelligence, that this person we are looking at wished this horrible infliction of pain upon himself, even to the taking of his life. If we say that God is all good, then we must realize that the concept of reincarnation is not just an academic question. Men come back to this earth to experience all of the pain and the sorrows that they inflicted on another individual in a prior life, and this is the only way God can be just and be good. This is the justice that God has decreed in order to say, 'I am just.' "

On his decision to begin picketing Grady, he says, "Assuming thoughts have no individual origin in man but are should I say preformed and handed down to man from good or evil, well, the good thoughts came to me, ideas of how to create tension at Grady Hospital. The only credit I could take is that I was a conduit through which powers greater than myself acted. When man gets to the point where he can dissect his thinking, that he can step aside and look at his thoughts and identify the origins of his thoughts, only then can man be free. So when you talk about Grady, anything written now will be written from the standpoint of the evils that were inflicted on black people. Well, that's very true, but if it could be proven beyond the shadow of a doubt that what we suffer and the racism we incarnate is dependent upon our prior life on earth, then to believe that after man leaves this world he disappears and is forever forgotten, that would be to deny God. I hate to sound philosophical to you, my friend, but these are some of the things that allow me to reconcile myself with Atlanta, and with the men in Atlanta.

"There are a whole lot of black people going to be white in the next life, a whole lot of white people who are going to be black in the next life. One of the things that determines what race a man will reincarnate in is whether or not he dislikes that race in his present life. That's an absolute certainty that you will incarnate into that race when you come back. If people were taught that there's abolutely nothing that a man can do that is not known, nothing, even if they do it behind closed doors and nobody knows about it, and the law is that whatever pain or suffering or happiness or joy that you elicit from your fellow man, this is your next life, then if you want to build a beautiful life, you be nice to people. But if you want to have pain and suffering, be ugly, cause pain and suffering. This is the only way that Christ can be just. If men knew this, see what a change it would make? So now if you were a horrific person in your former life and you did all manner of bad things to people and here you are coming back and you gonna cry out, as some poor little colored boy, 'Everybody is picking on me,' or, 'They don't like me. . . .' No, it's your ignorance that allows you to do this thing, and if you react as you are reacting now, you gonna come back and suffer worse things."

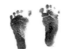

I Guess He Thinks He's a Man

Lisa Dean sat in her kitchen with her friend Lucretia and Lucretia's two children. The roar of airplanes flying overhead spilled in the windows and filled the apartment, but D'Lisa slept peacefully in a car seat on the kitchen table. Lisa's friend Marian Thurston walked in, from Cheryl's store next door, chewing gum. She said, "They sell three-cent gum for five cents."

Cheryl's son came in and picked up D'Lisa, cuddled her, put her back, and left.

Lucretia pointed at her son and asked Lisa how much her brother Franklin charged to cut hair.

"Four dollars for that age." Lisa picked up D'Lisa. "She's so nosy. See how she holds her head up and looks around. She can hold her head up by herself."

Lucretia said, "If I had it to do over again, I wouldn't have none, but now that I have two, I want two more." Like Lisa, she had her babies at Grady. "That old part was real nasty," she said. "The food was filthy."

Lisa said, "Just about everybody I know had their kids at Grady."

"I had my two kids there, and then some."

"Oh yeah, you had an abortion. I should slap you for that. If I could do it over, I would have waited until later. Until I was married." They got a big laugh out of that.

"That's what Shontelle said," Lucretia reminded them.

"Shontelle called me white girl," Lisa said, "because my skin is so light. She done got divorced?"

"Yep. She said she was happily married, then six weeks ago. . . ."

Lucretia stopped the thought, then said, "My oldest child's daddy, he helps a lot."

"Just imagine," Lisa continued, "how life would be different if we didn't have kids. We'd have it going on."

"We can have it going anyway," Lucretia said.

"That's right."

"I'm glad I had mine when I was young. I can get on with my life." Lucretia picked up D'Lisa and rocked her until she fell asleep. "I believe she likes me," she said. "Marian, after you have your baby, next year you'll be pregnant again."

Marian shook her dead defiantly. "Not me."

Lisa's son Rob and Lucretia's two children played loudly on the floor, rolling cars, moving superpowered action dolls, conquering a mighty foe.

Lisa recalled that when she learned she was pregnant, her sister was with her. In a squeaky-silly voice, Lisa said, " 'I'm going to have another nephew!' I said get out; I am not going to have this baby. She said yes you are. I didn't tell Dwayne; she told him. But I think he knew. He was sick before I was."

Marian said, "That's how Randall knew, too. He was sick."

Lisa said, "My mom said, 'I do not believe in abortion. You knew what you were doing when you were getting him, and you're going to pay the consequences. A child is a beautiful thing.' God makes a baby out of love, and all that kinda stuff. God is the only one to determine life and death, not you. Then I had to sit down and think about it. I cried, boy, I tell you. Marian said, 'I'll help you. I'll help you.' " She imitated Marian with a quick, nasal voice. "I thought I just wasn't ready for a baby. Rob was just turning five. And I didn't want it to be a deadend street, like when I was seventeen. And I wanted at least to be married. I guess God makes everything happen for a reason. But now I'm glad I did"—she spoke in a baby voice and smiled at her daughter—"because I got my little girl. I don't want to ever have no abortion, though. I'd be scared to do it."

Lucretia asked, "Are you morally against it, or you just can't do it yourself?"

"I can't do it myself."

"She's morally against it," Marian said.

"Yeah, that too."

"She is morally against it," Marian repeated.

Lisa turned adamant. "Most women, you *know*, use abortion for birth control, and that is not the way to go. That is not. I don't think I could have an abortion anyway. I sure didn't want to."

Marian said, "I knew she wouldn't have an abortion."

"And Dwayne was saying, 'If you kill my baby, you're going right behind it. I'll kill you.' But I didn't care because he wasn't going to do *nothing* to me. But I don't think I could have an abortion. I don't see how women can have one. I don't know. But that's other people's opinion. They have an abortion and later on in life they want to have one, and they won't be able to."

"I know a girl who had one at five months," Marian said. "That is murder."

"Even in your early trimester," Lisa said, "it is still murder because it might turn into a baby. When I was in the eleventh grade, this girl was in the tenth, she had an abortion at five months. They put in this salt water with a needle, and it will kill the baby. Why not keep it the whole nine months and give it up for adoption instead of having a dead baby? You know that baby was gasping for some air. That is cold-blooded. I cussed that girl out. Sure did. At five months! I had a book on abortion, and they showed how they cut it up into little baby parts. And they showed one in a trash can. That was disgusting. I couldn't do it. Five months! I'm gonna have my baby and give it up, if I'm going to do that."

The conversation rambled, then Lisa said that Jonathan, her new boy-friend, was locked up. "He went outside," she said, "and the Red Dogs came and he was with some people gambling. Somebody had drugs. He was charged. Because they were all in the same area, and there were a certain amount of people, they were all charged. All it took is for one person to have it."

A neighbor came in and wanted to use Lisa's phone. Lisa snapped. "You ain't fixin' to use my phone!"

Marian Thurston sat in the Grady Perinatal Center, awaiting an ultra-sound. Her younger sister, Jackie, was with her. Five women waited nearby, the normal vaginal delivery tape playing on the TV. One woman turned her back to the TV and said, "They offered me a mirror, and I didn't want to see it *then*." She was teased by a man with her, who seemed to think he was cute and funny, though none of the women in the room, who glanced at him grimly, thought so. Most women stared, rapt, at the TV, one grimacing all the way through.

Marian, who could change subjects quickly, began talking about her relationship with her mother. "I waited four months to tell my mom about my first period. She teased me. When I first grew breasts, I was watching TV on the floor. She said, 'Come here,' and pulled up my shirt, and touched 'em. She said, 'Oh, you got breasts.' She called everybody. I guess because I was her first one to have boobs. She called my grandmother, and she sent me a bra. But I didn't wear it. I didn't think I needed one.

"My father has a white wife now. They had this biracial baby. He acts like that baby's so fucking precious. I think he looks like Uncle Fester. I got on my father. 'Since you had him, it's like we don't count.'

"Some people ask me why I don't have a boyfriend, and I say because I'm pregnant. They say, 'And what?' I don't want a lot of people around my child, boyfriends it might get attached to."

The TV screen showed a C-section. "That's cool," Marian said, "having a baby in five minutes, but then you have that scar. It ain't worth it, so I'll try my best to push it out." Looking back at the TV, she said, "But that's so nasty. Some people say the human body is amazing. I think it's nasty on the inside. I don't want to see nothing." On the screen, a post-C-section woman struggled to walk. "Please, Lord, help me push it out," Marian pleaded.

"Marian Thurston?" the ultrasonographer said.

Marian's ultrasound went fast, the tech quickly spreading the gel across Marian's still-flat stomach, her left hand clicking buttons and taking pictures. The machine beeped as the murky photographs emerged. The little white arrow zipping around the screen, stopping momentarily under the tech's guidance, she fairly dashed from organ to limb to organ. She tucked the baby's indistinct picture into the cutesy folder and handed it to Marian. Walking down the hall, looking at the picture,

Marian said, "Shit, I don't know what's what." About the gender, she said, "I'm glad she didn't tell me. I don't want to know. It takes all the surprise out of it. May as well be buying puppies."

Sitting in her hotel room, her baby asleep in a car seat, the TV tuned to a daytime soap, Jan Dorman said she missed her baby's last appointment at the Grady AIDS clinic. Up all night with the baby, she had overslept. "It's a twenty-four-hour job. She starts fussing at night, and I start cussing. I feed her, change her, give her the bottle, and she starts fussing. I get frustrated. I got to give her sugar water when she has a lot of gas. I thought I would take care of her basically all day and sleep all night. I was wrong." She also quit giving the baby AZT. It made her sick. Plus, Jan no longer worried about AIDS. "I feel, I myself, personally, I feel, that I don't have HIV. That's the way *I* feel. My mom called the HIV hotline, and that woman told her a majority of pregnant women will test positive while pregnant. All the hormonal and chemical change going on. In January I'll get another test. I'm really hoping it will be negative. My chemical and hormones will get back to normal. They already did one HIV test on her, and that should be back soon. She's got my antibodies in her, so I know she's going to test positive to begin with because she's got my chemicals in her. If I'm negative, she's coming right off the bottle. Sometimes they won't take breast milk after taking a bottle so long, but I'm going to try it. This morning I was looking at her, and I started crying. I wanted to breastfeed. When that test came out like it did, it crushed my ego, period. I just knew I was going to get to breastfeed."

She said she was eager to leave the hotel. "It has roaches. The exterminator sprays, but they won't guarantee it because of the carpet on the walls. I sprayed the room yesterday. Where there's a crack in that part of the wall, you can hear everything that happens in the next room." She chuckled.

She was also feeling resentful toward the doctors for deciding on a C-section. "Once they got me in the OR they found her other leg. Any other hospital would have attempted to turn her around, but Grady, they didn't. I figure that was wrong. They could have attempted to turn her around, and I could have had her natural. But instead, look at what all I had to go through."

Her boyfriend, Carl, came into the room, on break from work at the hotel. He lay on the couch to sleep, apparently. Glancing at her sleeping baby, Jan said, "I used to be able to enjoy a cigarette. Now when I go to light one up, it's like she knows and acts ugly." Her pale arms had several small tattoos, the stories of which she began to tell, then stopped. "Yeah, uh"—she looked at Carl and snorted a soft laugh—"I'd rather not get into it. They were all stupid, let's just leave it at that. That one was just to cover another one." Later, Carl stirred from the couch and went back to work. She mentioned again the "rough life," to which she had often referred as the reason her family felt protective toward her; this time, she elaborated.

"My running away a lot. Living on the street as a runaway. Being raped. Their divorce. I got locked up at fifteen. I spent my sweet sixteen in a juvenile facility. I was arrested for theft by taking . . . my mother's car. I totaled it. I never finished high school. I was in the ninth grade about two, three years. Now I'm working on a high school diploma through a home school program. I finished one subject, got two As and a B. Now I go to general science. I need reading glasses, so that's a big factor in it."

The baby awoke and gurgled gently, "Ahht, ahht."

"They filed charges against me because I almost killed her. I'd had a very bad week, and all I needed was one more thing to tick me off, and mom called me a bitch, and I picked up a log and hit her up side the head. I didn't even remember doing it. When I get really angry, I black out. I was so angry, I was at a gas station, and I don't know how I got there, being blacked out like I was. Somehow, I managed to get there. I wouldn't go to school, and they just brought out the law that you have to go to school or you get locked up, or your parents have to go to court and pay a fine. Steadily fighting a lot. Being on the run, I was raped several times. The first time I was fifteen, and I had a miscarriage. My baby would be six years old now. My mama thought I was lying to her about being pregnant because I used to lie so much. She laughed it off, 'Yeah right.' The other day, she said, so you were telling the truth? Now

I don't lie to her. I used to lie about any- and everything, even the simplest little thing. She was like, I didn't know. When I lost that baby it hurt, because I wanted one.

"I was in my third month when I lost it. While I was pregnant, I was raped. He had a gun in one hand and a knife in the other. I had bruises all over my jaw where he grabbed me to stop my screaming. I had a thumbprint on one side and the other fingerprints on the other. I tried to break out a window and get the attention of someone outside. He grabbed me and bent my hand back. He did any- and everything he could, whatever he wanted to do. Except up my butt. I kept saying, crying and all, I'll go along with you. Just be careful; don't make it where I lose the baby, but he insisted on going harder. I ended up bleeding. I managed not to lose the baby. Later on the guy I was dating, I wouldn't let him touch me or kiss me and he realized I had been raped. We got into a fight a week later, and he kicked me in the stomach."

"Aaht, aaht."

"He didn't know I was pregnant. After that miscarriage, I got pregnant by him again and I miscarried at home with my mother. I've had a bad choice of men. I've always chosen men who would beat on me."

The door squeaked open, and Carl came in. Jan quit talking. He picked up something he'd forgotten and left.

"I continued messing around. I was with two guys in a car; they went down a deserted country road and one crawled in the back seat, to rape me. The guy driving was scared of the other guy, who had a gun, so he was doing what he was told to do. He was looking in the rearview mirror, and I could see in his eyes he wanted to stop him, but he was scared because he had a gun. They took me back to where the guy I was dating was and dropped me off. He asked me about my clothes, and I told him. We never saw the guy again, but we saw the guy who drove the car. At the time I sold drugs. He said, 'Jan, I'm sorry. You know I didn't want it to happen.' I said, 'I know but what could you do? He would have shot you.'

"Then one guy, he's still in jail for attempted rape. He snatched me into an abandoned building and tried to rape me. A friend of mine who was selling drugs at the same place I was, walked by and heard me screaming and he snatched him off me. He said to him, what are you trying to do, go to jail? So he left. The policemen came later and tried to lock me up. We were in an empty apartment, and someone called. I was scared to tell them what happened, but he told them. He described him, and they had arrested him just before they got us. He tried to break into a convenience store. So he's serving time for attempted rape and attempted robbery. He got the word out that when he got out he was going to kill me. So I left Conyers and Lithonia altogether. I was scared. He got the message all around.

"And when I got out of the girls' home, I got married. They were thinking about sending me back for another year, and we asked them what we could do to avoid going back to the girls' home, and the lady there said, 'I'm telling you this, but I didn't tell you this.' She could lose her job for it. The only way to get out of it was to get pregnant or get married. I wasn't ready for a child at the time, so I said I could get married, then get a divorce. So that's what I did. My dad met this guy who was getting ready to be sent back to Mexico because his green card was just about up. Our getting married kept him from being sent back. I was the type that believed when you're married it's forever, so I tried to make it work. But he was a Mexican, an alcoholic. The day we got married he started hitting on me. We fought every night. He put on a good act in front of my folks. I know he loved me. I know that. But the alcohol turned him into a different person. We got married on his birthday, and I left him on my seventeenth birthday, less than a month later. But we were married a year, two years. He still owes me a thousand dollars back alimony. I told the judge I didn't care about the money; I just wanted the divorce. I could go to the judge right now and he'd go to jail. From what I heard, I got out at the right time. His girlfriend, he beats her like a dog. She's got black eyes, fractured rib. He didn't beat her while she was pregnant, but after she had the baby, he beat the mess out of her. She was talking bad about me, and he said don't call her names; she's a good person. She may have did me wrong by leaving me, but she's a good person. He's beat two men up for talking bad about me. And I don't like people talking bad about him. He just don't know how to handle his alcohol."

She said selling drugs she made quick money. "I didn't use 'em; I just sold 'em. I thought about it, but I saw the people I was selling to. One woman was a very good customer. Very good. But she was using her welfare check. She had ten kids and seven had been taken. She was selling her food stamps and welfare check, every month, to buy drugs. One day she said I should come up to her house and meet her dad and kids. I went and saw the kids. She wasn't home. She was out getting high. Her alcoholic dad could barely walk. She would leave the kids with him all day. The baby wasn't no older than three, four months. He was in the crib, with a diaper that looked like it hadn't been changed in three or four days. A bottle of curdled milk. Thick, ruined milk. I was, like, nuh uh. All they had was powdered eggs and a little bit of bread, and the store was too far to walk, so I fixed them some powdered eggs and cleaned the kids. All of them had runny noses and stuff. When I saw that, it hurt me so bad that the next time she came to me, I would not sell drugs to her. I quit selling because of that. I quit for about a year or two, then got back into it for two weeks just to make a little extra money to pay my rent one time. But that was it. After I saw those kids, I didn't have the heart to do it no more. I'm not gonna lie. Sometimes I do feel like going back into it because it is fast money, but then I get to thinking about all the kids involved, that I'm getting the food and clothes they need because their parents are spending it on drugs. That's the only thing that stops me."

She reached over and held her baby's hand, gently stroking its small fingers. She said she and Carl were planning to get married in June, on his birthday. "We had problems when we first got together. He hit me in the nose. I think he broke it, but I couldn't do the X-ray because I was pregnant. He hit me on the side of my face, and I had a big ol' black eye. He hit my mouth and busted it open. Then I called the police, like in my fourth, fifth month. I didn't want to press charges, just scare him, but they locked him up because of the way my face looked. My face was so bad it wasn't even funny. I didn't want my family to see me. Since we've been back together, he hasn't raised a hand at me. He knows if he hits me again, he won't be locked up; he'll be six feet under. My dad and stepfather said if you hit her again, we're coming after you. Don't let us get to you before the police do. When it comes down to it, my family loves me. Lord help him if he hits me while my stomach's still open. If I'm healthy, he's got a good fight on his hands. The last time he hit me, I bit the hell out of him. They could have arrested me when they arrested him. He had that mark on his arm and knots on his head. Because I was pregnant, he didn't press charges against me. I told him he don't want to piss me off. I can fight like a man. He found out I was a dirty fighter. But since he got locked up, he hadn't done anything. My family knows I love him. They feel he loves me because some men nowadays won't stick with you if you're pregnant, but he's been with me. Even when we were separated, he was there by my side when I went to the hospital at five months, with premature labor."

She pointed at the baby. "I'm going to teach her when some guy says ooh you look good, you slap him and tell the principal you slapped him. If they suspend you, I'll take you to another school. If a female can't stand up for herself at school, she shouldn't be there. The first time somebody she's dating raises a hand at her, they're gonna have a bad mama on their hands."

She said she and her family had begun making small moves toward healing their damaged relationship even before she tested positive. "We were starting to talk more before I found out. When I found out, it made me open my eyes to how I had treated them. They showed me they loved me. I was so full of anger from my childhood that I didn't see it. I only thought of revenge for all the anger that had been caused. My father won't admit it. . . . All the anger is caused by him. As a baby, a psychiatrist I talked to said I was sexually abused by him. When I was nine, with the divorce, I saw a psychiatrist. My father beat me and my brothers. I always got the worst of it, I guess because I was the oldest. I started having these dreams, and the psychiatrist told me it usually means I was molested as a child and I blocked it out all these years, and it's just now coming to the surface.

"The only reason I started talking with my father a couple years ago was because my brother was staying at his house. I'd honk the horn for my brother, and my father would come out on the porch and cuss me out and all that shit. I heard he was dying, so I figured well, I love him because he's my father, but I dislike him as a person. So I wanted to tell him I loved him before he died. I told my brother to tell him I wanted to talk without us cussing each other out. He came over to the car, and I turned away. I thought, oh great what's he going to cuss me out about this time? He said, 'Aren't you going to say hi?' I cried. I got out, and we started hugging. He let me in his house. We've been talking ever since.

"I was scared to let her stay with him. If he could do it to me as a baby, he don't care how small she is. My stepmother knows when he gets out of bed, or even just rolling over, and that eased my mind. I can tell she don't really like him, but she loves him. She kept the baby right beside her. She gets defensive if you talk about it with her, but I think in her own mind she knows it's true."

Under a blood-red sunrise coloring a sky of mackerel clouds, Grady slowly came to life on Thanksgiving morning. Across the street a man slept in the entrance to the health department, protected from the cold wind by a makeshift cardboard wall. Down the street, a long line of men awaiting free breakfast stretched around Butler Street CME Church. The front of the clinic building was nearly empty; a few employees walked in and out. Inside the atrium, a portable heater kept the woman at the information desk warm. Back on the Pratt Street side of Grady, two new elevator columns were partially bricked, from bottom to top, like a condom being unrolled. Nestled at the bottom of the Grady parking deck, McDonald's was closed.

At the labor and delivery nurse's station, Renee Lindley said, "I wish I was home finishing my turkey." She began putting things on the counter in drawers. "I can't work with clutter." She checked on her patients, then made a quick call to her son, who had arrived from college late the night before. "Hey, I didn't get to hug your neck. I'm just so glad you're in this city. How was your trip? . . . That's it, just cool, huh? Happy birthday." She hung up. "He was thinking about not coming home. I said, 'I'm gon' kill you.'" Lindley received a call from home, about the turkey. "Don't touch it," she instructed. "Mimi's coming over, and she has all the instructions." She hung up and said, "I got to have forty-four hundred dollars by January twenty-seventh for my son's tuition. All he talks about is

Howard U., Howard Howard Howard. I say, 'What about lovely Atlanta?' " She gave money to Laura West, a nurse on her way to get breakfast. "I want meat, my usual junk."

"I'm going to the cafeteria. McDonald's is closed."

"All day? I'm going home. I'm just waiting to go to the OR anyway. 17's been in three days, they been inducing her, and she ain't done nothing." After a while, she said, "Where's my junk? I got to eat before I go to the OR." Just in time, her breakfast arrived.

West said, "Those biscuits were like this." She knocked on the counter. Instead, she brought toast, cheese grits, and boiled eggs.

Lindley carried her food to the break room and sat. She said, "I went to New York and ordered an omelet and grits and that waitress looked at me. 'You trying to be funny? Do you see grits on the menu?' She told me."

A nurse asked her how long she was working. " 'Til three. If the census goes down, I'm going to see if I can go home and promise to work sixteen hours tomorrow. I have to make my money back. I'm not getting financial aid from nobody for his tuition."

Along with administrative staff, pregnant uteri all over Atlanta were apparently taking the holiday off. The halls were quiet. Lindley told Annette Cagle, the midwife, she hoped the new doctor crew, which came on at nine, would let the patient in 18 go home. "Her cervix hadn't changed. She's obviously not contracting. There's a difference between safe and foolish. Keeping her is foolish. And I know this institution needs to save money."

Lindley took a call from the other end of Labor and Delivery. She hung up and said, "God almighty. They lost a baby over there. That's not a good way to start Thanksgiving. It makes you wonder if you're doing the right thing. She said the baby was alive when the mother got here. I wonder if that was Marie's patient." She called back. Marie Costley answered. "You knew I was calling. What happened? . . . Oh God, oh my God. She wasn't feeling anything? . . . She should have had some bleeding. . . . Yeah, a good *deal* of pain. . . . You know me. I got to find out every detail. Was she on drugs? . . . Uh huh, thanks, oh God." She hung up. "Complete abruption. One edge of the placenta was hard as a rock, big clot on the maternal side. She said she had no bleeding, came in for regular contractions. They put her on the monitor, the baby deceled, took her STAT to the OR. They got there and found it was one hundred percent abrupted. Fifteen years old."

Lindley took cranberry juice to the patient in 18. She told her, "We need to flush out your kidneys so we can get you to the house." She took breakfast trays to 20, 19, and 17. Dr. Rebecca Turner arrived to check on 18. She said she wanted to keep her a while longer. She left, and Lindley told the patient, "Cool out. Don't call your family yet. The doctor has a couple of things to do. We'll get you home. At the house, rest, drink plenty of fluids, cranberry juice. I didn't say nothing about eating a whole lot of stuff. Don't drink tea or coffee. Eat small meals. Drink cran-ber-ry juice. I got some for you. I don't want you in here Saturday having the baby. Keep it in there. Have you ever heard, 'The bread has to be properly baked'? Well, we want this bread properly cooked."

She went to the nurse's station, and later the patient in 18 beeped her. "It's been twenty minutes," she told Lindley in the room.

"She's got to make sure your culture is negative. Let us do things right so you don't have to come back. I'm an old lady, and old ladies like to do things right the first time. You sit back. I'm in the driver's seat. You're a backseat driver. Heh heh heh."

The patient used the phone she brought with her to call her mother. "Mom, come get me," she said.

"Is that your mama? Let me talk to mama. Mama? I'm trying to get her out of here. She has an infection, and we're taking care of that. She's OK. She'll be home just in time for that turkey."

She returned to the nurse's station and wrote on progress sheets. Patient transport arrived to wheel 18 away, and Lindley asked, "What did I say?"

"Drink cranberry juice. No tea, no coffee, no Coke. Small meals."

"And what else? Prop your feet up."

Lindley got another call from home. "Just pour it in there. You need that can of broth to moisten the stuffing. . . . That's fine, that's fine. . . . Just one to two, to hold it together. . . . Tell Doug to put the cans of cranberry sauce in the fridge. . . . Put two cans of corn, whole kernel.

Get Doug to help you. . . . Excuse me? Wake him up. Tell him to get on the phone. . . . Doug, go help Mimi, please."

"Talking turkey on the phone," West said, laughing.

Lindley's daughter called; Lindley spoke with her in a child's voice. "It did? And did the tooth fairy come? . . . What did it leave? . . . Good. Did you clean the bathroom? . . . Good. Are you helping Mimi? . . . When there are dirty dishes, help her clean them, OK? I love you. Bye." She continued writing patient notes. "I was up 'til one. I like things fresh on Thanksgiving day. If I cooked it before and put it in the fridge, no-o. All my sister has to do is stuff the turkey and cook it."

A resident sat at the nurse's station and dictated OR notes into the phone. One hand cupped over the phone to block noise, he spoke quickly, methodically, with the rhythm of a ninth-grader reading a poem, the end of each line a crescendo, breath, then the next line. ". . . Urinalysis showed only one-plus ketones. . . ."

The patient from 18 used the other phone on the desk to call her mother again, asking her when she was coming.

". . . continued on IV until blood cultures. . . ."

Lindley said to the patient from 18, "The doctor's finishing your chart, then I have a few things to add." The resident appeared with the chart and handed it to Lindley.

". . . contracting every five minutes."

Lindley wrote on the chart while talking. "You'll see the doctor next Tuesday. Come back when it's *time* to have the baby. We'll be here waiting on you. Where's your mom going to pick you up?"

"McDonald's."

"I'll take you." She pushed her wheelchair down the hall, passing two LPNs studying for a nursing test. "Hey, hey, quit that cheatin'," she teased. At the entrance, Lindley asked an aide to take her down to McDonald's.

After lunch, Lindley said to West, "Tomorrow gon' be a trip."

"You wouldn't think a baby would honor a holiday," West said.

"They don't. The moms do. So the ones that would normally come today will come tomorrow, *plus* the ones that normally would come tomorrow. Tomorrow gon' be a trip."

"I need a doctor to 14, STAT!" someone announced sharply.

Curious, Lindley walked that way; the residents darted into the room. She was told it was a placental abruption. She muttered, "That placenta gets completely separated from the uterus. It can happen from an injury, or from smoking crack or when the baby's in a low position." An EMT, wearing the all-black uniform with niches and pockets all over, exited 14. He must have brought her in. Three more doctors arrived.

"Thanksgiving turned out beautiful," Robin James said. "I was tired, but the children ate all the food, so it was worth it. I love to cook for them. When they cook their own, they say it ain't the same as at my house. I like that. We had Cheryl, the children, and Cheryl brought some children from over there, Melissa, Sandy, and some other little girl, maybe Sandy's sister. They brought her. And Shane's little friend, Big Boy, and Mr. Lewis's son. Cheryl always be doing things like that, taking them around with her, trying to do little things for the neighborhood. She don't do as much as she used to because their truck got broke down. She used to take all of them to the skating rink, as many as she could load up on the truck. Things like that. Hmmm huh. She was always trying to give little parties. This year we took 'em to the park for a little cookout. They really ain't got nothing to do over there and if Cheryl does it for her children, the other children would see it. We try not to make 'em think nobody better than nobody.

"I had turkey and dressing, and I cooked thirty pounds of chitlins and added some hog maws. I cooked some greens, macaroni and cheese, potato salad and Jello and a cake and strawberries, good stuff. Cheryl made three types of cake, three different pies, all from scratch. Apple pie from fresh green apples they picked. Her husband paid somebody to let him chop the Christmas tree down. He's from the country and likes things done the old-fashioned way.

"Then they sit around and told lies, you know. Like how ugly a boyfriend mama always get. Mama know she could pick 'em ugly, stuff like that. They got mad because I came on up early. I was tired. My blood was low. They cleaned up pretty good. I usually have something to say when they clean up, but they cleaned up after theirself pretty good this year. I guess everybody getting bigger, uh huh. You wake up at two o'clock in the morning, and go get some water and you have a nightmare, but they cleaned up pretty good."

"It was wonderful," Lisa Dean said. "We reminisced on old stories. I found out some things about when my mom was pregnant with me. My grandmother was saying my mom didn't tell her she was pregnant, right? She said, 'Are you pregnant?' She was losing weight. Mom said, 'No I think I have a cancer.' Grandmother told us. I asked Mom why you didn't tell me that?

"We ate everything. She made me cook. I cooked two cream pies, macaroni and cheese, and they cooked the rest of it. We also had, ooh, turkey, ham, all kinda stuff, candied yams, custard, dressing, gravy, all the good stuff. Collard greens, turnip greens. My grandmother came, and my aunt and her kids, and I met a cousin I never seen before. Heh heh. My mom is her first cousin. I'm her second cousin. 'This is your second cousin, Lisa, which is my oldest daughter.' And she met her third cousins, which is my kids and she met everybody. Just met more people."

"I was with Isabel and a friend," Azi Torres said. "We went to her house with Brazilians and we stay together. We had a lot of food. She make whole the food that Americans make and more some Brazilian food. It was delicious."

"Pppsh," Jan Dorman grunted. "It was alright. The only thing good about it was eating."

The day after Thanksgiving, Renee Lindley said, "We have an IUFD," then returned to room 17, where a young woman cried, "I want my mama." The patient's mother and cousin walked in and out of 17, sometimes needing to be out of there, sometimes in. The mother made a phone call at the nurse's station. "That baby's dead," she said. "They said it's dead." IUFD, intrauterine fetal demise.

"I offered to hold her hand," said Annette Cagle, the midwife, "but she was oblivious to me." On the computer screen next to her, the patient's strip was half alive. On the top horizontal grid, the black contraction line formed peaks and valleys, but below it, the fetal heart rate grid had no red line where normally there would be undulations gently creeping across the screen.

"Oh, please, help me," the patient cried.

Lindley and Cagle returned to 17, joining the first- and fourth-year residents. Cagle's voice could be heard saying, "Just let the baby come out. Big push, big push."

The patient cried and cried, cried once sharply, and abruptly stopped. The baby was out. Clinic aid Patricia Duncan brought a small stack of forms to be filled out and took them into the room. Dr. Ernest Miguez, the fourth-year resident, went to the nurse's station and called the county coroner, tersely giving the necessary information: age, cocaine use, name, address, phone.

"Do you want to see the baby?" was heard from 17, followed by several clicks of a camera. Later, the patient's mother and cousin walked out into the hall, where the patient's uncle joined them. They showed him the pictures.

"He's tall," the patient's mother said, gazing at the instant snapshot.

At the desk, Lindley said when dealing with an IUFD, she usually did not talk about the baby unless the patient initiated it. "I never say, 'I know how you feel,' or, 'This is God's will. You'll have another one.' I don't know her emotions that are built up. That shows you have no sympathy for what she is going through. That's cold-blooded. I've heard people say it's a good thing you didn't take it home and it die there. I focus on the patient. I teach her what we're going to do. I make her pain-free. Once it's born, unless the patient wants to see it, I don't force the issue."

Nurse Marie Costley added, "You think about the fact that the baby is dead. There's nothing you can do about that, but the mother still needs attention. You focus on *her*. As human beings we feel some emotional tug, but as a nurse I think about the fact that she needs the care. The baby is in the background. It is already dead, and there's nothing you can do. So you do the things for her, to make it more bearable. You support her.

You ask if she wants to see the baby, you offer. If not, you take it away, to the morgue."

Dr. Miguez hung up the phone. "They don't want it, so we'll do the autopsy." He said, "We tried pain reliever, but it doesn't help with a drug abuser. She said, 'That must not be a narcotic,' but it was."

A patient walking to stimulate labor strolled by holding her husband's arm.

The cousin of the patient in 17 used the nurse's station phone to call someone but got no answer. She began crying. Lindley asked if she was all right, but she said nothing and returned to the room.

"We just do labor, basically," Dr. Miguez said. "Watch for infection and bleeding. Do an ultrasound to confirm it's IUFD and to check the baby's position. Check the cervix for a cord prolapse. We investigate to see if we can learn why the baby died. Diabetes, drug use, hemorrhage, anemia. If there's cocaine use, we have to report it to the coroner. If there's anything suspicious, like if it was a home delivery and someone might have killed the baby, we call the coroner. Then we induce labor. Use prostaglandin to ripen the cervix, if it's needed, then Pitocin to start labor, and continue that through delivery. We want to get the mother into labor as quickly as possible. Once you know it's an IUFD, you don't wait for a spontaneous delivery. That risks infection. If there's been a placental abruption, it usually goes pretty quickly. There's not much intervention.

"We don't want a C-section. There will be some cases where we have to, if we can't turn the baby or it's stuck in the uterus. But we try our best to do a delivery. Sometimes it's in a breech position, and we can deliver with forceps. If the dead baby has a large hydrocephalus, water on the brain, we might be able to deliver if we can compress the head with ultrasound and a needle. If it's because of placenta praevia, she's likely to hemorrhage, so we'd likely do a C-section. You individualize, according to the situation."

He thought for a moment and placed his explanation into a sequence, a plan, as residents are taught. "So, first, assess the cause and assure the well-being of the mother. Deliver the baby; avoid a C-section. Have adequate pain control. And, reassurance. The mother is usually distressed. This is one of the most difficult OB situations. So you always confirm with ultrasound. Always call an upper level. Have at least two doctors check, so you're certain. When I tell the mother, I try to be empathetic. I give reassurance. I encourage them to cry, hold hands if they need to. Just be there. If her prenatal care was fine, I try to relieve their guilt. 'You were doing the right thing, taking vitamins, making your visits.' There's a lot of guilt involved. I try to convey that we are going to investigate and find out what went wrong. I always avoid saying, 'You'll have another baby.' It's a loss. It will always be their baby. I give them some time alone."

Miguez said all this in his usual steady tone. He spoke plainly, methodically, but genuinely. Nurses spoke well of him, that he cared, that he was very capable. He said he was not taught in medical school how to deal with a patient's grief and emotions, but that he read some helpful books. "It's not part of the formal education, the curriculum. I've tried to learn how to understand their situation. The worst thing you can say is, 'You'll have another baby.' That minimizes their situation; it's taking it lightly, not recognizing it was their baby. They usually want to know if it was a boy or a girl. Sometimes they want to hold the baby, get pictures. Sometimes I recommend they plant a tree at their home, take care of it, water it, as a symbol of that baby. Then every year you can have a celebration on the birthday.

"Later, they usually want to know if it will happen again. You have to discuss recurrence rates, which are usually inconclusive when they leave. The pathology report takes some time, so they might not know until their postpartum visit. There will be a lot of anxiety for them during that wait. Mostly, there's no final answer. If it's because of diabetes or high blood pressure, you can say that, but more than likely, we won't be able to tell."

"I had Katrina first when she was about a week old." In Marian Thurston's bedroom, Lisa Dean was telling about the second time she had taken care of an infant; it had been Marian's first time. The baby was neither of theirs.

"Didn't nobody in the family want the baby," Marian said.

"Her mother's on drugs, and I always wanted a little girl."

"She was so cute."

"And little," Lisa added. "First this other girl had her, and they couldn't keep her. I went and got her one day, and I told her mom I had her and she said OK. She said she'd give me ten dollars to get some things, but I didn't really need it. I used my money. How many months was she? Four? Five? I was in the PEACH program, and I went and got the papers to get custody of her, so I could put her in the nursery, but the family didn't want that. They didn't give me nothing, but they didn't want her. So I asked Marian would she keep her while I was in PEACH, and she just stole her."

"I took her like she did," Marian said, glancing at Lisa.

"We stole Katrina back and forth," Lisa said. "I used to take her to mom's house, and my mom said don't get too attached to her, and I was. I loved that baby. I cried. I thought, how could somebody do a kid like this? When so many people want babies and can't have 'em. And some that have them don't want them. I cried."

Marian went to her closet and pulled out a zippered black bag labeled, "Special Keepsakes." She removed a medical form. "She only weighed eight pounds. I had just took her to the doctor."

"Let me see that," Lisa said. "She only weighed five pounds when she was born. She was the smallest baby she had ever had."

Marian removed more items. "I took her in for her shots and all that. When that lady gave her her shot, Katrina just cried, and I started crying. Katrina was looking at me, like, 'How could you *do* this?' I lied to the WIC people because my name wasn't on Katrina's things. I said Katrina's mother was my mom and that she was going to have custody of her, but that I had her for now. They said OK. Me and Lisa were the two WIC proxies."

Lisa looked through Marian's bag. "Who took this picture?"

"Me," Marian said.

"They won't even let us see her now. We ask about her all the time. They don't even let her keep in touch with us. We *raised* her, practically, 'til she was almost a year old, eleven months."

"And she had everything," Marian said. "Everything."

"My grandmama gave a lot of stuff to her."

"And then I started working, and she had everything between me and Lisa. Then they came and got her. I got her those little open earrings. One week she was fat as hell, and when they had her she was skinny, hardly had any clothes, no earrings. I felt so bad for her."

"I cried," Lisa said.

"It was like she was my baby."

"I can't believe you didn't put my name over that," Lisa said, looking at a Christmas card Marian had given Katrina.

"You were at your mother's house. She was supposed to go with you." Marian laughed little snorts. "She was supposed to spend Christmas with Lisa."

"I was so mad. Marian snuck her away."

"I had her a little red Christmas dress. As she got older, I bought her clothes. Just like it was my baby, just like a mother raising her daughter."

"There's that black one I gave her," Lisa said, looking at a picture. She and Marian removed each item slowly and looked them over carefully.

"Uh huh. And her father started writing me, and we'd talk on the phone. He wanted the baby to stay in my care, but the family thought I wanted a check for the baby. But I didn't get a check. Only her WIC. I didn't need no check. That's when they came and took her. This is the last picture after they took her. She went from that to— Shawna had even had her, for a while, after they took her. All her hair came out and everything. I had just got a layaway out when they got her."

"That was about two years ago, two years ago about this time."

"She had a walker, swing," Marian said. "Somebody gave her a little pink suitcase."

"My grandmama did. She said this is her traveling bag. I should have kept it for my baby. My mom loved that baby." Lisa put down a picture and added, "She said, 'This is *our* baby.' It was a family baby. As the baby was getting older she was saying don't get attached, because I guess she was saying they were going to try to take the baby back."

"I always ask her mom when I can see her, and she says she was just out here, you missed her."

"She always says that."

"They say Katrina's got bad, too."

"Yeah, they say she's cursing and everything."

"She won't even remember who we are."

Chortling, Marian said, "I don't know who she with."

They began reminiscing about when Lisa was agonizing over a high school boyfriend and trying to convince a neighbor to teach her to drive. Laughing so she hurt, Marian imitated Lisa, " 'I haven't driven a car in a long time.' "

"You were just cursing," Lisa said.

"My mom's always saying, 'What's wrong with your mouth?' When I'm talking with her and I curse accidentally, I run across the room because I'm afraid my mom is going to get me. Like today I said me and Jean was doing some crazy ass shit! And I just looked at her and say, bye, and just walked on out." Marian shook her head and laughed. "I couldn't believe I said that."

"My boyfriend and I was on rocky ground," Lisa said, continuing the story, "and I wanted back with him so bad. He had a car, and he said, 'I will come back, but I don't have a license. If you will learn how to drive—' "

Marian howled with laughter.

" 'Then I'll come back and you can take me to work.' I used to cry every day about him. He hurt me so bad. I said, 'Please, I want to learn how to drive.' " Lisa laughed at herself. "And just when I let him go, that's when he start to come around. I didn't want him then. I just wanted to have sex and put him out."

A plane roared over, the first one in a good while.

Lisa then talked about her current boyfriend, Jonathan. "Remember when I was talking about not riding transportation to Grady and I got a ride? That was Jonathan. We'll be seeing each other six months on December fifteenth. We talked on the phone, and he said he wanted to see me when he got out of jail." She said he was out on bail now, that she had helped him raise bond money.

Just as Marian was walking to her closet to replace the bag in the closet, they heard a man shout, "I'll put a cap in your motherfuckin' head, nigger!" She carefully replaced the bag on the shelf and looked out the window. Lisa casually walked over to look. Two men stood on the ground below, one pointing a pistol at the other. The unarmed man stiffened his back and walked away, looking down.

"That Edward is stupid," Lisa said. "He's going to get himself killed."

"So Edward's got a gun?" Marian said. "I guess he thinks he's a man now."

"If you live by the sword," Lisa said, "you die by the sword."

They sat down and continued chatting.

Azi Torres moved in with a Brazilian woman and her two children, in an apartment complex with a small Brazilian community. On the phone, the animated Azi was subdued. "Jeff is back from Washington," she said. "Here with me for a while. We're going to see what we're going to do. Gonna rent some place. He could not be there alone, and it was hard, very cold weather and confused and everything." She stopped talking to give Jeff quarters for the laundry. "Hold on, let me make this little kid shut up because the mother is sleeping. . . . She used to live with her husband, but he used to get upset because she made more money than he did. He scream at the children and treat them bad and then she get rid of him, what I should be do with my husband long time ago."

She said they were living off the money from the sale of Jeff's car, an expensive sport utility vehicle. And they were looking for work. "He is looking for job, but is hard. After this money finish, we no have anything to sell anymore, so we gotta find work. Jeff is not getting money from family. He is not go over there because he thinks everybody tell him he screw up. And throw in his face. I think I gonna have wonderful place in heaven, because to put up with so much. James is pissed off with me because I am doing this. He is so mad I am put up with all this. He thinks I should throw him out and send him to hell. But I know what I feel. Nobody send him anything but me, so if I throw him out and send him to hell, I don't know what he gonna do."

Outside Marian Thurston's apartment, a wooden sign nailed to a parking lot telephone pole announced, "DENTAL PLAN 8.80 PER MONTH." A group of about fifteen young men walked in front of her apartment, across the dry, weedy clay ground. A man leading carried a metal pipe. "Give me my motherfuckin' money!" he demanded four times of a man they confronted.

"God damn!" he answered. "You don't have to get so upset!"

After several moments of staring, the group walked away, the implied threat hanging in the air. A boy in the back of the group said, as they left, "Somebody call Grady."

"Beep-beep. Beep-beep." The driver of a vegetable and fruit truck pulled into the parking lot. People appeared to buy squash, greens, cabbage, bananas, apples, and grapes. At 3:00 a school bus stopped in the lot. Chattering children, many with bookbags hanging from their shoulders, spread out toward their homes.

"Let me go, goddammit!" a woman's voice shrieked from a car in the parking lot. She sat in the front passenger seat, the man in the driver's seat holding her with both hands. A man in the back seat got out of the car and slid into the driver's seat as the other man slid over toward the woman. As the car drove off, she screamed again, "Let me go!"

"I'm back in school," Marian said in her bedroom, holding a brochure for Atlanta Center for Employment and Training. "I'm going to be the one in the book that does something. I told some people around here about this training. One said she needs to get her GED first. I said they *have* GED training. These people around here are sorry. They don't want to do shit."

She called a friend on the phone. "Is Tricia there? . . . Whatsup, girl? You don't know who it is." She talked a while, then hung up. "She said, 'I know it's Marian with that white girl voice.' Because I've been to college."

She heard her sister, Jackie, answer the door and went to see. Her sister showed her a box of food given to her by a church group. "They're feeding the poor," Jackie said. They all laughed.

"We're not poor," said Scottie, Marian's youngest brother. They removed two cans of yams. Out the window, they saw the group in teams of two and three. A man read a pamphlet to a boy.

"They always give yams to black people," Marian said. "Yams and collard greens. They think that's all we eat." Next came a canned ham, green beans, cookies, apple juice. "This is gonna be our damn dinner tonight." Marian went back to her bedroom and said she would rearrange the room when the baby came. "It'll be like when I had Katrina here."

She again insisted she would have privacy when she delivered her baby. "Cheryl is going to videotape me screaming at home, when I go in the ambulance, when I get to Grady, in the room waiting, then *after*, when they clean the baby. Under no circumstances will anybody but the doctor be looking between my legs. My book says I can refuse anything, and I will." She flipped through her book on pregnancy. "I think I'm going to make a list and tape it on my titties. Don't do this, don't do this. I'm going to train my mom to say, 'She don't want that shit.'

"This one boy asked me what I wanted and I said it didn't matter. He said what if it's born with both girl and boy genitals. I said I'll have the dick cut off. He said then you want a girl. I hadn't thought about that."

Someone knocked at the door, the church group again, with another box of food. This time they wanted to talk about a Spiritual Interest Questionnaire. Jackie and Scottie called for Marian. She was greeted by a white teenage girl and a black teenage boy. "We'd like to ask you a few short questions," the girl said to Marian. "Do you think God cares about you?"

"Mm huh."

"Do you believe that Christianity is worth investigating?"

"I already go to church. Yeah."

An airplane roared over. The girl raised her voice.

"What could the church address that would make you want to go to church? Family concerns or race relations . . ."

"I go to church and everything. Teach the Bible and relate it directly to what is happening today."

The boy stepped in. "If you could find out about a *genuine* relationship with God through Jesus Christ, would you be interested?"

"I already do. I've been baptized."

He read from a tract, "God wants to have a relationship with us. That's what Jesus came for. To bridge the gap between you and God. Sin is the problem, and Jesus came to crush sin. For he so loved the world that he gave his only begotten son that whosoever believes in his name shall not perish but have everlasting life. Are you interested in knowing God personally?" Another deafening roar from a plane heading to Hartsfield Airport. The boy continued reading. "We were created to have fellowship with God, but because of his stubborn self-will man chose to go his own independent way. Fellowship with God was broken, and this is what the Bible calls sin. If God tells you to stop something and you don't—"

"Right," the girl said.

"—that's called sin. God said the wages of sin is death; that means spiritual separation from God. But the gift of God is eternal life. This diagram right here"—he showed Marian a page in the tract—"illustrates that God is holy and man is sinful. A great gulf separates the two. Man is continually trying to reach God and establish a personal relationship with him through his own efforts, such as philosophy or religion, but he inevitably fails. Do you understand that?"

"Uh huh."

He ad-libbed, "It's like if you're with a kid and you have a lollipop, and he reaches up to it, but you won't give it to him. He's gonna keep reaching, but you're big, and he's down there. But God genuinely wants a relationship with you. He doesn't hold it up. He put it on a cross for us."

"Uh huh."

"All we have to do is accept the fact that, um, Christ came and died for our sins." He resumed reading. "Jesus Christ is God's *only* provision for man's sin." He read three Bible verses from the pamphlet, then showed her another diagram. "It demonstrates that God has bridged the gulf that separates us from him by sending Jesus to die on the cross in our place to pay the penalty for our sins. Do you understand that?"

"Like I said before, I do go to church."

He kept reading. "We must individually receive Jesus Christ as our Savior and Lord. Then we can know God *personally* and experience his love."

The girl intervened. "You say you go to church, but God wants a *personal* relationship. You really need to feel a personal relationship with Jesus. If your church does not give you what you need, then ask God to send you somewhere that you can find a personal relationship with God. Obviously, God wants to show you what is good for you."

The boy read three more verses and added, "Once you give your life to Christ, God is looking down on you and saying, 'This is my child. This is *my* child.' This is a gift of God, not as a result of works so that no one should boast. You don't have to kill a pig or sacrifice a virgin, none of that." He read again, "We receive Christ by personal invitation," then ad-libbed, "If you are open—and you seem to be open right now—you can ask him right here, right now, and he will come into your life." Back to the pamphlet: "Just to agree intellectually that Jesus Christ is the son of God and that he died on the cross is not enough. An emotional experience is not enough to be saved."

The girl added, "Like he said, it's faith. Right now you don't feel God in your heart. You must have faith that he will enter into your heart. He wants to change your life and fill you with love, so much that you're gonna have to give to others, so much that you can't hold it all. God loves you so much, you cannot imagine."

"It's as simple as this," the boy said. "If you sat in a chair, you would have faith that chair will hold you. That's all believing in Christ is. You have faith he will save you. And he will. Would you like to, um, at this moment, you know, pray to receive Christ as your personal Lord and Savior?"

"I've already done that."

He nodded. "You've already done that?"

"Uh huh."

"That's good. A lot of people need to see that. They need to see Christ in you. Jesus is coming soon. After he comes, this place is gonna be wild. We did our best to hook you up."

"OK."

"Thank you for your time."

"Thank you."

"You have a great house," the smiling white girl said. "Good-bye."

They left, and Jackie laughed. "We got the same box again. The same box. We hid that first box."

"Now, obviously," Marian said, "he didn't even hear the first thing I said when he walked in. He didn't hear a thing I said." She chuckled and said, "When I was baptized three of my plaits came out. They were floating in the water. I said to that minister, 'I got to get my hair.' "

They jumped at the sound of someone banging on the door. "Please let me in!" a boy pleaded. "Please let me in!" Marian laughed. "Don't joke around with this! She's coming! She's coming!" Marian opened the door, and her brother Russell ran in, to the kitchen sink, and began running hot water.

Who was this ferocious person he feared? A thief? A crazed neighbor? Worse—it was Mom, and he was a son who had not done his chores. She entered the apartment, looking stern. Seeing the water running, she said, "What's that?"

Scottie said, "He's going to wash the dishes."

"He should have already washed them. I've been working eight hours."

"That's right, eight hours," echoed annoying little brother Scottie.

Azi Torres's roommate's two children, plus a neighbor's child who was there until his parents came home, played a video game in the living room. The game blipped and blooped musically as manic creatures skittered around and the players, with spattering bursts of electronic flashes, scored points. Azi was still talking about Jeff's return from Washington. "My friends were very upset with him because know he married me, left, and think I have to take care the baby and not care if I have a place to live. He was out of money there. He ate just bread, just whatever he find to eat. I sent him money so he pay the campground and get his car because something broken, and he needed to pay repair. I borrowed money from my friends and sent to him, and then he could get his car to sell. He was upset because, when got he here, I didn't make any party for him, like, 'Oh, dear, I miss you so much.' " She mocked his voice. "I was so upset with him, three months there. He took about twenty-five hundred dollar, but he expends money like a crazy. He starving so long there that I think he learn a little bit, but he still bad with money. Starving, sleeping in shelter and doing whatever, I don't think he learn enough. If you give me twenty-five hundred dollar I can survive for three months well. He thinks his mother gonna deposit in his account, and she was tired of this, pissed off with him. She was 'Aacht.' " She ran her finger across her neck. "When he ask her to send money, she send only little bit. I said I give up.

"I said to myself, this is no going to work out, this relationship like that. He no have repair any more. You cannot fix something that you grow up like that. What I can do is let him free. Let him go back to his family, live his life. If I put this cross on my back, I no go anywhere because it's too heavy to me, this cross. I did so much to him. And what I have? I have a son to take care, what support I have?" Thinking of James, she said, "I gonna lose somebody that love me and care about me and wanted marry me and take care myself and my baby. I no have any support from Jeff's family. They treat me like nothing. If I stay with him, I will make his life miserable because his mother get him out of money completely."

She picked up Robert, who looked ever more like Jeff. He squirmed in her lap and cried. "I went with him everywhere to take application. He get no job. He said I will even deliver Domino's. He fill up the application, but he no do really like that job. You know, just leave there, and he talk too much with people that was not supposed talking. He ask anything, everything, like a politician. He talk about growing up in Atlanta. He talk about everything, come and talk and talk and say my wife is from Brazil. What I am trying to say, he no go to the point that he got to do. If he wants to go to Europe, he go round whole world first and get to Europe the last thing, understand?" She drew a circle in the air. "And I am very straight. He wants what is easy for him because he have everything in his hand. He no want fight for anything."

She also said they argued about his aloofness from her Brazilian friends. "He talk little bit, then go to bed. He said he is educating himself, reading some paper that have news about Cobb County. I said educating about what? Cobb County? He drive me crazy. He want tell me that I no read newspaper. I said I have a lot to think about. I have a son to take care. I have to work in short time. You need to worry about how you gonna find work to support your wife and son, not worry if your wife is educating herself about Cobb County, understand? I want squeeze him and say, 'Go to hell, please.' Throw him out. I have to say, God, be patient." She looked skyward.

She moved to the table and fed Robert. Holding him in her lap, spoonfeeding him, she called him Jeff, then corrected herself. Robert.

She said she had had very little contact with Jeff's family, but one day she decided to try the woman who, according to Azi's sister's vision, should be her one support in the family: Jeff's grandmother. "I went to her house and I told her I was moving out and Jeff have a big problem, but I didn't want to ask her for money. I was saying to her that probably I was about to sell my car to send him money because he was out of money there and live in shelter. I told her everything, and she just said, 'Oh, I am sorry.'" Again, Azi used that mocking high tone. "Then she go back to the time that Jeff left his job and went to Brazil. She said he left a pretty good job. I said I didn't say to him to leave his job and go to Brazil. Don't blame on me. She's very nice lady, but she say, why you didn't make abortion? I said, What? I said I didn't make because I was not preparate to do something like that. I said I gotta go, and I left her house. I said that's enough."

Grandmother's support was gone.

"Then Jeff call his brother, too, and his brother said I'll send money if you send receipts, like from the campground, but he wasn't at the campground. He was far away by then. He want the receipt before send the money! He have one brother in Montana and one here and one sister, and who help him? Me. I borrow money from my friends. His family is cold. They are very artificial with him. They never ask about his personal life because they know it might be something they no want to hear about. And when he talk about me, they criticize. His mother ask me, the way I used to use my hair. Is straight but if I want more curl, use some stuff, can see not natural. She ask if my hair was like that. They ask him if my hair was like a black hair because she could not say I am black because probably she look me and say well, what she have, like a black people? I no have face features like a black. She ask me if I was come from Indians or something because she could not say I was come from black. She probably want to know if my family come from black people, because my lips is kinda big. Jeff ask me if I make any surgery on my nose, playing with me, but in reality they no think that white people can have— They probably think every Latin is like Mexican face and nose.

They was looking for my past, oh she come from black people. I am foreign to them. They try make him believe I was with him because his money. He never gave me any money."

And there was still James.

"He is waiting. He is not angry. He is giving me a lot of support. He thinks I should say go to hell, I am not going to put up anymore. He thinks I should look for lawyer and make up the divorce papers. I not gonna sue him for nothing. I only will make him have his responsibilities by his son. When I say this to Jeff, he say, 'I love you. You are the best thing in the world.'" The mocking voice, again. "He no leave me, but he no want me. He sometimes says we are not made for each other. 'I think we got married without thinking.' He thinks I didn't think, and he didn't think. He took me there; he didn't ask me. But I let this thing happen. I don't know how say this in English, is like the more you try solution, the more screw up you be. James is saying, 'If you become available, you just come and live with me.' But I cannot think about the future right now. I have to organize my life right now."

Crazy Without Her

Grady had not won in several years. Once they had delivered so many babies a month that timing one *just* after midnight, and making the headlines for having the first newborn of the new year, was not a difficult challenge. The Grady babies just didn't stop. Grady had filled the rooms and lined the halls—and sometimes the staff break room—with bulging-bellied, laboring women. Now, they delivered babies in spanking-new rooms with only one patient apiece, rooms that were designed for two patients in anticipation of the multitudes that did not show. Indigent patients were accepted, even enticed, elsewhere because of higher Medicaid obstetrics payments. It was a fight.

"Two are possibilities," said Karen Olsen, the third-year, looking at her board. "Payne will probably deliver before midnight, Kennedy maybe."

On the television in the corner, a newsman reported on the abortion clinic shootings in Boston. "Turn that up," Pete Myers, the second-year, said. "I'm going to do more abortions because of that," he said, glaring at the TV.

At the bottom of the board someone had written the number of days left in residency for each year. Fourth: 181. Third: 546. Second: 911. First: 1,275. The fetus doll was curled up nicely inside the model pelvis, except it was butt first—a definite C-section. The fourth-year, Mary Lowry, entered the room and poured herself some coffee in a urine specimen cup.

"Is that a clean-catch?" Myers asked.

She chuckled, said, "No protein in it," and sipped away.

Myers passed around a box of Whopper malted milk balls and Chex party mix. Olsen returned from checking on Payne, and updated her from 5 to 7 centimeters on the board under "Cervix." A clerk wrote NP, for new patient, on the lines for rooms 11 and 12. The departing third-year showed off the sparklers he was eager to light at midnight, then left. Jodi Reeve came in, wearing a white turtleneck under her scrub shirt, strode right up to Olsen, and said, "We're"—meaning the midwives— "gonna have the first baby of the new year."

"No, *we* are."

Reeve pointed to the line for room 6. "She might be the one."

"Do they get a tax deal?" Olsen asked.

"She's fifteen. I doubt she itemizes her tax return. And you can't cut someone to win."

"I won't even vacuum," Olsen said. "I'm going to win fair and square." She turned to Myers. "This is not a friendly rivalry, so don't go near her."

"These kids need the gifts, so don't let Northside win." Reeve said *Northside* with a sliding sneer. They all compared times on their watches and synchronized them.

"I just want my picture with the baby," Olsen said. She looked at the newspaper she had brought with her. "Can you believe someone else was killed at an abortion clinic?"

"Doesn't that piss you off?" Reeve said.

"This is crazy," Olsen replied. "Pro-life, right."

"The one in 4 might do it," Myers said. "Or 2. She's got a small baby."

In room 6, Reeve said, "Hi, I'm Jodi. I'll be with you to the bitter end. We were saying yours might be the first baby of the new year. You get more stuff if you're first. It doesn't mean we're going to do anything different, OK?" She looked at the strip. "You're contracting *great*." She went to the nurse's station, sat next to the OB tech, and wrote on the chart. She turned to the tech and said, "Olsen said she's going to beat me fair and square. I trust her."

"What do they get?"

"Something. Savings bonds, diapers. I don't know."

Myers walked by, headed to 4.

"Don't do any cheating," Reeve warned.

"She'll be out of contention if she gets an epidural," he said. "It'll slow her down."

In 6, an epidural providing calm, Clarice Vance, Reeve's patient, lay on the bed, accompanied by her mother, Rolanda, and sixteen-year-old Tyrone, the father of her child and one year her senior. Rolanda sat in a chair at the foot of Clarice's bed, presiding over the room. She had a round, freckled face. Tyrone sat next to Clarice, joking and teasing her.

"We've been going to Grady all our lives," Rolanda said. "It became my home away from home. I was born at Crawford-Long, but I've been coming here ever since." She stroked Clarice's leg. "I wasn't happy when they put in that epidural. I had an experience with it, but it's her choice. It seems to be helping her a lot. There's always something going on at Grady," Rolanda said. A young woman slipped into the room. "She's back. That's Clarice's cousin. She sneaks out, then comes back to see if she's still here. You need to call your kids."

"I already did."

"You got a brain on you after all." Rolanda, who had been there with her daughter since 5:30 that morning, yawned. She watched the strip emerging from the monitor. "Your contractions are coming regular."

"I want to be able, by the time I'm forty," Olsen said to Reeve at the nurse's station, "to do clinic work, raise my kids, and do some good things."

"It's hard," Reeve said. "I work, have two kids, pay bills. We should take three months off, and, oh, go to Mexico and learn Spanish."

"Yeah, this residency's for the birds."

"When some finish," Reeve said, "they're emotionally at the bottom. My husband was."

"It's hazing. It's against the law if you do it in a fraternity."

"Some people end up bitter and cynical, thinking I'm gonna get what I can get."

"Yeah, cynical."

Looking at Clarice Vance's chart, which included the baby footprints taken when she was born on the thirteenth floor of Grady, Reeve said, "Her entire medical history is right here at Grady."

A nurse walked over from 8 and said to Olsen, "I think 8's about ready."

"Already? Is she ruptured?"

"Yes."

"I'll come in and check her."

The nurse looked at the screen, then said, "Yours in 6 is contracting."

"Uh huh," Reeve answered, scratching on yellow progress sheets—covering her ass again.

"My family's in Chattanooga shooting off fireworks," Reeve said. "Anybody feel sorry for me?"

"My out-of-town boyfriend is by himself," a nurse said.

"My in-laws have a house on a ridge," Reeve continued. "We sit in the hot tub and shoot fireworks and watch everybody in the city do theirs. Actually, New Year's is not a big deal to me. I'd just as soon be here." Reeve called her family in Chattanooga. "I'm trying," she said. "One of mine is three, four centimeters. But the doctors are trying, too. They're serious about it. They have several. Actually, we just want our hospital to get it, doctors or midwives." Her son got on the phone. "Did you take your second dose of medicine? . . . Good. I miss you. I just wanted to call. Have fun. . . . Do you have some good fireworks? . . . Good. Bye."

Second-year Myers came by and sighed, "These two over here will deliver before ten."

Reeve returned to 6. "What are we aiming for here? Boy, girl?"

Clarice shrugged. "Her name is gonna be Veronica."

"Oh, you know it's a girl. Ultrasound?" Clarice nodded. "So you didn't see the turtle, huh? That's what we like to call it."

"That's my mom's middle name," Clarice said, meaning "Veronica." Rolanda stuck her tongue at Tyrone, whose middle name, Michael, was altered a bit to make the new baby's middle name, Michelle: Mom came first.

Looking at the strip, Reeve asked, "Do you have the house ready?"

"God, yes," Rolanda said. "My husband bought everything."

"When did you last pee?" Reeve asked Clarice.

"An hour and a half."

A baby cried down the hall.

"One down," Rolanda said. "Someone's out of contention."

"That is a tax write-off," Tyrone said.

Reeve asked him, "Are you ready to be a dad?"

He grinned. "Yeah. I'm used to it. I have a child."

Rolanda rubbed her daughter's foot and looked at the strip. "They're coming regular now." Clarice nodded. The cousin slipped back in and reported, "Donnie said he hopes you have it on the New Year. He'll come see you tomorrow. Oh, I forgot to call Kate." She went back out, Reeve behind her.

"It seems like yesterday y'all were babies," Rolanda said. She spoke softly, rubbing Clarice's feet. "Now you'll be getting child support. I remember making a pallet for you when I worked at K-Mart."

"I remember reaching up to the counter."

"You loved to leave your fingerprints on the glass. I'm thirty-six years old. I can't believe I'm gonna be a grandmother. I'm still trying to party."

"I went back to K-Mart, and they remembered me touching the counter. I touched the glass, and she said, 'Don't start it.'"

They both laughed lightly. Tyrone left to go to McDonald's to get food.

"Just a little nostalgia," Rolanda said. "I remember you were born the same day as my nephew. My sister-in-law that afternoon and me in the morning. Both were born here at Grady. He's something else, always wanting to know what he's going to get for his birthday. All y'all grew up fast. That was a big one there," she said, looking at the strip. "It went all the way off the page."

"I didn't feel it."

"But it's there."

"I'm so glad I got nice nurses."

"That nurse this morning did your footprints when you were born. And she was almost here for *your* delivery." She paused, then said, "Did you hear about Bill Bennett? The police cuffed him, and he ran. His friend can undo cuffs."

"That's not a good thing."

"The next day, they arrested him again. There's two big ones back to back. They're getting stronger. Oh yeah, that one's off the scale. Nine-fifteen, two-forty-five to go. Are you excited about being a mother? I thought I was Eve when they put you in my arms." She laughed at herself. "I thought I was Mother Earth. That was the most gratifying thing I ever felt, like I was the only one that ever had a baby. It took me a long time to come down from that high. Yeah, they're regular now. Are you going to let him sign the birth certificate?"

"No, I just don't want to."

"It's your choice."

Reeve returned and explained they were putting antibiotics in her IV. "When your water's been broken a long time, there's a chance of infection."

At 9:30, more baby cries, from next door.

"She's getting there now," Rolanda said, looking at the strip. Tyrone brought Rolanda a hamburger and fries, which she put on the bed next to Clarice's feet. Tyrone ate popcorn he had bought and microwaved in the snack bar.

The anesthesiologist came in to check the epidural. She asked, "Has she been checked?"

"Yeah, she's six, seven," Reeve said.

Clarice writhed and breathed hard. "Where are you uncomfortable?" Reeve asked.

"Down low."

"That means your baby is moving down." Reeve left and returned to the nurse's station.

"In five minutes, it'll take effect again," the anesthesiologist assured the grimacing Clarice.

Tyrone licked salt off his fingers.

Rolanda said, "Come on, breathe. Don't hold it in. Yes, that's it."

The anesthesiologist said, "That's mean, eating popcorn in front of you. You ought to kick his butt out the door."

"Come on, breathe." Rolanda stood and held her daughter's hands.

The anesthesiolost said, "You might not be able to move your legs for a while, but it'll make the pain go away. You'll feel that pressure in your bottom until the baby comes. Just think if you'd have done this natural, ugh!" To Rolanda, she said, "Did you have yours natural?"

She nodded.

"You're one of those ones, huh?"

"It was not easy."

"Oops, I did it again," said the anesthesiologist, who had knocked the monitor cables loose. "The baby's gone. She's gonna come in."

Reeve was right in. "What are you doing, messing with my baby?"

"See?"

The baby in 7 cried again, loud.

"That's a strong healthy baby," Rolanda said, "screaming his lungs out."

The anesthesiologist said, "I'll be back in an hour. This will feel better to push and let the natural thing take over. I speak from experience. They didn't give me *any* medication."

Clarice picked up the cup of ice chips with melted water at the bottom.

"You can't have water," her mom told her.

She drank it quickly and said, "Now there *is* no water."

Covered with a jacket, Clarice's cousin went to sleep on a sofa. Yawning, Rolanda sat on the other sofa. "I'm going to try one more nap." She picked up the empty popcorn bag from the sofa, handed it to Tyrone, and reclined. She curled up under her coat. "If anything changes, wake me up."

The nurse peered in and said, "Your cousin said he's coming."

"OK," Rolanda said sleepily. "I wonder which one."

The nurse shut the door, and the room became quiet, except for heavy breathing as they all slept, the machine's watery thumping, and a baby's faint cry down the hall.

At the nurse's station, Reeve said she was leaving Grady in two weeks. "I need to make more money, work more regular hours, full-time. I'll see a wide range of patients. I've been here a long time. Eight and a half years." She looked at the screen. "I don't think mine's going to make it 'til midnight. Maybe."

"I need a doctor to 3 for a decel," someone announced.

Reeve peeked in 6, where they all slept, the niece snoring softly. Tyrone slept on a stool, his head resting next to Clarice on the bed.

"Please set up the OR for a vaginal repair."

"Congratulations!" Dr. Olsen said in 9.

When Olsen walked out of the room, Reeve said, "Another one out of contention."

"I know."

"They'll all deliver before midnight," a nurse said.

"Not mine, necessarily," Reeve said.

Just before 11:00 Reeve said on the phone, "Is she having contractions? ¿Dolor? . . . Water's flowing out? . . . No, not if she can't talk to me. . . . She thinks maybe the water's broken? If water's coming out of the vagina and she's having contractions—her belly's hard and tight—she needs to come in and let me check her. Tell her to eat something, then come in."

At 11:00, Clarice was listed on the residents' room board as 6/7, the doctors' patient in room 4 measured five centimeters. No others on the board were higher than five. It would be between the two of them. Reeve peeked in 6, where all still slept. In the hall, she said, "We only have an hour."

"The papers will be looking for the first baby," Myers said in the residents' room. "Maybe we'll have a STAT C-section, cocaine use, abruption. That was the first delivery in this new building."

"If my patient would wake the hell up," Reeve said, "she'd have a baby."

"Whose magazine is this with the article on cruise ship doctors?" Myers asked. No one knew. He said, "That's what I should be."

Reeve walked to 6 and squeezed by the sleeping Tyrone. "Let me get in here and see what's going on." Rolanda awoke and sat up. It was 11:22. Reeve checked her cervix and said, "She's complete."

Nurse Ella Davies came in and said, "If somebody comes in and delivers in six minutes, like that one over there just did, *they* might have the New Year's baby."

Reeve hurriedly darted outside and snagged an anesthesiologist. "I need you to lower the dose in 6. She's complete." She returned to 6 and explained to fifteen-year-old Clarice how to push while on an epidural.

"You won't feel the contractions. We'll tell you. So push down and out your butt."

Reeve and Rolanda became a team, Rolanda at the side of the bed watching the needle on the monitor and announcing when a contraction was coming, Reeve guiding Clarice through the delivery. They spoke in soft even tones. The epidural having removed the pain and scroaning and ferocious grimacing, Clarice said little.

"OK, you're having a contraction," Rolanda said. "Push, that's it."

"Push only when you're having a contraction," Reeve said. "Don't wear yourself out. We need to set up for a meconium."

"That's what I'm doing now," Davies said.

"Long and steady," Reeve instructed.

"I see one coming," Rolanda reported.

"Long and steady. Take a break now."

"Easy," Rolanda said to her daughter. "Rest now. I'm so proud of you."

It was 11:39. Tyrone sat on the stool, his arms crossed. The niece sat on the sofa under the window.

"Here one goes."

"Long and steady," Reeve instructed. "Now push right away. Quick breath and do it again right away."

"It's coming down, Clarice. She's got a lot of hair." She smiled at her daughter.

"Rest while you can," Reeve said.

"It's coming now," Rolanda said. "Come on, let's get this done."

"Long and steady, quick breath."

"Come on, one more. She's got a little pony tail like you. Ha ha. It's all good. It's right here."

"Push it, push it, quick breath. That's the way. Long and steady."

11:43.

"Out your butt," Reeve said, "long and steady."

"It's coming," Rolanda said. She squealed, "My *baby!*"

"You're looking goofy," the niece said to Tyrone, who stood by the bed, his arms crossed, saying and doing nothing.

"Is one starting?" Reeve asked Rolanda.

"Yep."

"Another push, that's it, more more more more."

"You're almost there. You're a big girl now, ain't you?"

"Is it starting?"

Rolanda craned over to look at the strip. "Yep."

"Push it push it push it push it push it. Real hard, come on."

Breathing right with her daughter, Rolanda said, "I'm here, I'm here. Whew, child, you hadn't worked that hard in a long time. She's right there. Believe it or not, you can see her."

"More more more more more more more."

"That's it, baby, let's get it out. Big one."

Clarice said something understood only by her mother, who laughed.

"What'd she say?" Reeve asked.

"'Just snatch it out.'"

"Down and out," Reeve instructed. "That's it."

"There she is. I can see a little face. Get that sister out of there."

"OK, good, take a break."

11:50.

"Is it coming?" Reeve asked.

"Yep."

Grunting while she pushed, Clarice tightly squeezed Rolanda's hand.

"Roll over this way," Reeve said. "Sometimes it helps to move around. More more more, push. Quick breath. Down and out, that's it. Quick breath."

"It's OK, baby, we're right here."

11:53.

"Down and out, long and steady, down and out your butt. Let yourself open up. More more more more, let it go. That's a way, one more. That's it, stretching open." Reeve explained that the baby had had a bowel movement.

"Meconium," Rolanda said.

"Yeah," Reeve said, suctioning quickly. "We need to suck it really clean and then they'll check its lungs to make sure there's none in there." She told Davies, "Tell someone to call peds. That's it, nice and easy." Two pediatrics residents came in. Reeve told them, "Three-plus meconium, term."

They positioned themselves and suctioned the part of the baby's face that had emerged. "Stretch yourself slowly," Reeve said. "Take a deep breath and let yourself stretch. I could have done an episiotomy and had that baby right now, but I'm not going to change my management for the new year."

"Why not?" an incredulous pediatric resident asked.

"Take a breath, this is it."

Rolanda said excitedly, "You got it going, girl. We got it. Her arms out! See? Hey hey, you did it, girl."

The new baby cried, the cord was quickly clipped, and Reeve took it to the baby warmer, where peds checked her lungs, which were fine. The new baby cried in protest when they suctioned her throat.

"Check my beeper," Reeve told Davies. "I pushed it when she came out."

"Twelve-oh-two."

Reeve examined Clarice and told her, "Girl, you got a small tear where you pee. Not that bad. I don't necessarily need to stitch it, if you keep it clean. Wipe front to back when you have a bowel movement." She helped Clarice push the placenta out and explained it to her. "Can you believe your body *made* this and grew a healthy baby?"

Peds said, "She looks great, Mom. I'll hold her up so you can see."

"Look! Look!" Rolanda said, both hands holding her face.

"She weighs thirty-two ten."

Rolanda asked, "What's that in real weight?"

"We'll have to translate."

"You pushed beautifully," Reeve said. "You stretched slowly. That's the way to do it."

Davies came in and said, "They're calling the supervisor since this is the first official baby."

Reeve massaged Clarice's belly. "I think your uterus is starting to firm down now. Feel right here. It needs to be hard so rub it. Now let me get you cleaned up, darling."

Rolanda cooed, "How you doing, grandmama's baby? Yeah, it's a big girl. Hello, sweetie, whatchoo doing?" And so on.

Reeve asked Clarice, "Are you going to breastfeed?"

"Yes."

"No," said Tyrone, his first word in over an hour.

"Yes."

"No."

"What's your problem with breastfeeding?" Reeve asked him.

He shook his head and said, "Similac."

Reeve walked to the nurse's station, where Olsen asked, "What time?" Reeve raised her hands in triumph. "Twelve-oh-two."

"I would have done an episiotomy," Olsen said, "and delivered at twelve and fifteen seconds, but I'm not a midwife."

Reeve called her family. "Hey, I just delivered the first Grady baby of the New Year. . . . I don't know. They're gonna call around." The phone rang. "This is Jodi Reeve. . . . Yes, I did it. Has anybody called around? And make sure my name is spelled right." In 6, she said, "OK, doll-baby, the administration knows." She did the baby exam, then Clarice finally held her baby.

Reeve returned to the nurse's station, where the phone rang again. "Nothing at Gwinnett, huh? That's one out of the picture."

The nurse next to her shook her head. "Look at this competition."

Lowry, the fourth-year, came by and congratulated Reeve. "I hope Northside didn't beat you."

"We know Gwinnett's out of the picture. My friend called me from there. She said she was getting her patient to pant and blow, but it delivered seventeen minutes before midnight."

"You didn't do anything?"

"Nope. I could have done an episiotomy, but I didn't. We should know soon. The night administrator is calling the paper."

A new patient was brought by in a wheelchair. She clutched a stuffed Piglet doll. Her husband massaged her back. The front desk called. "I *believe* it's the first one," Reeve said into the phone. "Everybody's on pins and needles, wanting to know." She hung up. "They said when he called the paper, no one else had reported anything."

The next day Channel 2 news showed Clarice's baby sleeping. "A new Atlanta resident won the first baby of the new year honors," the perfectly coiffed news coanchor said in his smooth baritone. "Born at two minutes past midnight. She weighed in at seven pounds even. Her mother and the baby are doing *splendidly*. Mom says she hasn't come up with a name yet. Any suggestions?" he said to the grinning weatherman holding a pointer.

"No," he said, still grinning.

"Too cute, too cute," said the other anchor, a heavily made-up woman with big white teeth. She turned back to face the camera and nodded her head.

"Yeah, beautiful baby," the first anchor said.

"I want to show you something on Radar Scan that I didn't get to show you earlier. . . ."

Channel 11 had two women anchors. "She was due to arrive *tomorrow*, but Veronica"—somehow they got the name when Channel 2 did not—"and her mother are doing fine, and she looks precious." "Precious" oozed out of her mouth in a gooey, smothery voice. The baby squirmed slowly on the screen.

"A-a-aw," the other anchor said.

"Looks good."

"She looks good."

They grinned at each other.

"See you at 11."

The daily newspaper told the story of the second Atlanta baby, born at a suburban hospital fifteen minutes after Clarice's. The story hardly mentioned Grady and Clarice. It said she "could not be reached for an interview." Jodi Reeve was not pleased. "PR wouldn't let them take a picture or talk with the mother because she's fifteen. I guess they don't want people to know, but 25 percent of their births are teenagers. I bet they don't want the teen patients to know they're embarrassed to have them." She snorted, "The powers that be."

As for Clarice, who lay in postpartum, her chart stuffed with still and video photography release forms, she was tired. "They wanted to see the baby," she explained. "They didn't talk to me a lot. I guess I was asleep when the paper called. They never actually said the paper called. I was up all night. The nurses thought I would get a free one-year supply of milk or diapers, something, but there was none of that." She pointed to a large wicker basket of samples. "I'm planning to get back in school, when I find a babysitter. Tyrone works two jobs. I used to work, but I quit when I got pregnant. Mom was here all day Sunday, then went back to work today. She's a manager at Wendy's. She works so hard all the time. She had to go do payroll. That place would go crazy without her."

"Arctic Blast Hits Georgia," the newspapers announced in early January. The woman at the round information desk in the atrium wrapped herself in coat, hat, scarf, and gloves. A portable heater hummed next to her. The wind blew cold outside; the front of Grady was empty. Atop the building thick white vapor emerged from air vents and quickly dissipated. In Labor and Delivery, muzak in the hall—a new addition to the floor—played Jimmy Buffett's "Margaritaville," a flute version. Jodi Reeve came by the nurse's station and invited the nurses to lunch in the conference room—her goodbye present to the floor. She brought spaghetti, salad, and cake. "It's tofu spaghetti," she said, "so you'll remember me." Reeve asked Renee Lindley about her son.

"My baby needs me to work twenty-four hours a day." She squeezed a dollop of lotion in one palm and rubbed it in her hands. "Ooh, that feels better. Howard University is looking for me now. As well as a bunch of other people." Through the door to 8, standing ajar, Lindley could hear a TV. "Soap operas," Lindley said. "That's a buncha crap that messes up your mind. My mama used to call 'em 'soup.' She'd say, 'I'm watching soup in the kitchen.' I'd say they were soaps. She'd say it was soup, what they got on there. I'd ask why. 'Because some of it is *hot!*'"

A man wearing scrubs and a white coat walked by holding a small ice chest, the kind used for small picnics. "Placenta man!" Lindley cried. A nurse must have obeyed the pathology department sign requesting placentas worthy of study. She walked with him down to room 16 and went in while he waited in the hall. She came out carrying a plastic blue tub. He put on gloves and used tongs to lift the placenta from the tub and put it in a rectangular Tupperware container. He dropped it in the ice chest, which was half-filled with ice, and clicked the top shut. The nurse returned the tub to the room; the placenta man removed his gloves, washed his hands, and left.

Reeve walked to the conference room, where her food was spread out. She taped to the wall a yellow Progress Report sheet and wrote on it, "GOOD-BYE EVERYBODY I'LL MISS YOU." A nurse warily forked her spaghetti, not sure about that tofu. She ate it and said, "This is delicious." A nurse came in and said, "Slice some cake for me."

Reeve pounced. "You have to have vegetarian spaghetti to get cake."

"Uh, well, OK, I'll get some."

"Always have an open mind."

"Is this low fat?" a nurse asked.

"None of it is," Reeve assured her. "You just have to get a low amount."

Most of the nurses wandered in for lunch. Another midwife came up from the OB clinic. They reminisced, telling old Grady stories. Reeve turned grim when Lana Vickery, a first-year resident, peered through the door, spying the dwindling supply of food.

"I didn't invite any damn doctors," Reeve whispered. "When they have food in the doctors' room, they're a herd. I don't recall one time the doctors inviting nurses in for food."

Vickery came in and said, "What do we have here?"

"Vegetarian spaghetti."

"Oh, good." She helped herself. "I'm a vegeterian."

After she left, Reeve told a nurse finishing her spaghetti, "If you want some cake, you better get some now. The doctors are coming."

"Oh, well," the other midwife said, "maybe in three years when we start our birthing center and ask her to be our backup, she'll remember the tofu."

A nurse looked through the doorway and asked the midwife if a patient could eat. She nodded. This evoked a farewell sermon from Reeve. "If they want to eat, eat. I'm changing my tune. This is my political thing. We're told only fluids, but that's antiquated. Stupid. A healthy woman who is hungry should eat. Plus, it might keep anesthesiology away. We have them feeling like they're invalids, like something's wrong. 'I can't do this myself. I have to have this monitor, epidural.' If she's hungry, let her eat. Labor is an intense experience. You need energy. Some say it makes the gut slow down blah blah blah. We're not using common sense. We do it because we've always done it. I don't operate that way. If they get general anesthesia, they could aspirate the food and die, but I've never seen that. And it's very rare that they get general anesthesia. Usually only those that they rush to the OR. Anesthesiology is our ball and chain. If people are hungry, it's not a bad thing to eat. The ones that are just piddling along, we leave them three days without feeding them. That's ridiculous! I'm practicing by my own common sense. I may get in trouble with anesthesiology, but it makes sense. That's the whole thing. How many things do we do that don't make sense? Like leaving the monitor on all the time. Like that's going to help them progress."

By the time Vickery returned to the residents' room, word had gotten around among the residents, who were always alert for free food.

"I heard there's some food. Where is it?"

"Down in the conference room, but there's not much left."

That did not stop him, or the others.

"I'll see what I can get."

Reeve watched as they filtered in. The muzak played Billy Joel's "Uptown Girl." Two more residents, one anesthesiologist, another resident. Soon there was no more sauce, only a bowl of white spaghetti. A lowly medical student came in and plopped a mound of plain noodles on a plate and dug in.

"He's claiming it's not his," Lisa Dean said, speaking of Dwayne. Lisa sat in a worn, thickly-padded easy chair in her kitchen. Clean laundry dried on a cord stretched across one corner, just above the washing machine. "He's upset because we broke up, but he's welcome any time. He might be hurt, but he can't take it out on the baby. I wish she wasn't his, but it's too late." Of her new boyfriend, Jonathan, she said, "He gets me whatever I need. We have our ups and downs, but it's mostly minor stuff. He be there for me." Looking through the kitchen window, Lisa watched Dwayne walk by. "He won't speak to me." Softly, she mockingly called his name, "Dwa-ayne." She added, "Our relationship was kind of abusive. When Dwayne was locked up the first time, when he was caught with drugs and all that stuff, Jonathan was there for me. He took me to see Dwayne, to Grady. I grew attached to him. When me and Dwayne got into it, Jonathan came to see me. We would talk, especially when

Dwayne was locked up. Then when I was eight months pregnant, one thing led to another, and we had intimate relations. It was protected.

"Me and Jonathan, we don't fight. Me and Dwayne used to fight. He would hit me, and I would hit back. I don't even remember the first time or how it got started. It was a shock so I tried to stab him after he hit me. Jonathan would break us up. He didn't like the way Dwayne treated me. Sometimes men have a good thing going and mess it up. Dwayne started messing around. Remember that time Lauren Foley gave me a prescription? Dwayne gave me trichomoniasis and gonorrhea. I told Dwayne after I had the baby I was gonna leave him. I guess he thought I was joking. He wanted to see if it would work out after the baby, but it changed for the worse. I met Dwayne on May 28, 1993. He used to give me money. I didn't like him at first, but then I did. He had different sides to him. My friend was going with his friend and told me to talk to him. Then I guess I just grew attached to him. There is no reason for us to fight. I tried to give him a chance. He said, 'I'll stop. I'll stop,' but I knew. They have you where they want you. They know you won't leave them. But if a man beats you, he don't care about you. When I got to where I hated him, I couldn't stay with him, but it takes some women longer. Some of them think he's joking when he says he's gonna kill you, but I know better. I think it worked out best. I'm happy. He's out of my life. I don't want him out of my daughter's life, but mine.

"On my birthday Jonathan gave me roses and balloons, delivered to me. Tammy fixed my hair, and someone knocked at the door. He said it was for Lisa and could go only to her hands. The card said, 'Happy Birthday from a Friend.' Jonathan was across the street, and I didn't think of him. I asked Dwayne if they were from him, and he said, 'Uh, yes.' I could tell by his look. I said, 'You a damn liar!' My mom can't stand Dwayne. She can read somebody from the first meeting."

A neighbor came in to borrow Lisa's phone. "I'm trying to get somebody to take me to pay my pager bill."

Lisa nodded OK and said, "I wanted to take those childbirth classes, but I didn't have no coach. I couldn't get Dwayne to go. I bet Jonathan would have gone. He wanted to be in the delivery room. If Dwayne hadn't been around, I would have let him."

Rob came in from playing and said, "I want to eat."

"Want some cereal?"

He nodded. She poured him a bowl of Cheerios.

"I want some milk."

"You don't need any milk."

He took his cereal outside.

Her friend Nikki dropped by to visit, with her two young children. She sat at the table and began eating a Big Mac. A truck pulled into the parking lot and honked. "Excuse me," Lisa said, "I got to get my baby's milk."

Nikki said, "They go to all the projects. There's no store around here. They come every Wednesday. They give you some Pampers, too."

Lisa returned with two boxes of formula and a bag of disposable diapers. Rob brought his cereal bowl back, put it in the sink, and left. "I want to send him to military school," Lisa said. "He is hard-headed. He needs a change of environment. I'll save my money for that. He'll come back a man."

Lisa asked Nikki about her brother, a teenager who spoke to school groups about abstaining from sexual activity, an effort supported by Grady's teen counseling program. "He's so smart," Lisa said. "He's so, so mature. He has a deep voice, like a grown man."

Nikki said, "He's a virgin, and he'll tell you in a minute. He says he wants to marry a virgin. He says he doesn't want to marry an open woman."

"I wish I was still a virgin," Lisa said.

"Me, too. He goes to middle schools to talk about sex. I'd tell 'em that, too. 'Don't do it. Don't do it.' "

"Me, too," Lisa said, "but I love my kids."

On the phone, Jan Dorman's mom, Teresa, said Jan had moved in with her, but had later decided to return to Carl. "She's gone back to that . . . guy." She said "guy" with a sneer. "His mother's getting him a little bitty house somewhere around the motel. They're sleeping at the motel; the house was a mess." She said Jan had a stitch removed that had worked its way to the surface and was keeping her C-section wound from healing.

The baby, Deanna, cried into the phone. Teresa soothed her, "Yeah, yeah." She said, "She's not taking her formula good. She has colic real bad. Otherwise, she's doing good. The HIV preliminary test was negative, but we won't know for sure for six months." Teresa said she had taken care of Deanna often. "To be honest, other people have had her more than Jan has, and I've had her the most."

Robin James sat on the sofa in her small living room, a large King James Bible open in front of her on the coffee table. Yellow highlighter in hand, she marked certain verses. "I don't like it when they change the words," Robin said, "so I look 'em up." She closed her Bible, put down her highlighter, and scolded a grandson who left dirty clothes lying on the floor. She said she had recently seen a bag of crack cocaine while at a laundromat and was drawn to the powerful little packet—then walked away. She remembered living in a Salvation Army shelter—she called it Sally's—and hoping her grandchildren never saw her like that. She began recalling the history of drugs in her family.

"My other brother on drugs, he got delivered. I'm delivered. We're praying for the other two. There was nine of us. Megan, Nadine, Shannon, Tremaine— Hmmm. Is that it, Lord? Out of nine, they was the only ones that wasn't on drugs. Now all of us is delivered except two. That's Rochelle and Thomas. Tonya got saved; I got saved. Stanley went from one thing to another, from drugs to alcohol, from alcohol to wild and crazy women. The best thing I know for anybody to get off drugs is to get saved. Them programs, they send you from one trip to another."

Robin stood and pointed at a painting on the wall. She had begun painting while in the psychiatric hospital, to help her emerge from her confusion. "I haven't finished it because I don't know the end, but in that picture there is a lot of my pain, a lotta little happiness, and a lotta hope. A lot of danger and drugs and the people that I met. You can see they ain't got no faces. All the people that be homeless and stuff, they always got some hats and things over their face because they don't know who they are. When I was amongst them, the only things that held me together was, I knew who I was, and I knew where I didn't want to go." She pointed at a corner of the painting. "This is Gabriel's horn. See the blue pipe with the orange flame? That's the dope. That's the people all around. See the confused people? These is people who no longer know what's happening with them. This man here, he still has hope. Hope is here, always here, but the people don't see it. Ain't nobody saying, you can do it, you can do it. Here is Satan looking, seeing everything. See the red dragon? But in the midst of all this evil, there's still hope. The fruit's blooming on the trees, the birds building their nests. Still got hope. Still got hope. Even when Gabriel come and blow his horn, hope will still be here. I couldn't finish my painting because I really don't know what the end is gonna be. I don't like to rush because I be thinking of things. And the music notes, that's the sound of the trumpet. When the trumpet blow, that's it. See the hand of God right here? Crushing the tail of the dragon. He's not as big and bad and tough as people think. He's gonna really be showed up when God show us how small he is and insignificant he really was in the end. But right now he's a big monster, causing chaos everywhere, but later on we're gonna really see he's just a little ol' thing, not even important. Ha ha ha."

Carrying her baby, Jan Dorman stepped off the bus and walked up a small hill to the Infectious Disease Center of Grady Hospital. At the pediatric AIDS clinic, the clerk, who wore a red AIDS ribbon on her Grady nametag, told Jan to get a new Grady card; hers had expired. She followed a series of signs with arrows pointing down this hall, then that one. "I don't know why they moved it," she said, of the Grady card office. She sat in a curved plastic chair and held Deanna. "I don't know what sleep is like. I'm living on coffee." The baby cried. Jan pulled a bottle from her green vinyl bag and fed her, rocking gently. "I must have lost some weight. Every time I try to eat, she wants to. She's eating real good again. She had a real bad cold and wasn't eating right, but she is now." Watching Deanna suckle rhythmically on the rust-colored nipple, Jan said, "She's cute as a jaybird. Negative as one, too."

She and Carl had moved into the house, she said. "It's a little two-bedroom, three hundred a month. It's not bad. He's working now doing inside construction work, tearing down walls and putting up new walls."

"Miss Dorman, is this card for you or your baby?"

"My baby."

Jan picked up her purse and walked back to the clinic, where she was told, "They gave you the old card back. You can't do anything with this card. I'll run down there and see what happened."

Grateful it was not she who was running down there, Jan sat in the waiting room. "That's Grady for you. If I had known it would take this long, I would have brought my cigarettes." Changing the baby's diaper, she said, "My stepmother thought I was beating her. It looks like a bruise on her butt, but it's a birthmark. Most of the time they fade, but her daddy has one on his butt, too." She gave the baby some juice and burped her. "I know it hurts, baby," she said soothingly. After the soft "hic," she fed her again. "If they give her more iron, they're going to have to lock me up. At the hospital in Rockdale, they said too much iron makes her constipated." Saying that, her face briefly quivered with anger. Jan removed the bottle and said, "Now you're going to spit up on me." Deanna did, on Jan's leg. "I should have just worn what I slept in." She wiped her leg clean and gave the baby a warm hug. "You nasty girl," she said in a bouncy light voice, "just like your stinking daddy. Yes, you are." She nuzzled Deanna's ear and kissed her face. Jan made clucking noises, which made the baby laugh. "His mom is opening a boutique, and she's gonna put me in charge of running it, so I can get off welfare. Are you going to throw up on me again?"

Blurp.

"Yes, you are."

To a woman sitting across from her, Jan said, "Is yours mixed, too?"

She paused, and answered softly, "Yeah."

"She's got that pretty hair."

"I hope he doesn't lose it. It's falling out."

Jan stroked Deanna's hair. "She lost a little."

"His is coming out on the sides here."

Jan pointed Deanna's face at the other infant. "There's one of your people. You'll have a lot to talk about. You'll go through a lot, in this crazy world." To her new acquaintance, Jan said, "She was about that dark when she was born, but she's lightened up."

"He was lighter, and he's gotten darker."

"I wish I had brought my cigarettes," Jan said.

"I may go smoke one, but about the time I go, they'll call me."

Jan wrapped Deanna in a coat and rocked her in her arms. She put a pacifier in her mouth. The baby drowsily closed her eyes, opened them, closed them. "I'll be glad when her hair gets longer, and I can put bows in it."

The woman covered her baby with a blanket, picked up the car seat, and headed out the door. She told the clerk, "I'll be back in a second."

Jan remained, biting her nails. "Our appointment was *two hours* ago." A nurse came to get Deanna; Jan went along. The other woman was called while she was outside smoking. When she returned, the clerk said over her shoulder, "She's back." Deanna's exam finished, Jan went back to the Grady card office to get a new Grady card for herself. A sign at the window said, "Gone to Lunch."

"Oh well, I'll get it when I come back. All her tests are still negative," she reported. "There's one test pending, and it most likely will come back negative, too, they said. They'll test her every month for six months, then every three months. Then once a year to make sure."

In a car riding to her small brick home, Jan watched a thin young woman walking along Sylvan Road. " 'Ho'," Jan said flatly. "She's a whore. I can pick 'em out just like that." She snapped her fingers. "I met enough of 'em. I never did it myself. Thank God I didn't have to."

At home, she brewed some coffee and lit a cigarette. She spoke in her usual high soft voice that matched her soft pasty cheeks. "Carl's mother owns two or three condominiums. She bought this house across the street, to make into the shop. She has over twenty thousand dollars in the bank. She said, 'And that ain't nothing.' I looked at her like, 'To *you*, it ain't nothing.' "

About Carl, she said, "I love him to death. He loves me. We haven't gotten along as well as we should have. And Mom doesn't like us living in Atlanta, in a drug area. He hit me once. Because I hit him in the arm. He says I hit him in the face, but I didn't. I have two witnesses. But he didn't hit me as hard as he has, before. The other night he threw me against the wall. He said I was aggravating him. We've gotten to where, since we're in this house right here, we don't even argue. In the hotel we didn't have a room to get away from the other. We saw each other day after day in that one room. When I get mad at him, I go in the bathroom and lock the door. I like the house better because we can smoke in here and it won't aggravate her. I can go to another room, and in the hotel you can't do that. Even the vent in the bathroom at the hotel didn't work. Him—" She pointed across the street. "Him" meant Carl, who was renovating the house his mother bought. "You asked me how I could spot out a prostitute. He used to be a pimp. He don't too much lie to me about what he did when he sold drugs and was a pimp. He taught me where I could spot 'em out like that. A lot of times you can tell by the way they walk, the way they wear their makeup, how they carry their pocketbooks. Sometimes they'll have a change purse connected to their belt loop, and that's where they keep all their money and drugs. I'd say ninety-five out of a hundred prostitutes do drugs. That's how they support the habit. You can tell. He wanted to get back into it, but I won't let him. I can't handle the thought of him being around a bunch of women, wanting to touch him and tell him they love him. They make the girls fall in love with them in order to get them to do what they want them to do, go out there and make money. I got a friend who loves to give it away. I told her if you're going to give it away to all these men, why don't you start charging 'em? Forty, fifty dollars, something. Don't get a pimp. Work for yourself. Keep your money. They usually have a quota to meet. If they're good, and the pimp knows they're good, they have a high quota, and if they don't have that quota, most of the pimps beat them. Some will take only sixty percent, but some only give you ten percent. It's the same with selling drugs. Your drug dealer gives you drugs to sell; you got to bring him a certain amount. It might be a seventy-thirty deal. I was lucky. I got fifty percent. That was in Lithonia, then in Conyers. I was always too scared to do it in Atlanta. You don't know who's a cop and who's not."

She said most of her customers were middle class. "The media is always on the low-class people, on welfare and food stamps. The media always classifies the blacks being the only ones on welfare, when there are more white people on it, like myself. . . . I'm not going to sit here and deny it. And the main ones they show doing drugs is the black people. They don't focus on the white people that do drugs. They focus on blacks and Hispanics. And it's wrong. Most of my customers were white. I only had a handful of blacks that came to buy. If you can get rich people to buy drugs, it's unbelievable. Most of my customers had jobs, they had their own place, one or two kids, and they still took care of home. They didn't spend all their money on drugs like the lower class does. I get offended when doctors ask me if I use drugs. Look at how healthy I am. A hundred and eighty-two pounds. I asked 'em once why they kept asking me that, and they said it was a question they have to ask all their patients. But I've been to some that don't. I don't think I could be friends with the media. They turn around what you say, to put it in the paper a different way. And it ends up being the lie that gets put in the paper. I think it's wrong. They're stereotyping poor people."

She took a puff and tapped ashes.

"My T-cells dropped. I cried because I knew I was positive. I was crying because I was hopeful. . . ." She said she still planned to get a GED. "I'm sure I can pass that. I've done two pretests. My English isn't very great, so I need to take a couple classes in that. The only problem with getting into school is I can't get financial aid because the credit bureau's got me, from some hospital bills I had. The only way I can get the money to do that is if me and him go ahead and get married, then his mom will probably pay for at least half of it. I know my mom ain't going to give me no help because she ain't got it. Getting ahold of the lady in Savannah who tried to adopt me is like finding a needle in a haystack. She would do it, but she's always going back and forth between Savannah and New York. It's hard to catch her. She wanted to adopt me when I was sixteen. I was in a girls' home down there and ran away from it. I kept running away, and they finally realized they couldn't hold me nowhere. That's when the caseworker at the welfare office almost lost her job because she told me what I could do to keep from having to go back, either get pregnant and have the baby, or get married." She pointed across the street. "Him, he drinks every day, but he don't get drunk."

Little sleeping Deanna turned in the crib and whimpered. "I'm gonna let Mama keep her this weekend. He don't know that yet. He doesn't want her around Mama, period, because of the interracial issue. I was given an ultimatum, the last time. Either to stay there and she'd help me or come back and she wouldn't. I didn't like being given an ultimatum. You don't give me an ultimatum. I'm a grown woman, and I love this man. I love him. And we're gonna get married when we decide we're ready. It's basically up to me. I'm not sure, more than he. I give her an ultimatum when I was younger. To either be with us kids or get married. And she got married. I tried everything in my power to cause a divorce. I didn't want her married. When she divorced my dad, she swore to us she'd never get married again. When it popped up on us, we didn't even know the man. She dated him for two years, and we had never met him. We didn't like it at all. To this day, he can't get over the fact that I tried to cause a divorce. But you got to understand I was a child, about ten. I wanted my mama to myself.

"It was like she devoted all her time to him. His word goes. That's why I don't feel she had the right to give me an ultimatum. Stay there and she'll help me. I couldn't live in her house because he didn't want me there, so what right do I have to be given an ultimatum? None. As much as I love her, I couldn't take it. If it wasn't for me needing rest, she wouldn't be getting the baby this weekend. Carl wants my dad-n-'em to keep her." She tapped her cigarette. "I love my family because they're family, but there's part of my family, I love 'em, but don't like 'em. And to me, Mama's getting to that point. I love her, but I don't like her."

She recalled being beaten by her father. "Me and my brother, too. That's when they sent me to a psychiatrist. I didn't like it. I would not talk to her. I'd go, but I would not talk to her. After a couple of months of seeing her, I started opening up to her. Then she thought she could bring my dad and his wife in, but when they came in, I wouldn't say nothing. I knew once we got home he would beat me again. So I wouldn't say nothing. Then in the girls' home, all the girls had to see a therapist. I never told her about the problems I had growing up. I told her about school and stuff. I thought, well, it happened, there's no way they could change it. So there wasn't any use in talking about it.

"When me and Carl first got together, I started having dreams about when I was a baby, being molested and raped as a baby, and it startled me. The first couple of dreams I couldn't see the face. After a while I was able to see the face, and I ended up more mad than startled because it was my father's face. I talked to my mom about it, and she was mad. She was, like, 'I didn't know. I coulda stopped it, but I didn't know.' If it wasn't for my father supposedly dying, I still wouldn't be talking to him. I didn't want him dying not knowing I loved him. I hate his guts, but I love him, because he's my father. It's just hard for me to believe, even though I seen it in my dreams, it's still hard for me to believe. A lot of people ask me why don't I ever date white guys. The only thing I can figure is that experience, as a child, my father, then his so-called friend trying to get it on with me. Then my stepmother's father, then another white dude come through my bedroom window, trying to force me. With all that going on at such a young age, that's going to put a block right there toward white men to me. Even though I've been raped by black men, it didn't start off with nobody in my family. Nobody black in my family did anything like that."

It's One

Outside Lisa Dean's apartment, a group of young men held money and threw dice against concrete steps. Each either exulted or groaned at each throw. Next door to Lisa's place, a boy stepped out of Cheryl's apartment—store—shaking a steamy bag of microwave popcorn. A young woman entering Cheryl's apartment told a little girl, who held her hand, "We're going to see the candy lady." Lisa sat in her kitchen, Jonathan's new Rottweiler puppy tied to the barber chair and nipping at her feet. Her washing machine turned rhythmically. She said she was taking her two children to stay with her mother that weekend. "I have to do my community service, picking up trash by the side of the road. I got eight more days before I'm finished. It happened a year ago. I was hanging out with the wrong people. They were stealing in a mall, and I was with them." She said Dwayne had come in once last week and asked to hold the baby. "He's held her two times since then, but he still doesn't come to see her like he should."

Child support?

"Nah." Her friend Tiny came in and began washing dishes in the sink. "Jonathan buys her Pampers. He's more like her father than her biological father. I'm ready to go back to school, as soon as I finish my community service. I'm going to this place that has GED classes."

Someone knocked on the door.

"Who *is* it?"

A boy came in and asked for change for a ten. She gave him a five and five ones. "I would have graduated in 1990. I should have gotten my GED a long time ago. I was stupid. I just didn't like school. I hung around with people who don't want to do nothing. They quit school already. It'll rub off. My mom told me, 'You're too stupid to go back to school and too smart to go back.' She said I acted like I was the smartest person in the house. Right, Tiny?"

He scrubbed a frying pan. "Yeah, you thought you were highly educated."

"Heh heh heh. Mom kept trying to get me to go back to school. I didn't want to get up early. I wish I had now. My principal told me to miss one quarter since it was so close to my due date, and come back the second, but after missing the first, I didn't want to go back. If they had let me go back that first quarter I would have finished. I was hanging with people who didn't say, 'Get back to school, or I'm not your friend.' They said forget school. Now, I am twenty-three, and I ain't got shit."

"Yes, you do," Tiny said. He finished the dishes and left.

D'Lisa cried. Lisa picked her up and kissed her face. Lisa cradled her, looked around the room, and said, "I got a secret I'll tell you some day." She looked out of the corner of her eye. "Believe this or not—No, I'm not going to ever tell you. I can't. Yes, I can. No, I can't. I'll tell you . . . one day. You're going to say, 'How could you?'" She moved to a metal folding chair and put D'Lisa in the big soft easy chair, where the little girl sat upright well. "Sit up there," she said and went upstairs to her room, then returned. She picked up D'Lisa and sat in the soft chair. "She can really focus on stuff now, like she knows she's looking at something. And I bet she'll be talking before she can walk. My mom was real upset with me in high school. Now I wish I had done what Mom told me. I would have a high school diploma. I would have learned a trade, and I'd be doing better." D'Lisa cried again. Lisa gave her a bottle, looked around the room and said, "Jerry, I think I'm pregnant again. I believe I am. I will be getting my tubes tied if I am. We used condoms, and the time it burst last month, that's the last time I seen my cycle, and this month is almost over with. He wants me to go to the doctor, but I don't want to. I was sick last week, and my mom was here. She asked me what was wrong. I said I had the flu. She said, 'Yeah, the nine-month flu. This time you're on your own.' I burst out crying when she left. If I am pregnant, I want to get my GED before it's born.

"One thing about it, Jonathan graduated and has one year of college. He'll keep after me to get my GED. He was working for a factory, but he said he was just standing up there falling asleep. He wants to do something where he moves around. So he's been getting up early looking for a job, ever since he quit a few weeks ago. I just hope he's not in jail when I deliver. Back in November he was out with a group playing craps, and you can get arrested for that, plus somebody had hid drugs over there. He was in the wrong place at the wrong time. He goes back to court in February. His mom put up some money to get him out. I put up a hundred." She looked upstairs toward the bathroom. "I feel like I'm going to get sick."

Labor and delivery nurse Renee Lindley looked at the monitor at the nurse's station. "I better up that Pit." She went into room 4, then returned. "That baby's withdrawing. The doctor let me give her some juice and she knocked it all over the floor. I guess she said psssht on all o' y'all. Heh heh." She sat and wrote a progress report, glancing at the screen. "Look, that's a big one." A steep craggy black hill arose where the contraction line crept across the screen. She talked as she wrote, chewing her usual wad of gum. "I thought I could get an extra thirty minutes of sleep this morning, but Doug said he was going to work early, so I had to come on in. And I had to come up with an extra fifteen hundred dollars for my son's tuition. They went up. I cancelled my Christmas savings and vacation. And I can't borrow. I'm at my max. I had a good bit for vacation, too. I don't know about nobody else, but fifteen hundred is a lot of money for me."

Michelle Horn, the nurse working the station with Lindley, arrived from room 2. They began talking about residents. "The fourth-year we got today," Horn said, "some nurse said she's a good doctor." She and Lindley exchanged blank looks. "I said, 'Would you go to her?' She said, 'Uh, er, ominy, ominy, ominy.' And the third-year has a nice personality, but, Renee, would you go see her?"

The same look.

"Ooh, look at that face."

"I think Southern nurses are slier," Lindley said. "We just give 'em that look. We don't call a fool a fool. We just look at 'em."

Lindley finished writing and went to the break room. She got a Yoo-Hoo soda and sour-cream-flavored potato chips. A red label on the soda crowed, "99% FAT FREE CHOLESTEROL FREE." She sat at the table and called home. "Are you doing your homework? Be finished by the time I come home, OK? . . . Y'all can have some ice cream. . . . OK, bye-bye." She hung up and said, "When I got home from school, my mom was *there*, and we went straight to the garden. It was as long as this hospital and just as wide." She finished and returned to the station. Horn squinted at Lindley's hand. "I like your wedding band," she said, "but it looks like a man's."

"It is," Lindley answered. "I wear his, and he wears mine. To confuse the evil spirits in the house. When they do something, my ring usually gets tore up or something, so we switched to confuse 'em, and since then, things have been better."

"Take it *out!*" a woman shouted in room 1. "Oh! Oh! Shit!"

Lindley said, "My husband Doug had to go through so much to get his kids back. He had 'em by someone he wasn't married to. They eventually were put in foster care, and it took him a long time to ever get them back. When they act up, he'll say, 'You're doing this? After the hell I went through to get you back?' I say, 'Doug, chill on that.' I think he conned me. Heh heh. He used to talk about getting his kids back when we were dating. I thought that was such an admirable quality. Heh heh. And when we got our daughter from the county, I made chicken, raisin-apple salad, potato salad. She crammed food in." Lindley made shoveling motions into her mouth. "She couldn't breathe, her mouth was so full of food. I said, 'Doug, she was deprived, wherever the devil she was.' She was afraid she wouldn't get nothing else."

Loud scroans echoed from room 1.

At the other end of the hall, Marie Costley took the vital signs of a patient in room 11; the patient grabbed her and said, "I'm afraid." A patient's fear, grasping a nurse—these happened routinely. But looking into the woman's face, Costley's intuition told her, Get somebody in here. The panic on her face—it seemed like oxygen depletion. Remain calm, Costley told herself. She shouted toward the hall, loud but controlled, "Get a doctor in here. Now."

A flurry of announcements paged doctors to room 11. First, the third-year, the fourth, the attending. All were called STAT. Nurses and doctors rushed in and out. A crowd of nurses and clerks and clinic assistants gathered in the hall. A sign on the door warned,

STOP
RESPIRATORY PRECAUTIONS
YOU MUST WEAR A MASK TO ENTER THIS ROOM

"She's HIV-positive," someone said, "with twins, preterm. And positive for TB and asthma."

From the room came a flurry of words: "Is there a heartrate? Is there a heartrate?" "Get a cup of ice!" "Tell Nancy the patient coded." "Get anything we'll need in case we do a C-section!" "We're trying to stabilize her now."

Patricia Duncan, newly promoted from clinic aide to clerk, stood next to the nurse's station. "If someone coded, I'm supposed to stay right here. That's what I was told." She grasped the counter. A doctor exiting 11 said, "It's hot as hell in there." Inside, a crew worked on the thin patient, surrounded by a crowd of OB, pediatric, and anesthesiology residents, learning about something they may never see again. An LPN at the nurse's station looked in the patient's chart for family to call. She announced, "She doesn't have a phone. Only one in the Bahamas."

Over the intercom came announcement of another emergency. "Set up the OR for a STAT C-section, breech, from 6!" From that end, a small entourage quickly wheeled a bed toward the OR. Fourth-year Mary Lowry knelt on the bed between the patient's legs, her hand in the vaginal canal, keeping the awkwardly positioned baby inside, saving its life.

"Slow down, slow down," someone instructed as they turned into the OR.

"If I get her family," the LPN said about the woman in room 11, "what do I tell them?"

"We'll get a doctor to explain it to them."

"This is the third time. She's done the same thing twice before. We just had a baby of hers in NICU for fifteen months. She's got papers to have her tubes tied. Maybe this time she won't be back."

"How much blood do you need?"

"Two."

Strapping on a mask, OB department chief Dr. Wayne Denson strode into 11.

"I got the patient's mama on the phone, long distance."

A nurse left the room and quickly rummaged through the crash cart, which, with its drawers and compartments flung open, looked like a burglar had frantically rifled through it in the dark. A resident, speaking into the phone, explained to a mother far away that her daughter might require an emergency C-section. "Everything happened at once. I need to get your verbal permission. Right now we have her on a machine. You may want to call back in a couple of hours, and we can tell you more. . . . OK, bye."

"We need some goggles in here!"

"We need an IUC."

"I'm going right now."

Word filtered down that the emergency-breech C-section from the other end had produced a good baby. The action in 11 slowed. She was stable. A decision was reached to do a C-section. Clerks and nurses began rehashing the episode from the moment they had heard about it. Marie Costley emerged from 11. She had been in there the whole time. Her sweaty hair was matted to her head. She looked weary. Third-year Dr. Griggs announced, "Prepare the OR for a C-section," then sat and wrote furiously on progress sheets. After the patient was wheeled to the OR, a housekeeper, covered in white protective clothing—boots, overalls, gloves, goggles, mask, hood—entered 11 to clean it. Gauze, torn paper and plastic wrappers, progress sheets, and bits of tape were scattered all over the room, deathly quiet after the massive rush to save a woman and the two babies inside her.

"You look like you're going into a blizzard," a nurse teased.

"Are you going on the space shuttle?" Duncan asked.

In the residents' room, a medical student asked about the breech C-section. "At first I thought they might try to deliver vaginally in the OR," second-year Melissa Avery said, "but there's no way she could. We had to cut a lot of the uterus. She's going to have a big scar, but—"

"The baby's out."

"The baby's out."

The pelvic model had been moved over to a desk by the small refrigerator and microwave oven. The brown fetus doll lay next to the model, on its side, balled up, staring at the refrigerator. Food was strewn all over the desks: Diet Coke cans, an empty milk carton, two large empty aluminum foil pans, bagels, a brown McDonald's bag, sliced carrots in a Ziploc bag, small tubs of coffee creamers, a Dole pineapple can, and a bag of microwave popcorn. Dr. Denson returned from the C-section on the HIV-TB patient with twins.

"How'd it go?" Avery asked.

"Like clockwork," he said. "They're little, not too little."

The phone rang. Another emergency. "Who has a prolapse?" Avery said into the phone. She hung up and said, "Thirty-two-weeker from 4B, ruptured, C-section STAT. She's on her way over." The residents hastily put things down and dashed into the hall.

Griggs shouted, "Hold the door open so they can come right in!"

A team of doctors waited at the entrance. Here they came, turning out of the elevator, pushing the frightened young woman, on her bed, through the doors. "Slow down! Slow down!" they shouted as they wheeled her around the corner at the registration desk, and pushed her toward the OR. Third-year Karen Olsen ran beside the bed, her hand in the woman's vagina, holding the baby's head and the cord in place. The cord had entered the birth canal; if pinched by the head, it would supply no more oxygen to the baby, killing it in moments. Olsen's face was ashen, terrified, only slightly less so than that of the patient, who stared ahead, frozen in terror.

"Call peds, STAT!" Griggs shouted to the clerk at the registration desk. Nervously, quickly, the clerk read the instruction sheet next to the phone, running her finger down the words. "Oh, Lord, please, how do you do this?" She punched in the code. "OK, I did it." The code was normally entered at the nurse's staion, not here at the front desk. Two pediatric residents slammed open the stairwell door. "Another STAT?" they said, running down the hall toward the OR. "Good, it went through," the clerk said, and sighed, relieved to have completed a task she was rarely called on to do.

A nurse trotting by said, "It's STAT C-section day."

Soon, Avery and Griggs returned to the residents' room. "We saved that baby's life," Avery said.

"Yep."

"And it was crying strong."

"We cut her immediately and had that baby out in thirty seconds. Sleep time was twelve-forty-four, and delivery time was twelve-forty-five."

A physician assistant who had come in the residents' room to eat lunch said, "I asked this one patient her number of sexual partners. I told her I had to ask her. She said she used to work the streets, so I asked for an estimate. She said twenty a week for ten years."

"Whoa!" Avery said.

"Set up the OR for a C-section from 2," someone announced.

A nurse leaned into the room and asked, "How are all those emergency babies doing?"

"All four are doing well."

At the nurse's station, Lindley said, "Whew, when I get home tonight, I ain't gonna do homework with nobody." The muzak chimed the melody to the old Kenny Loggins hit, "Danny's Song." "Even though we ain't got money, I'm so in love with you honey . . ." oozed out of every speaker on the floor. An LPN came by and told Lindley she had won money in the state lottery by looking at how much she spent on groceries that day, her social security number, and her husband's car tag number. "They all had three numbers in common, so I put down those three, and I won. I wish I had *known* I felt lucky. I would have put down more money and wouldn't have to come to work today." Lindley received a phone call from her husband. Her face grimly set, she listened, then said in a soft but firm voice, "Did you tell them? . . . Tell them I don't play. Say don't mess with my chillun." She hung up the phone. "These kids were trying to get mine to fight. You can burn my house down, but don't mess with my chillun."

Lindley answered the phone again; it was the mother of a twelve-year-old girl in labor, who was alone in room 2 and who had received no prenatal care. Using her steady I'm-a-nurse voice, Lindley explained, "She's doing fine. We gave her an epidural for pain. She's contracting nicely. It should be later this afternoon or this evening, but she's doing fine. . . . OK, OK. If you haven't heard anything by one or two, give us a call back. . . . OK, bye."

Lindley had at least three voices: the soft firm voice of a nurse talking to a mother or a patient, the snappy down-home-Louisiana-girl voice that sassed in the break room, and the educated-nurse voice of a woman who could remember book information by closing her eyes and recalling what she had read. The muzak from the intercom speakers in the hall ceiling played Billy Joel's "I'm Only Human."

Clerk Roberta Lilly walked by, and asked Lindley, "How's your baby?"

"He's still in classes, but we couldn't come up with the dorm fees. He was gonna move in with friends and look for an apartment, but he took his stuff to a friend's room two floors up. I said, 'Lance, you can't do that. It's still the same building.' They said he couldn't get back in even if we came up with the money. They said they'd have to go back in the *computer*"—she rolled her eyes—"like that's a big deal."

"He's going to make it," Lilly said, "if he's trying to get back in that dorm after they said he had to leave."

Lindley turned grim-faced and said, "I'm trying to work something out with the financial aid office. If it don't work out, I'm gonna have to go get him. One good thing, since he's in college out of state, they can't throw him out until I come get him. That'll give me time to get some money." She slapped the monitor. "She's complete. Call the doctor." The twelve-year-old's mother called. Lindley told her, "She's contracting well. I'd predict a baby by four o'clock. She dilated to seven or eight, only two more to go. She's doing great, and the baby's doing great. . . . You're welcome." She did not tell the mother that a urine test had shown large amounts of ketones in her blood, which meant she had not eaten well for a pregnant girl. Her body had turned to itself for sugar. An IV dripped a sugar solution into her bloodstream. Lindley went into 2. Before shutting the door, she said, "Stop that pushing. If you're not really complete, it can hurt you."

In thirty minutes, the doctor returned to 2, and Lindley began instructing the twelve-year-old to push. The muzak played the tune of Firefall's old song, "You are the woman that I've always dreamed of. I knew it from the start," on synthesizer and horns; then a flutey version of "Don't Be Cruel." "Push, push," Lindley instructed. "Push the burning away."

"You're doing beautiful, beautiful," the doctor said. And in a few minutes, a baby cried.

Lindley returned to the nurse's station and said of the twelve-year-old, "Her mama found out last night when they brought her here. If that was me, you'd have to throw me in jail. She said she's thinking about not keeping the baby. They haven't had a chance to talk about it. She wants her mom to see the baby, but she's not here. She was here earlier but not now." Above, horns played a bland version of "Jailhouse Rock," then Earth, Wind & Fire's "September" ("never was a cloudy da-ay"), then John Lennon's "Imagine." "She keeps asking if her mama called. Her mama said she couldn't believe it. I said I can only *imagine* what it's like for her. My family had a relative deny it all the way up 'til she fell out at school." She scratched her arm. "Whoo, between the stress over my son and these scrubs, my skin is drying out. I'm worried about his school, and I'm allergic to the soap Grady uses." Scratching, she said, "My kids say, 'Mama, we got you something for Valentine's,' and they be like this." She held her fists tightly under her chin, widened her eyes, and looked around. "They're dying to tell me. That tickle me."

A woman using the nurse's station phone said, "Yeah, this one's pregnant, too. They're driving me crazy." She hung up and dialed again. "I better call my job. They'll wonder where I am." A nurse carried the baby from 2 to the nursery.

"Mom'll have to go to the nursery to see the baby," Lindley said. "We couldn't wait any longer for her to get here. Oooh look, she's a big baby. Look at those fat cheeks." Lindley went outside for a smoke, then returned in time to take a call from the twelve-year-old's mother. "You didn't get here," she said in her soft voice. "The baby's doing fine. She's at the nursery. When y'all come, if she's not here, she'll be over in 4 A, in front of the old Grady. . . . She's doing great right now, just hungry. . . . A girl, a big ol' pretty girl. . . . I know it's hard. . . . OK, uh huh, you're welcome. Bye, bye."

Later in the afternoon, in the break room, Lindley said to Ella Davies, "I thought the old Grady era is gone. We used to work like this on old thirteen hundred. The gremlins are out today. Our nicely planned nursing schedule is shot to hell." They were talking about the tension of the day, with its constant stream of arriving patients, three emergency C-sections in an hour, the harried staff. The phone in the break room rang. Lindley listened a moment and said tersely, "I'm at lunch." She returned the phone to the hook. "She hung up on me. She wanted me to come to the ICU. I haven't finished my OR report yet, and I haven't had lunch yet. These are old thirteen hundred days, honey. We just forgot to tell the patients, 'This ain't old Grady no more.'" She took a bite of her lunch. "You know, Ella, I don't usually fuss, but when I feel like I'm being taken advantage of, I raise hell."

In the hall, a nurse snapped at an OB tech that he had not set up a room correctly. "Let's go in here!" he snapped back. They retreated into a conference room to finish talking. The tension had reached the residents' room, where a resident complained about something, "Why the fuck weren't they doing anything during that time?"

At the atrium information desk, the clerk sat without her coat and scarf and gloves on, and she was fine, even though it was frigid outside. A heating unit had been installed next to her booth. Nice warm air blew gently toward her. Additional heaters were being installed above the front doors, the blowers aimed into the atrium. In the OB waiting room, Lisa Dean said, "Well, here I go again. I'm going to get my tubes tied this time. I sure am. Then I'll be happy." She sat next to Robin James's daughter, Pauline.

Pauline was pregnant again, too.

Ms. Griff walked by and waved at Lisa. Lisa waved sheepishly. She told Pauline, "She was so nice to me when I first came here. She told me what to eat, what not to eat. And she said don't come back next year. She should have said that last time, too."

Ms. Griff walked back by, smiling. "Don't—" Lisa demanded, holding her hand up.

"I didn't say nothing."

Pauline said, "I wanted to go to a private doctor, but I was afraid they might miss something. But when I have an appointment I expect to stay two or three hours at the max. Lisa said be prepared to stay all day, but I don't have that much time."

Lisa was called to the desk and referred to an HIV counselor, for a routine information session. She sat in a small cubicle. A poster above her head reminded, "AIDS You Can Protect Yourself." Another said, "You Can Get A New Man, But You Can't Get A New Life." A bumper sticker on the wall said, "No Glove No Love." The counselor told Lisa her blood test would be confidential. Results would be told to her face-to-face, not through the mail or over the phone. She said they would test her for HIV only if she gave permission. She was shown a consent form and asked to read it and explain it in her own words. Lisa read it and said, "If the test is negative, I should come back in three to six months. I'm not in the clear yet."

"And if it's positive?"

"I am HIV positive. But I take the AIDS test every six months anyway."

"Is there a Georgia law that says you should tell your sexual partners?"

"Yes."

"What kind of condom gives you the best protection?"

"Latex."

The counselor held up two condoms, a pink one and a blue one. "See how thin this one is? It will tear, so use latex." She was shown a female condom. "See how soft this is? It'll tear, too."

Lisa was handed a questionnaire. She read each question and made check marks to indicate her answers. She asked, "It asks if you've had sex with a person who's in prison. What about jail?"

"They mean *prison*."

"I'm gonna change my answer, then." She finished and was told to wait for her name to be called for her medical interview. In the waiting room,

Lisa said, "I'm not going to tell my mom. My sister says she's six months pregnant, and she still hasn't told Mom. She ain't really big. She wears big clothes. I think she's retarded for not telling her. When she goes into labor, what's she going to tell Mom? And she stay with Mom! She *act* like she on her cycle." About her own pregnancy, Lisa said, "Jonathan was happier than I am. I don't like that shit. It's just so *soon*. I'm just glad I'm not younger. That would be like having one right after Rob. And I will get my tubes tied. I don't care what anybody says. They can take my insides out, for all I care."

Two teenage girls sitting next to her made fun of a woman walking by, whose facial skin was deep red. "Fried chicken wings," one said. They giggled.

"Don't say that," Lisa scolded them. "That's wrong. You might hurt somebody's feelings.

"Tameeka was so mad at me. 'We had so much planned for this summer, and you got pregnant.' I'm not trying to get my phone hooked back up. It gets on my nerves. It rings rings rings. And I will not go to my mom's house. I'll try to lie, and I will not be able to. She'll look at me and say, 'You're pregnant, aren't you?' I'll say, 'No.'" She said the "No," in a pouty, little-girl voice.

At the OB desk, Pauline James checked out after her prenatal visit, clutching a blurry ultrasound picture of her baby. "I'm due one day before my birthday. My mom's not excited yet. I guess she's afraid it might turn out like the other one."

Robin James was happy, but wary, about her daughter Pauline's pregnancy. "I just don't want her to be disappointed this time. Been too many times. She got a lot of happiness right now, and I would hate to see it all change." She also had mixed feelings about the father of this child. "I hope I'm not bearing false witness, but that's my opinion. I'm not happy about him, but you can't pick nobody for 'em. He's from a family with a whole lot of money, and he is spoiled to death. Only his feelings count. That's what I pick up. That ol' lowdown boyfriend, I told him he better not call me. If he call me, I'm going to call him what he is. He ain't righteous at all. He's one of those guys that's undependable. And Pauline do not need one of those in her life. Pauline needs a dependable person. He been with her more than five years and, my Lord, he can't be dependable when she gets pregnant? That's terrible."

She said she was most pleased when she was in the kitchen cooking, and Pauline called, hungry. "I'll be cooking stuff, and she'll say she's got a craving for something, and that's what I got on the stove. I love that."

In the Perinatal Center, Lisa Dean waited for her ultrasound. The TV/VCR played a tape on delivery, this time dubbed in Spanish. Black and white Americans walked around and moved their lips on the screen, but Spanish words came from the speaker. As the woman's delivery became imminent, everyone in the waiting room turned toward the screen, even those who spoke no Spanish. Some chuckled. One woman stared hard, squeezing a pencil against her nose with her top lip, her forehead furrowed. At the climactic moment of delivery, even the three clerks at the desk turned to watch. Once the baby was out, conversations resumed.

"I can't wait until this is over with," Lisa said. "The whole thing." She said Jonathan was back in jail. The original judge was on vacation, and the substitute had revoked Jonathan's bond. "I sure hope that judge is back next Tuesday," she said, "and reinstates his bond. His lawyer said the DA had it in for him." She said D'Lisa was at Jonathan's family's home. "I think he and I will tie the knot, but we haven't reached that point yet. He said all it takes is a little love and trust." She snickered and watched the TV. "Her water done broke. My water never broke. Jonathan's upset because he wanted to be here for the ultrasound. Twins run in his family. Twins. He said, 'I hope I'm there for the delivery.'"

Lauren Foley, Lisa's midwife during her last pregnancy, called for a patient over the intercom. Lisa recognized her south Georgia twang. "If Lauren Foley sees me, she'll say, 'What did you do? Why did you do that?' My mom told me she already knew. She set me and Jonathan down and asked us what we were going to do. Jonathan said, 'I'm going to take care of mine, D'Lisa too, if her father don't.' Mom didn't want to talk about it at first, but she's like that whenever I first get pregnant. She was kinda mad then got over it. She never liked Dwayne, but she loves Jonathan." She watched the TV again; a new tape was playing, this one in English. Lisa said, "She's crying, she's crying, she's crying. I didn't cry." She listened as the people on the screen talked about delivery. "They crazy to be talking about that shit."

"Lisa Dean," an ultrasonographer called, standing in the doorway.

In twenty minutes Lisa returned to the waiting room, dancing. "It's only one," she sang. "It's one. It's one. It's one."

A More Permanent Basis

"They say it usually goes up after you have a baby," Jan Dorman said about her T-cell count, which was in the seven hundreds—well into the healthy range. She sat in the den of her little house, her boyfriend Carl working at the house across the street. "And I haven't had any thrush in a long time." The house, she said, was getting crowded. Carl's sister and three-year-old son had moved in. "And her boyfriend's here a lot. Her and her boyfriend don't get along when they're together. They've been together three years. He comes by about every day." She noted that the room did not smell of smoke. "I don't let anyone smoke in here, and I quit all smoking in the house. She inherited allergies from me. It smells up the furniture, the carpet, the curtains."

She said she was likely not going to work at Carl's mother's boutique, as she had anticipated. "Some Chinese want to rent it and start a nail place. They already hired a receptionist, so I don't know. I still got this house to take care of. And the baby. My mom wants me to come there more. I ride the bus, and she meets me somewhere. She still doesn't like me living around here, but she's worried more for the baby than me. I'll be so glad when she"—she looked at her baby sleeping in a crib—"gets out of these sleepless nights. Carl's just now getting to where he's playing with her a lot. I let her sit in the room and cry instead of picking her up. I use reverse psychology on him. He just expected me to do it." She said she quit taking her AIDS medicine and would let the disease take her if the HIV turned into AIDS. "I could take the medicine, but I don't want to. I took it while I was pregnant. When I get sick, I ain't going to take nothing." She shook her head. "When the Lord thinks it's my time, it's my time."

"We're in mourning, Jerry," Lisa Dean said in the kitchen of her neighbor, Cheryl, whose kitchen was also the store. Marion Thurston sat at the dining table, rolling coins for Cheryl. A sign above the sink said, "Christ is the head of this house, the unseen host at every meal, the silent listener to every conversation." Lisa continued, "Our friend lost her baby at birth. The cord was wrapped tight around its neck. She went in for an ultrasound, and it had a heartbeat, but between then and the operation the baby must have died. I can't imagine having a dead baby inside you."

Neighbors came in, bought candy, sodas, bread. Lisa and Marian took their money and put their purchases in brown paper bags. Cigarettes were fifteen cents apiece, two for a quarter; a roll of toilet paper was fifty cents. Marian said, "My best friend said he would be my labor coach, but he don't want to watch those tapes, when they show women having babies and shit."

"Marian," Cheryl asked, "are your legs getting bigger or smaller?"

"Bigger," Lisa said. "And her booty, too."

The fruit truck pulled into the parking lot; the driver gave a long blast on the horn. Lisa went out to get some apples. She returned and said she was mean to everyone these days. "Don't mind me. Seriously. I don't know why."

"You're not mean to me," Marian said.

"You a damn lie," Lisa answered.

Cheryl settled it. "You always been mean."

Lisa said, "I feel like my attitude's messed up. Oh, Cheryl, you got Summer's Eve. How much is it?"

"Fifty cents."

A woman buying candy asked Lisa if she was going to have this baby at Grady.

"Yeah," Lisa said. "All my babies are gonna be Grady babies. If I have twelve." Marian, still pouring coins through a plastic slot into paper tubes, slashed a sharp look at Lisa. Lisa roared laughing, then said, "Children are the best drugs you can have. You'll be deprived and that baby'll look at you, and you'll feel so good. That's why I don't see how some people can give away their baby. Every time Jonathan came over, he said he wanted me to get pregnant. I just hope he's out of jail by the time I have the baby. He got four years. He might only have to serve four months if he goes to boot camp."

"What about your brother?" the woman asked.

"That is his baby all the way, but she won't let him see it. She's trying to say it's that other boy baby. He felt so bad. It really hurt him. He was so depressed."

"Mm huh."

"She's gonna end up needing him. The baby's doing fine now, but I think she'll be a little slow. She was in the hospital a while for brain damage. I don't know what happened. I don't know if they dropped the baby, threw the baby or what. Her head was so swoll', girl. When she does need Franklin, I'm going to try to get custody of my little niece. She called me from the hospital and wanted my help, but then later she tried to say it wasn't my niece. But she looks just like Franklin. Her hair is just like his."

"What about your case?"

"They closed the case, girl. I was so happy. The probation officer was going to lie and say I didn't *want* to do community service, but I was sick. But the judge knew I was trying, so he closed the case. I'm off probation. I don't have to do nothin'!"

"Good."

Lisa said she now sees Dwayne almost daily. "He comes to get D'Lisa. They go off. He takes care of her, for a good while now. He got it into his head that I got somebody else and it's over, and he's got a little girl. He wasn't around at all for a while. His little boy's mom wouldn't let him see his boy. He just didn't want to be around, I guess, at that time. But now he comes around. I was getting on him. A lot of people were getting on him. I think his mom was getting on him. And D'Lisa looks just like him but with my complexion."

She repeated that she wanted to get her GED. "For my kids. I don't want to stay in the projects all my life, like a lot of these girls do. I'll pass it then take up a trade and do something other than sit around. Put my kids in a nursery and try to better myself. With or without their fathers there. It doesn't matter to me, as long as I'm there. My mom raised five kids by herself, and I know damn well I can do it. I know I can do it. My grandmother raised six kids by herself, after her and her husband got a divorce. So why can't I? I'm a strong woman, just like my mom and my grandmother. I can do it. I'm not doing it just for me anymore; that's just the thing. I have kids to do it for now, and I love them a lot, and I need to do something for them, too, instead of just for myself. I can't think about just Lisa. It's Rob, D'Lisa, and another baby now. I can't just think about myself. One day you're going to see me, and you'll say, Lisa, you did it. I'll say I did it all with God. Anything is possible with God. With God anything is possible, and I need him on my side because he wants me to get my life together."

Rob came in the door. "Mom!"

"Yes, Rob."

"Mom, I got me another toothbrush. I ain't gonna lose that one."

Lisa laughed. "OK, don't lose it."

She was still not sure what to think of her sister's pregnancy. "That's a loony tune. I said, 'Tell me. You weren't really pregnant, were you?' I love her, but she's crazy. If she was pregnant, I don't know what happened to it."

"My urine is not yellow," Grace Lewis announced to the childbirth class, which Marian Thurston attended, her mother Ginger sitting next to her. As usual, Marian arrived early and prepared. She had read all the literature distributed the weeks before and correctly answered every question Lewis put to the class. Mother and daughter waggled their feet as they sat listening. Lewis told them the importance of drinking plenty of water, giving herself as an example of someone who drank water so regularly that her urine was diluted. Ginger knew it all, too. She would whisper under her breath what Lewis was about to say. "Amniotic fluid," she mumbled when Lewis mentioned the "bag of water." Lewis began talking about foods they should avoid when they reached labor. "Don't eat what will stay with you. Fried foods, dairy products. What do you think you should eat?"

"Toast," someone volunteered.

"Salad."

"Good," Lewis affirmed.

A young man who accompanied his sister asked, "What about oatmeal?" Grimmacing, his sister turned and flashed him a look.

"If your water breaks in public, does it make a big mess?" someone asked.

Lewis answered, "It is no respecter of persons. When my water broke, I was pumping gas back when people first started pumping their own. I tried my best to make it look like I had spilled gas. I was so embarrassed."

Ginger and Marian laughed when the boy who asked about oatmeal asked if the baby tore the bag open. He illustrated by furiously kicking his feet and pumping his fists in the air. They laughed harder when he asked if the baby came out feet first, does it have anything to do with the sexual position during conception. His pregnant sister smacked the side of his head.

At the break, Ginger put her head in her hands and yawned. She had been at work since seven that morning, and had not yet been home. Lewis resumed the class by telling them to find something to concentrate on to help them through contractions. "Anything but the clock," Ginger whispered. Lewis asked them to get comfortable on their blankets so they could begin practicing relaxation techniques. Marian lay on her back, waggling one foot, her hands on her big belly. Ginger picked up Marian's arm, to see if she was relaxed. Lewis told them, "Breathe in—I am—breathe out—relaxed." Sitting next to Marian, Ginger breathed in and out with her daughter. After the exercises, Lewis asked if there were any questions, and a patient asked how someone's belly button became either an innie or an outie. "It's just heredity," Lewis said. "Some people tape a silver dollar over it."

"My mom did that," a young man volunteered, "and we're all innies."

"Tell her that's not what did it."

One woman said, "I've been thin, and now I've gained forty-two pounds being pregnant. And in this dream, I've had the baby and I've lost weight, but I have fluorescent yellow stretch marks all down my legs. All my friends are saying, 'You look great.' And I say, 'You're lying to me. Look at these.'"

Lewis continued by reviewing what they had learned the week before, all of which only Marian remembered. "We no longer do enemas," Lewis said, "unless you need it." Someone asked what an enema was.

Someone said, "It's when they make you doo-doo."

"That's about the best way I know to tell you," Lewis said. She had a drawing to illustrate that, too. "We used to shave pubic hair," she continued, "but we don't anymore."

"That was awful," said Ginger. "Whew, and when it grew back!" She shook her head.

Every face became serious as Lewis listed the things that could go wrong for no apparent reason: cord prolapse, placenta previa, placental abruption. Silent and motionless, they stared at her as she recalled a patient. "She did everything right. She went to all the classes, all her prenatal visits, read everything. She went to sleep one night and woke up in a pool of blood. The placenta had pulled away, and the baby was dead." She continued: cephalopelvic disproportion, fetal malpresentation, and so on. The class finished with breathing exercises. They watched and listened carefully, believing that correct breathing somehow made everything all right in labor. Lewis suggested that their labor coaches give them a ratio of so many inhales to so many exhales. Demonstrating for them, she said "Hee" on each inhale, "Hoo" on each exhale. Three-to-one went, "Hee, hee, hee, hooooo." Soft breathy hees and hoos flittered in the room. "Do short breaths, like you're blowing out a thousand candles. Don't breathe like a dog. That's just on TV. It dries your throat. If you feel faint, you're breathing too hard, you're hyperventilating. Then what do you do? Anyone?"

"Breathe in a bag," Marian said.

"Right."

"So far all the news is good," Jan Dorman's mother, Teresa, said, in her home. "I'm going with her tomorrow to ask questions. It's six months now, so they should know." She spoke of the baby, who was with her.

The baby cried long and loud. "So far she's been good and healthy. Jan asked me to keep her. She can't make up her mind if she wants me all week and her weekends. She wants to get a job." Another long cry, this one punctuated with hiccups. "From eight 'til five. She's talking about a baby superstore. And she may work weekends, too. I would keep her more, and I don't mind at all. I'm pretty much open to anything. I'll keep her all I can." She said Jan's health continued to be good. "The doctor said she was in excellent health and not to come back for a year unless there are some unforeseen problems. Her T-cells are in the seven hundreds, and anything over five hundred is normal and healthy. I didn't know when you lost 'em when you're HIV-positive that you could recover. None of these booklets explain that."

Carl she could do without. "I don't talk to him. One time she'll tell me he's the father, and sometimes she'll say it might be this other guy. So I don't know one way or the other. As long as he treats Jan good, I don't have anything to say. But with the baby, if something happens, I will have something to say. He's hit Jan and stuff. He's not dedicated to the baby. I'm not impressed at all and never will be. Jan said Carl has been paying more attention to Deanna, but at first he wouldn't pick her up or talk to her. She said she thinks one of the problems is Carl wanted a boy. And, excuse my language, but I said, 'That's too damn bad.' If he treated Jan right and loved her like he's supposed to—her personal life is her personal life, she's grown; it's none of my business—but when he treats her bad, it is my business. I don't trust him, and I never will."

She looked at the baby, who squirmed in her arms. "She doesn't know what she wants, sleep or eat. She'll wake up in the middle of the night sometimes; she won't even be crying; she'll just wake up and stare at me and play with my face. She's had some pneumonia, and that's one of the things they tell you to watch for, so whenever I think there's nothing to worry about, something happens. But anybody can get pneumonia. She's gaining weight, and they say to look for that. And she's strong." The baby gurgled happily. "She knew I didn't like her being with black guys, and at first she didn't know if it was Mexican or black, and when she figured out it might be black, she quit calling me altogether. And she'd move every few weeks, so I never knew how to get in touch with her.

But when it came close to time for the baby to be born, she started contacting me again. The further along, I knew it didn't matter. Especially when she was born. Like right now, we don't know if she's Mexican or black, and it doesn't matter. She's been trying to contact the Mexican guy because she's thinking it might be him. She knows he will want a blood test."

More gurgling. Teresa began feeding Deanna with a bottle. She said, like Jan, she never graduated from high school. "I quit a couple of weeks into the ninth grade. We both say we're going to get our GED, but we never get around to it. She had so much to deal with, and I didn't know about it, and I think she blames me for not knowing, know what I mean? We're different, too, total opposites in a lot of ways, but we love each other. She's my daughter. And I've noticed with her growing up some, too, that's making a big difference. I see things in black and white; it's right or wrong, and she's been more, I don't know, before it was like she did everything to shock people, the more shock value the better. Now she's settled down into a real life, I guess you could say. But now, I'm ashamed of my feelings I had about her being pregnant." She laughed softly, then smiled at the baby. "I'd take her in a minute. She's a sweetheart, isn't she?

"My husband was fighting feelings of getting close to her, because of his relationship with Jan, plus he was scared of HIV, scared to let himself love her and end up losing her, but one time she had a hard time digesting milk, and she was screaming in pain. I was in the kitchen washing dishes, and she was in here in the car seat on the couch, and he got to her before I could get my hands dried, and he sat down rocking her, and she quit crying and stared in his eyes. She'll do that, she'll just stare and stare in your eyes. And he fell in love with her. Now, he adores her. He was just trying to protect himself, but that one incident broke down his barrier. He's a good man; he really is."

She said she hoped to get temporary custody of Deanna while Jan got her life together. "It's mutual," she said, "and you get a lawyer to draw up the papers. I'm concerned about her growing up in a stable home. She shouldn't have to worry about going back and forth. I want full custody. I hope Jan will come around to it. But I know not to push her on it but let her make up her own mind. If I say black she says white; if I say hot she says cold. She needs to be in a stable home where she's gonna be loved, and is wanted. Jan loves her, there's no doubt, but she hasn't bonded right. And it wouldn't be a thing where we'd have her call us mama and daddy. She has a mama and a daddy. But they fight and fight and fight."

Deanna cried again, loud and long.

"I sure wish she'd have enough self-respect to look for somebody who'd treat her right. Shhhh Shhhhh," she cooed to the baby, looking in her face. "They can see pretty well at six months. They're a lot smarter than people think. Used to be they thought they couldn't see for a long time. They thought they were blind at birth, but now they know they can see up close." The crying continued. "Sometimes it helps to walk around."

Robin James said she credited God for Pauline's pregnancy. "I was worried it might be another miscarriage. She called me scared to death. I had been praying, asking God to help her and let this baby live. I was looking at Benny Hinn one morning, after he had prayed for this boy with a blood disease. He said stretch your hand toward the television. I believe in faith healing. For a long time I didn't because I didn't see no evidence of it, but it wasn't for me to see no evidence of it. It was for the people who was sick. For their faith. I had to be convicted of it. So I believe God helped Pauline. The devil was really kicking at my face. She called and said she was spotting. I said no you're not. She said yes I am. I said oh, God. It was almost like shattering my faith into little pieces of glass. Here I am praying with a man I feel is annointed of God and I'm thinking my faith is all this, and then she called me the next day and says she's spotting. I said, uh uh uh. We rushed down to Grady. I cried, and she was fussing, 'I told you don't be getting your hopes up, Mama. Don't be getting your hopes up about this baby.' I said but God told me. She said let us just wait and see. She's nervous about talking about faith. We got down there, and she said you can go on home. I said the baby's all right, and she said, 'Mama, you don't know that. Don't be saying that, hear?' I was about to cry. I finally went on home. A couple of hours later, when

I got my feet laid back in the bed, she called me. 'Mama, come and get me.' She said, 'I only got a yeast infection.'

"Another day I went again with her, but I said I can't keep running down here when the Lord said the baby's going to be all right. I can't be acting like I'm worried when she's worried. I got to keep having faith, no matter how it look. Then the third time she said, 'I got to go to the hospital!' I said I ain't going. 'We got to go! The baby's coming out!' I went down there and tied a white string up under Pauline stomach, like my grandmama-n-'em did me. Didn't tie no bow, just tied a knot. Supposed to tear the bottom of a white sheet off, the hem, then you lay it across the baby, then you tie it around, and the baby will automatically—I don't know why—but the baby will move up in the mama womb. And that's what the baby did. Today she said her back was hurting. I said you ain't got that string on what I put 'round you. She said, 'How do you know?' I said you keep that string on. With all her other children, she never would let me do that. This one she did.

"When we saw the ultrasound picture of the baby, it looked like the baby said, 'Hey Grandmama!' Pauline said what's going on? She said turn this screen around, so I can see what got my mama looking like that. And the baby looked like it waved at her, too. We left out there happy people that night. We called everybody in the family and told them about how the baby said, 'Hey Grandmama.' That baby did do that to me, I'm telling you."

Marian Thurston's mother, Ginger, talked about Marian's pregnancy one morning in her Floral Acres apartment. A sign on their front door said, "WANTED BY THE FBI: A DRUG FREE AMERICA." Another said, "No Glove, No Love."

"I have some suspicions about if he really is the father," she said, of Randall, "because of the length of time he was gone. It doesn't add up to me. I mention it to her, and she doesn't acknowledge it, and she doesn't deny it. I've never talked to him on the phone. It's like she's trying to do everything on her own. I don't know. She had a perfect situation, and I wouldn't think about having a baby if I was her. She was making eight dollars an hour, on her first real job. A car and a job. I'm still thinking about that. She is the first in our family to have a child out of wedlock, so I wasn't real happy. The father should be more involved. Their father was there all the time. Scottie is the only one. . . . He was two when we got divorced. But it's mostly been the two of us raising them. I just feel like all children need male and female influences in their lives. That's my only disappointment. Nobody in the family has had a baby without being married."

She said that for a time she worked at the same job as Marian, in the evenings, after working days at the hotel. "We called people. They told us one thing, but once you got into the job, it was more like phone solicitation. This one looked at their credit rating and if it was good they sent a card. If they use it, they activate the card automatically. A lot of people turned it down because they had cards from recognizable banks. But if they used the card, we would call and sell them insurance for the card. I liked it; it was good money. But I started having doubts because of what we were told. A lot of people said they didn't sign up for the card. I thought, these people signed up for it, but I guess anybody can send you a card, and if you activate it, it's your card. It was good money."

She said her hotel job was good but boring. "I've been there eight years. I don't want to keep doing that job. I would like to go to the front desk, but I'm not going to try to do that until I get a car. I see us moving from here in two years. I'll have less kids. We used to live near the hotel but the rent, trying to keep clothes on their backs, I had to work two jobs. It was getting tiring. So I came to this apartment after we divorced. I've been here six years. I'll save up some money, then by that time my next oldest son will be on his own."

Huge planes roared overhead. Outside, a grimy garbage truck loudly picked up the dumpster across the yard, upturned it so that the contents slid into the back of the truck, then clanged the empty dumpster to the ground.

Her oldest son, Russell, who was sixteen, had a pregnant girlfriend, and Ginger could foresee herself caring for the baby. "She was pregnant before, and her mother gave her an abortion, then she turned around and got pregnant again. Russell's not a responsible person. This is going to be my responsibility and her mother's. They can't really get any jobs."

She recalled that when Marian and Lisa took care of the baby they had taken from the neighbor who was on drugs, Marian tried to foist the baby's care off on her. "Marian started getting tired. She would want to go out, and I would wake up. She'd be done brought the baby and put it in my room. I'd be like, 'Marian.' 'Marian gone.' I'm like, 'Oh no.' Then the baby started teething, diarrhea, colicky, and she had to take it to the doctor, and she didn't want to do that. I tell her now you can't give this one back; you got to keep it. I'm going to keep my doors locked. *I'm going to be gone*. I had to buy Pampers. Then when she got a job, it was a little more hectic. We had to find somebody to keep her, and I had to pick her up. I was like, wait a minute. This is wearing me out. I had to come straight home and get her because Marian would still be at work. She worked at night, so I had her all night. So we already had that little trial, but this one is on a more permanent basis."

"I didn't want to hurt anybody," Lisa said, carrying D'Lisa, walking toward Marian's apartment with Marian. Tameeka's sister, Tammy, drove up in a car packed with children. She offered to take D'Lisa to her place, so Lisa handed her over. In the apartment, Marian was stretched out on the love seat against the wall in the kitchen, near the stairs. Lisa continued, "But I didn't like that abusive relationship we had. Dwayne really was hurt. He even asked Jonathan to give me back to him. He cried."

Marian laughed. "It's funny now, but it wasn't then."

"I laughed at him to his face because he hurt me so bad. Any time somebody would catch him in a different girl's apartment, I would tell him one day you're going to find yourself by yourself. He told somebody regardless of what I do or what I say, Lisa will never leave me. Never say never. I heard about that after we broke up. I'm happy now. I don't care what anybody says, as long as I am happy. My mom is glad I have left him. Marian is glad. A lot of people are happy. My friends are happy for me."

Marian said, "Both of us were abused, at the same damn time, heh."

"Oh yes," Lisa said, "and I couldn't stand neither one of them. I told Marian I'm going to leave him. I would cry, and Marian would be sitting there like, I don't give a damn. I was like, how can somebody fight somebody they say they love? I had been through it before with lil' Rob's daddy. And then to go through it again? It really hurt. While I was going with Dwayne she was going with this dude named Mr. Conley."

Marian guffawed.

"At the time," Lisa continued, "Mr. Conley used to try to get it on with our friend, Susan. One day he felt on my breast, and I tried to kick him down the steps. I told you about it, didn't I?" She looked at Marian. "He was going to make it look like I was trying to hit on him, but it wasn't like that. He wasn't no good. Nobody liked him, nobody. Nobody. Just like Dwayne. Both of them were unlikable."

"Walking devils."

"Demons," Lisa echoed, then added, "They used to call us bitches and all kind of shit." Lisa's brother Franklin came into the apartment with D'Lisa. He said Tammy had brought D'Lisa to him; he handed her to Lisa, then left. "She must have gotten tired of her," Lisa said. So, why did Marian and Lisa stay with their men so long? Lisa said, "Love is blind, sometime."

"Then one day you just wake up," Marian said. "I don't know why with women, they can't get out of it. It took something drastic for me to get out of it. But some women don't give a damn."

"Even though Rob's daddy fought me, I didn't talk to him. I would ask people, and they would say, 'Leave him alone.' Dwayne slapped me so hard when I found out I was pregnant with D'Lisa, and hit my head on the side of the brick wall, and I got stitches. That didn't make any sense to me. Then Jonathan said, 'You don't need that.' He said real men do not fight a woman. He right. I'm glad I'm out of it. Dwayne was already fooling around, and Jonathan liked me. He helped me, gave me rides. Eventually one thing led to another. When we used to fight, Jonathan used to break us up. Even before me and him started messing around, he used to break up our fights. Jonathan used to be real mad, and I used to wonder why, and I found out it was because he liked me. Then, with Dwayne, it was, kicked to the curb. Over." Lisa added, "It's so funny to see Marian pregant. She has always been small, no belly, and now she's got the pregnant walk. You don't want anybody in there to coach you in labor?"

"No."

"Forget that, you crazy."

"It's my moment, with my baby."

"It will *still* be your moment. Nobody to hold your hand?"

"No."

"Shoot. She's going to be acting the fool, and she don't want nobody to see her."

"I'm not going to be acting no fool. I just don't want nobody in there."

"I could not be by myself."

"Cheryl's going to film it."

"So she'll be in there with your behind. I was glad Rob's daddy was there, but I would have preferred my mother because I couldn't stand him at the time. When I delivered D'Lisa, I said Dwayne bring me some water. He said, 'Are you OK? Just breathe.' I said, 'Shut the fuck up; bring me some damn water.' He was like, 'Just breathe.' "

"That's all anybody remembers. Breathe, just breathe."

Lisa said she was still skeptical about her sister's pregnancy. "She is supposed to have her baby May 11, and she is no bigger than I am. That's less than two weeks. She don't even have a pudge. I was looking at her the other day, and I thought, did she have an abortion? It might look like it sometimes, but I'm not going to believe it until I see that baby in her arms."

Last night, Marian Thurston said in the OB waiting room, she had dreamed her baby was a light-skinned boy. "It was about like my complexion. It had a flat head full of hair, and he was looking too mean. I'm going to beg them for an ultrasound. I know I'm having a boy, but I want to be sure. I just know. I dreamed I had a boy." A woman sitting across from Marian said aloud to a friend, "I'm getting those shots or my tubes tied." She munched onion-dip-flavored potato chips. "Too Good to Eat Just One," the bag crowed. Marian said her mom did not want her to put the baby in daycare until it was a year old. "Mom said at first she wouldn't keep him, but she says she'll watch him every other weekend. I guess so I can go somewhere." Marian also said that Tameeka and her sister Tammy got tattoos, so she and Lisa decided to get tattoos, too.

After her vitals were measured, Marian went to McDonald's to get a McChicken sandwich, fries, and a Coke. She walked with a waddle, her small frame distorted by her big belly. She wore baggy elastic-waist short pants, a large loose sweatshirt, and soft sandals on her swollen feet. She returned and walked past the "No Eating in the OB Clinic" sign, right when Dr. Culliver called her name. During her prenatal visit, Marian congratulated Dr. Culliver on his new baby. He showed her baby pictures, and she grimaced and snorted "Ugh!" at one picture of the slimy, just-born infant. Culliver said his wife would take some time off, then return to her residency.

"She's a doctor, too?" Marian asked, surprised.

"Yeah."

"Lucky kid."

Culliver shrugged uncomfortably, and said, "Yeah, if he ever sees us."

Culliver left and in walked a medical student, whom Culliver was instructing. He laughed too much with Marian, artificially adding a little snicker at the end of every sentence. "Back again? Ha ha ha." "How far are you? Ha ha ha." "We're going to check your cervix today, OK? Ha ha ha." At the last statement, Marian sneered. After he left, Marian said, "He's a student. He doesn't know what the hell he's doing."

Culliver returned and said everything was normal, after asking her the usual questions and looking at her lab report. Before she left the exam, she reminded Culliver, "I don't want *any*one else in the room."

"It's supposed to be a happy moment for you," Culliver said, "so whatever you want."

A few days later, Marian lay in a Labor and Delivery room, an epidural in her back. Next to her were: neighbor Cheryl, sister Jackie, mother Ginger, father, and a friend of Jackie's. Cheryl's video camera lay on the window sill. Marian, who had arrived at 4:00 a.m., sat up in the bed, her eyes drooping. Her father slept on the sofa, his mouth gaping open. "You lay down," Ginger told Marian, and reached for the bed controls to lower the part of the bed Marian reclined against.

"No-o-o," Marian replied, shaking her head.

Ginger acquiesced. She leaned to Marian's belly and said, "Your grandmother is tired. Come on out so we can go home."

At the nurse's station, Renee Lindley said, "When she first came in, she was adamant that she did not want an epidural; she changed her mind at nine-thirty." She looked at the strip for her other patient and said, "She may not have an adequate pelvis. Most teenagers don't. That's why they have those cute little hips, and we look like we do. Heh heh." She slapped herself on her hip.

Nurse Holly Eberhart asked about her son in college.

"Lance and I laughed and cried. We wrote three hundred sixteen people asking for money. We wrote AT&T, everybody. I told him we should write Hillary Clinton."

"So, you don't qualify for Pell grants or anything?"

"No'm."

Ginger's boyfriend arrived and joined them in the room. Rubbing sleep from her eyes, Jackie walked out of the room to the water fountain in the hall, got a drink, and returned. Lindley went in and came out dancing. She snapped her fingers and sang, "I am complete." A frowning patient in a gown walked by the nurse's station, having apparently been instructed to walk her labor into action. She passed by, and Lindley said, "When she's ready, she's going to kick some butt. She looks serious." Marian's father's second wife arrived and entered the room. The second-year entered and soon called out to Lindley, "Things are happening fast in here." She quickly joined him. Before the door closed, Ginger's voice could be heard saying, "Marian, we love you." Before long, Ginger was squealing, "You did it, baby, you did it." The entourage applauded. "Thank you, Lord," Ginger said. "Oh, look at the baby! Thank you, Lord. Yes, yes, yes. It's a girl!" They applauded again, louder. The baby cried, and Ginger responded, "Yes, I hear you."

A week later, at home, Marian narrated the night before she went to deliver her baby. "I told Cheryl, 'I'm fixing to have this baby.' She said, 'No, you're not. Get out of my house.' " Marian went for a walk and timed her contractions. A dog barked at her and chased her; she quit timing and ran home. When her contractions were five minutes apart, she took a bath. "I knew to eat nothing; I didn't want to have no bowel movement on my baby. My water was leaking, but I took a bath anyway, even though they said not to. I went to my room and closed the door. I was still having contractions. I thought, 'This baby's coming.' I put my bag by the door, lay down, watched TV. Cheryl sent me a half a watermelon and I ate all that, and I ate some fruit cocktail, but I wouldn't eat no food. I drank water, drank juice. They came every five minutes. I wanted to stay home as long as I could. I kept going to the bathroom. Mom was in the bathtub once and I needed to use the bathroom. She said, 'Are you having contractions?' I said yes. I hadn't told her before, even though Cheryl told me to. Then I woke up at four in the morning. I was all calm, cool, and collected. I said it's time for me to go the hospital. My mom said, 'Really?' 'Yes.' Mom tried to wake Cheryl, but she wouldn't get her ass up. I didn't want to call the ambulance because I didn't want everyone to come outside. I walked around, then sat down on the porch and my water just gushed out." They tried Cheryl's apartment again, but they slept soundly, oblivious to the knocking on the door. Marian relented and called an ambulance.

Her baby cried, laying in a crib. "What? What? You want all the attention, don't you?" She shrugged at the memory of a room full of people, when she had insisted she wanted a private delivery. "I don't care. It was like they weren't in there because I had the curtain pulled." She said the childbirth classes prepared her well. "My daddy was laughing. He said they should use my tape in childbirth classes. He was saying how I wasn't screaming and stuff. I was on the phone when they were stitching me. I breathed like the teacher said, 'Hee hee hee hoooo.' "

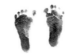

Childhoods

"I don't even remember. It was OK. It was kinda hard; I was the oldest and my mama was working, and I sometimes had to babysit. Until I was seven my dad was still with us, then they got a divorce. It wasn't traumatic. If I could, I'd forget my dad. The last time I seen my daddy I was ten. I was going to visit, and his mom was so mean to me, to us, me and my two brothers. I thought the old hag died because she was so mean, but she had a brain stroke. It was around Christmas; I have never seen my daddy again, and I really don't care. I called him and said I was pregnant with D'Lisa, to let him know, and he was like, How could you? I said I am damn grown. He missed that part of my life, so whatever he said really didn't matter to me. I'm not going to talk to him anymore, and he knows it. If he wants to see his grandkids, he knows where I stay. When he die, he will die alone. I am grown. All of his kids are grown. What in the hell would he do? Get beat up. Trying to tell us what *not* to do? Oooh. I mean, I love him as a person, but being a daddy, he never was.

"I loved high school. I skipped school and everything. I did everything any normal teenager did, but after I got pregnant I didn't go back for my last year. Like a dummy. I'm trying to tell kids now it's not like— education is the best. I am going back to school and get my GED. I want to go ahead and take the test, instead of taking classes, and what I fail—*if* I fail anything because I feel I am a smart person—I'll go and study for it. But I want to go ahead and get my GED. If my kids say, 'Well, Mom, you didn't go to school,' I can say I tried and I have my GED. If my kids don't do what I say, I'll put 'em out. You can't stay in school, you're not gonna stay in my house. I wish my mom had did me like that. But it's not my mom's fault. It's my fault. I didn't want to go back to school. Me and my mom's relationship got on rocky ground then. She wanted me to leave and that's why I went to get my own apartment and moved here. I love my mom to death. My mom has taught me a lot. She helped me grow up. I had to grow up, and I feel that my mom did a lot of good things. Whether I use it or not, my mom was a good influence on me. That's my backbone.

"We used to argue, now. I wasn't the best child there was. I wish I was, but I wasn't. Nobody is Miss Goody Two Shoes. Now I say I thank you, Mama, for what you did. You helped me grow up. She told me, you earn your womanhood with blood, sweat, and tears. And she never lied. It wasn't only my not going to school. I was trying to be too grown and when you're staying in somebody's house, you have to follow by *their* rules. You can't do what you want to do, grown or not. I wasn't grown. I was grown in age, as they say, but other than that, I was living off my mom. Believe you me, we have the best relationship apart. I love my mom."

"We didn't relate, basically. Some of the stuff that happened to Jan, I wasn't aware of, and so when the behavior problems started, it was like when puberty hit, she turned into an alien or something. I had no idea what a lot of it was related to. It just pulled the rug out from under me, and every time I'd get back on my feet, something else would happen. It was a real, real rough time. She kept running away from us, and I couldn't afford therapy. I tried the free therapy, and it just wasn't working. I ended up giving up custody so she could be placed in a home for girls in Savannah where she could get plenty of therapy, but she kept running away from there, too. There was long stretches when I didn't know where she was. Since the baby's been born, we've gotten closer. She's done a lot of growing up with this HIV thing. She's got a lot to go, but she's grown a lot. Now, she's a lot more truthful. She had a terrible problem with telling stories. She's more willing to accept responsibility for some of the things she's done. Where she's always tried to blame everything on everybody. That's a big step. Jan's done a lot of things totally against my ways, but when it comes down to it, she's my daughter, and she always will be. The times when we haven't spoken, that's been her choice. If you didn't agree with her, it would make her furious. And she was so mixed up. She really needed therapy, and she wouldn't let anybody help her. The harder you tried, the harder she pushed you away. That was real hard to deal with."

"My mom could not handle all of us too much, so we did what we want. It was very happy. We was in a big city, but we used to play in the street. The street was dirt, and would play a game like you call hopscotch. In Brazil, we have a street we call lazy street. It means doing what you want. We close the street and play. We do this a lot to play games. And we play a game in the field where you have to hit someone with the ball. When you are hit, you are out. I was very good at that. If you catch it, then you can try to get another person, on the other team. You always have to run and wait and you can grab the ball. I was good at grab the ball, and the people are the enemy, and if I have the ball, I can be very fast and get him. I have so much fun.

"I was kinda quiet. We was poor. We could not afford to go to parties. My mother could not afford to take us to a movie or take us to shop, anything like that. I remember my sister get married when I was thirteen, and she bought a dress to me and was a store like a K-Mart, cheap clothes. But the dress was pretty. The only time I remember my mom went to the store with me. But my sister paid for the clothes. My oldest sister started making money. She went to law school, economy school, and engineer school. She have degree three schools. She has her own business that makes projects to the big companies, and then she makes projects to the government part-time.

"My Dad was very straight with things. If anybody do anything wrong, he would prepare to get spank, everybody. Everybody sit, and we stand up one after another to get spanked. It was too much kids, and he punish everybody for one. Everybody try behave. I was small, so he never hit me hard. He used to hit my older sister harder. Here, he would go to jail, but no in Brazil. I have heard that some people kill people with spanking, and I never see anybody go to jail for that. The financial situation make him very crazy. My Dad, after a long time he realized it was not the right thing to do. He stopped to do that completely. After 1981 my dad start making more money, and my sister make money, and things got better, better."

Driving through the neighborhood of her childhood, just south of downtown, Robin James recalled the area before I-85/75 was built through it. "I used to sit on those steps right there and smell them cooking sweet bread. See that apartment building back there? Them been there a long time. I used to play all around here. One time I was riding my bike, and I hit that tree right there. I still got the scar. We lived in a two-room shack. This right here was a gr-e-eat big grocery store. They used to give everybody credit and everybody wasn't on no. . . . All these was big houses with the columns, old big, big, used to sit around here. They was a little well-to-do. Those people may have moved out to Cascades, because they were black. All the black people lived kinda together, the ones what had money lived in the same area as the ones with no money, but there was no such thing as everybody running to the welfare office. That welfare office kinda became popular with my generation. That welfare thing. They had it, but my mama and my daddy both worked. A lot of time I would have to stay after school to keep my sisters and brothers while they worked. Wasn't no whole lot of nurseries. That wasn't no big thing in our neighborhood. Was no daycare. If it was, I didn't know anything about it."

Robin said it was important to her to remember what happened in her childhood. "I try to write things down because I'm trying to leave a legacy for the grandkids, so they'll know about our family. That's why I try to keep up with everything going on in the family. I been writing down stuff ever since '65, after Cheryl was born. I started writing about the changes that was happening. I remember when Kessler's used to be downtown, and I remember we would come from Grady and then down there get your prescription filled where that Big B Drugstore is. I can't remember the name of it. I probably got it wrote down. Didn't nobody want to get in that long line at Grady to get your pills filled. It wasn't as cheap as it was at Grady, but at Grady, boy, you had to wait just as long for your medication as you did to see the doctor. We would stop down there at Kessler's to get some water at the water fountain, and they would have a sign saying 'Colored' on this water fountain and one over here saying for whites."

She returned to the subject of recording the family history. "I write down things, stuff my grandmama told me about her husband, my daddy's daddy, where they used to live, how they pumped water from the well, and where my great granddaddy buried at down there in Eatonton, Georgia. I try to do family history. What they tell me. I remember things. They used to wouldn't talk so I started asking questions. If you want to know anything, you better ask it. Then they'll act like, what she want to know that for? I just want to know. I used to be wanting to go down and get some land we used to own in Eatonton. This white man who gave my great granddaddy his last name, which was Shurden, gave my granddaddy property down there, like sharecroppers do, but he gave him land and the white folks down there didn't like it. I got all that wrote down. My uncle and them won't go down there with me and get it. Everybody scared to go down there because the white folks ran my granddaddy and my grandmama—she died at a hundred and something—they ran them off from down there. The Masons helped them get away. Some of them was white. It has always been some white people would try to help black folk. Like there has been some to harm 'em. They didn't like it because my granddaddy didn't go to the back of the stores. My granddaddy's man who gave him his last name had it fixed where he didn't have to go to the back door, and they called him 'Mr. Shurden.' The white folks called him mister. They didn't like him giving my granddaddy that land. They didn't like him being able to come in the front door like they was. He would take my uncle and my daddy in there with him. My uncle said they kept saying, 'I don't know why you ever let this nigger come through the front door. He ain't no better than the rest of them.' Stuff like that.

"My grandmama was working in the fields during this time, chopping cotton. One day she was working and she heard some noise. They said, 'He's dead.' She dropped her hoe and asked Uncle Joshua did you hear that? Uncle Joshua said, 'Yes ma'am.' She said head for the house; something wrong with your daddy. When he had got there, one of those white men had hit him in the head with an axe. He had been making moonshine for the white man. When she got there he was all bleeding and everything. He couldn't go to the hospital. I don't know why he couldn't go to the hospital, but they took spider webs and turpentime and put 'em in the wound and tied his head up and it healed like stitches. I don't know how, but that's what she told me. About three years later he died from that wound. My father's father.

"Then the Masons came and told them that it would be best if they leave because they wasn't going to stop until they killed all of them. They hooked up a buggy and two horses, put all what they could on it and moved up here, but they didn't like the city. I need an adult to went down there with me. I wanted Uncle Joshua to go because he knew where they lived and everything. But he's scared. Even to this day, he won't even go down there to visit great granddaddy's grave. I can still picture it in my mind, where his grave at. If I could go, I would just like to go, to just see. I wouldn't try to get the land back or anything. I would just like to see so I could write it down and everything like that because maybe somebody else know something. I kinda know where you're coming from, on liking to know stuff. That's how I am, too. That's why I like helping you."

Epilogue

In the fall, Lisa Dean's boyfriend Dwayne was at Floral Acres at 1:30 a.m. when a red Mustang drove up next to where he stood in the street. No witnesses were close enough to see what happened, but police think it was robbery. Or attempted robbery—Dwayne had no money. Onlookers saw the Mustang tear down the street, and they found Dwayne dead with a bullet in his chest. A car matching the description given by the witnesses was seen two hours later in downtown Atlanta, and three men in the car, all in their twenties, were arrested for Dwayne's murder.

The front cover of the funeral program at the Workhouse of Faith Missionary Baptist Church featured a picture of a smiling Dwayne, baseball cap on backwards. Relaxed, his arms crossed, he wore a Los Angeles Raiders T-shirt. As the family proceeded down the center aisle to view the remains, the minister read the Twenty-third Psalm. Dwayne's father and mother sobbed loudly as they leaned over the casket. His father's strong, broad shoulders quaked, as the pastor read. An associate pastor prayed, quoting Ecclesiastes that there is "a time to live and a time to die." He added that it was still sad to lose someone. "Lord," he cried, "allow us to reason with one another before we kill each other."

"Amen, yes, Lord," came the reply from the congregation.

A soloist sang "Precious Lord, Take My Hand," and "His Eye is on the Sparrow." His pretty tenor filled the small chapel, sobs punctuating the lyrics. The pastor gave the eulogy, his voice thundering, then whispering, thundering, whispering. "I'm praying for all you young people," he preached, "that you will reach up and hold God's hand. He'll hold yours if you do."

"Amen!"

"That's right!"

He recalled Dwayne coming to the church when he was six years old. The pastor said he rode the van to Sunday School. He was good at softball and baseball, and the church came to love him. "We live in troubled times," he roared. "It's a mean world. Especially for black Americans. We have come a long way, and God has blessed us, but it seems like things are going back. Some people treat their dog better than they treat other people. Some people will kiss a dog and shoot a man. If you are out on the streets, they'll kill you, and you might not have any money. We owe God," he announced. "God is like Georgia Power. If we don't pay the bill, they'll turn your electricity off. We owe God." He recounted his own life of dancing, drinking vodka and Jack Daniels, running numbers, smoking reefer, selling illegal liquor. "I was a fool!" he shouted. "We are on life support for now, and I don't mean Grady Hospital. God keeps us alive. I don't understand everything in the Bible—I'd be a liar if I said I did—but I know God allots us a space of time. Ecclesiastes says there is a time to live and a time to die, but why die before your time? Time is running out! God gives us time, but it's not *our* time. It's *God's* time! So learn about the Lord. When you eat collard greens, you need to learn about the one who put it in the ground. Time is running out! Some people do right by their boyfriend, their girlfriend, but not by God. Time is running out! If God says it's my time, I'll be dead, but I'm not worried about where I'll go. So get right with God! He'll show you how. If somebody has your social security number, they can tell about your past, present, and your future. Well, God has our number. He knows where we go and what we do. Time is running on! Don't let time pass you."

He extended an invitation to anyone seeking salvation, then led them in singing "At the Cross." No one answered the altar call. The service ended with the congregation recessing out the back door, among them Dwayne's relatives, Lisa, her friend Tiny, her brother Franklin, Cheryl and her daughter, Lisa's mother holding D'Lisa, Lisa's friend Leslie, little Rob handsomely dressed in a dark suit. The last man exiting the church said to a companion, speaking of D'Lisa and Dwayne, "She look just like him, don't she?"

"Yep, sure does."

Azi Torres moved into a nice two-bedroom apartment in Marietta, then filed for divorce, although Jeff said they meant too much to each other and should work things out. "He want to blame it on James. I said you did the same thing with Kenneth. He said I was having affair with Kenneth, and I was Kenneth's girlfriend, and all bullshit, and then he get in touch with Kenneth and make sure I was just his friend. He did the same thing with James. He called James. James said to Jeff, anything that gonna happen, or will happen with me and Azi, is going to be after you be over with her. This is not my fault, and I am not in your way. It is your problem with her, not my problem. I say to Jeff I no want to have to kiss his mother ass every month so she leave the money that is supposed to go to him, so me and Robert can have food to eat every month." Azi said she had visited Jeff's mother once more, to say she, the mother, should help Jeff more. "This marriage was mistake, I said to her. But everybody commit mistake, so I am just more one. She ask me things like, 'Why you did that?' 'Why you no did?' But what is the point of going back to the past? What is the past going to help to the future? Nothing."

She said her last argument with Jeff was over her lack of appreciation of his help for her. "He the father of this child. I no have to say, 'Oh thank you so much,' all the time. I get really upset with him, when he said I am not appreciating things. You no have to say thank you forever. I come from a country where we never sent a thanks note in life. You appreciate your friends by saying come over whenever you want and whatever you need, you have a friend. Friends are friends. You no have to write a letter"—she wrote in the air—"'Thank you so much. It was so nice.' They know you love them. We have a different way of appreciating them. He doesn't respect that. I said tell me right now if you want to be married, or whatever it gonna be. You keep telling me I am sleeping around. One day I was in love with Kenneth and I sleep with Kenneth, the next day you tell me I love James and I sleep with James, and the next day you tell me I sleeping with someone else. I must be somebody really bad to open my legs to anybody."

She had a speech prepared for when Jeff and his lawyer would begin talking money. "I gonna say even if you have all the money in the world,

I no want your money. It's your money. It's your problem. Give it to somebody else. Marry an America one, then she gonna get tired of you, not gonna put up with you, and she kick your butt and sue you. I'm gonna say that to his face and his lawyer face."

When the divorce was final, as predicted, she asked for no alimony. She only asked for, and received, child support and assurance that Robert's college education would be paid for by Jeff.

Finally, the six months passed, and Jan Dorman's baby tested negative.

Two months after her baby's birth, Marian lay on the sofa in the kitchen watching a videotape of a party she had missed. Marian laughed hard at Cheryl, Lisa's neighbor, dancing close to her husband. The party tape finished, and, for the first time, with no one else home, Marian retrieved from the top shelf of her closet the tape of her baby's delivery and inserted it into the VCR. She watched it all the way through, then she wept.